F. S. Weill E. Bihr P. Rohmer F. Zeltner

Renal Sonography

Completely Revised Second Edition

With 355 Figures in 836 Separate Illustrations

Springer-Verlag Berlin Heidelberg GmbH

Professor Dr. Francis S. Weill
Chaire de Radiodiagnostic, Radiologie A
Hôpital Jean Minjoz, Avenue Fleming
F-25030 Besançon

Dr. Edmond Bihr
Clinique St. Vincent, 3, Rue Jean Macé
F-35000 Rennes

Dr. Paul Rohmer
Radiologie A, Hôpital Jean Minjoz
Avenue Fleming, F-25030 Besançon

Dr. François Zeltner
8, Place Kleber, F-67000 Strasbourg

ISBN 978-3-642-70419-2 ISBN 978-3-642-70417-8 (eBook)
DOI 10.1007/978-3-642-70417-8

Library of Congress Cataloging-in-Publication Data. Renal sonography. Bibliography: p. Includes index. 1. Kidneys–Radiography. 2. Diagnosis, Ultrasonic. I. Weill, Francis S., 1933. [DNLM: 1. Kidney Diseases–diagnosis. 2. Ultrasonic Diagnosis. WJ 302 R393] RC904.R39 1986 616.6'1'07543 86-10102

Originally published by Springer-Verlag Berlin Heidelberg New York in 1987
Softcover reprint of the hardcover 1st edition 1987

Typesetting and bookbinding by Brühlsche Universitätsdruckerei, Giessen
Printing by Appl, Wemding
2121/3130-543210

Preface

Renal sonography forms a basic part of routine diagnostic strategy. This textbook summarizes eighteen years of experience in diagnostic ultrasound. We want it to serve as a guide to both imagers and mere consumers of information. That is why we shall emphasize practical advice and diagnostic pitfalls; it is also why we shall often deal with the relations of sonography with other diagnostic procedures, which it may complement or replace, precede or follow, the purpose being to achieve efficiency at low cost.

We shall limit our subject matter to the kidney itself and the neighboring retroperitoneal compartments, dealing only briefly with the lower urinary tract, which requires specialized procedures.

We devoted considerable space to renal sonography in our book *Clinical Atlas of Ultrasonic Radiography,* published in 1973. Since then, nothing has changed and everything has changed. Nothing, because even then the differential diagnosis between a solid and a cystic mass, the etiologic diagnosis of a nonsecreting kidney, and the positive diagnosis of a traumatic juxtarenal hematoma were quite reliable, making possible drastic reductions in the indications for instrumental roentgenologic examinations. Everything, because improved resolution and grey scale imaging (already partially achieved in 1973, thanks to real time) have profoundly refined both anatomic and pathologic ultrasonic studies. And now high resolution real time imaging has revolutionized renal examination techniques, whereas Doppler is entering routine ultrasonic diagnosis.

Our Lord Almighty, when creating the liver, the pancreas and the gallbladder, only created, in his infinite wisdom, one of each. Alas for the sonographer, He stuttered a bit when dealing with the kidneys, doubling the opportunities for abnormalities, and therefore for diagnostic difficulties. Please forgive Him – but never forget.

I would like to express my deep gratitude to the colleagues who kindly agreed to contribute their own documents to this book: Professor Tran Minh of Lyon, France, Professor Diard of Bordeaux, France, M. Lafortune MD, M. Crevier MD, J. Y. Quellet MD, J. Bourgeault MD, and S. Ethier MD, of Montreal, Canada, P. L. Cooperberg MD, of Vancouver, Canada, Dr. Barc from Vannes, France, and Dr. Petigny, from Audincourt, France.

I wish also to thank most warmly my wife, who once again managed to find all the documents I keep losing daily, and my secretary, Miss Cheval, for her permanent help. My thanks go also to Messrs. Gaudron and Bernard, photographers.

Last but not least, we must also thank our friends who kindly took care of our wives during the long evenings we spent dealing with rotten kidneys and secondhand bladders.

Besançon, Autumn 1986 FRANCIS S. WEILL

Contents

1 Echoanatomy: Tissue Echopatterns

We shall deal first with the kidney itself, then consider the kidney with regard to other retroperitoneal structures. Subsequently we shall examine the organ's less-direct relationships. We shall also review briefly the basic tissue echopatterns.

1.1 The Kidney Itself

The gross echopattern of the kidney is quite similar to the pattern of anatomical sections. The similarity is particularly evident for the organ's shape (Figs. 1.1, 1.2). It is also evident when one observes the juxtaposition of the parenchyma, which is rather sonolucent, and the sinus, where echoes from the pelvis, major calices, related vessels, and surrounding fat give a pattern of strong reflections (this is the pyelovascular central area, PCA).

Shape

On sagittal or coronal sections the kidney's shape appears so similar to what it is on conventional X-ray images that it does not deserve a detailed description. It should nevertheless be emphasized that the outline of the renal capsule is smooth and regular. There is no local bulging, with just a few exceptions to be mentioned below. The two renal poles taper regularly.

On transverse sections, the shape of the organ differs according to the level of section. The upper or lower third of the kidney has a round or oval shape, but in the hilar area the internal contour is deeply indented by the renal sinus (Fig. 1.3).

There exist a few nonpathological variations: a local bulge is often encountered on the left side, at the level of the lower pole of the spleen, on coronal sections. This corresponds to the classical *dromedary hump* (Fig. 1.4a). Another variation is that of fetal lobulation, with multiple bulges, a pattern which we shall study more in detail later on.

Hypertrophy of the margin of the renal sinus can bulge enough to mimic a tumor (Fig. 1.4b, c). Lastly, internal sagittal scans often show an anterior indentation, due to the anterior aperture of the renal hilus. This pattern should not be confused with the true retraction of chronic pyelonephritis (see Fig. 1.5).

Size

The vertical length of the kidney varies from 11 to 14–15 cm (Meschan 1966). Length discrepancies between right and left kidneys classically should not exceed 1.5 cm, providing that the orientation of the sections is similar on both sides. Ultrasonic measurements are, however, true measurements, without the drawbacks of the geometrical projection that has to be taken into account in conventional roentgenology. When one compares the size of the two kidneys on transverse sections, their differences in situation must be kept in mind in order to avoid confusing a mere difference of level of section with a real size abnormality.

Pyelovascular Central Area. Renal Pelvis

The renal pelvis can be visualized as a small pouch, of liquid echopattern, well delineated by the pelvic walls, with a diameter of 1–3 cm (Fig. 1.6). The shape and size of the pelvis vary according to hydration and urinary bladder repletion (Morin and Baker 1979). On transverse sections, the pelvis can extend outside the sinus (Fig. 1.7).

With normal hydration and proper oblique sections, the *major calices* are differentiated from the neighboring *arteries* and *veins* and are well individualized within the rich echotexture of the PCA. The outline of the PCA is star shaped (see Figs. 1.2, 1.11). Its radial branches mark the columns; apart from these radial expansions, the general shape of the PCA is smoothly rounded without particular local bulgings or indentations. It may be divided into two separate areas of reflection. This does not necessarily mean kidney duplication; the division

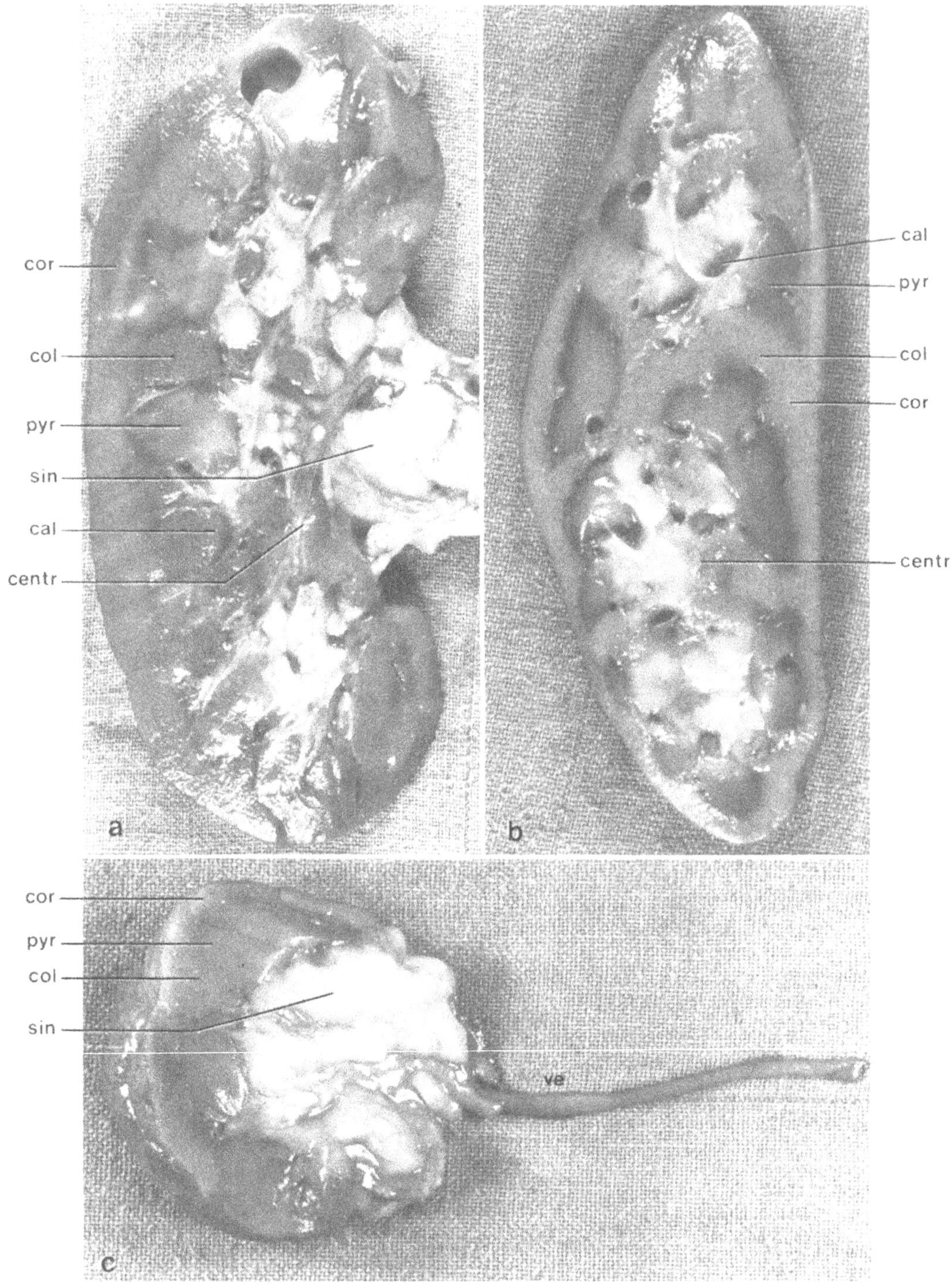

Fig. 1.1 a–c. Renal anatomical preparations: **a** Frontal cut, **b** oblique cut, **c** transverse cut. *cor*, cortex; *col*, column; *pyr*, pyramid; *cal*, calix and caliceal infundibulum; *centr*, central area, with sections of major calices and vessels; *sin*, sinusal fat; *ve*, vein. Note the rounded pattern of a pyramid when obliquely cut

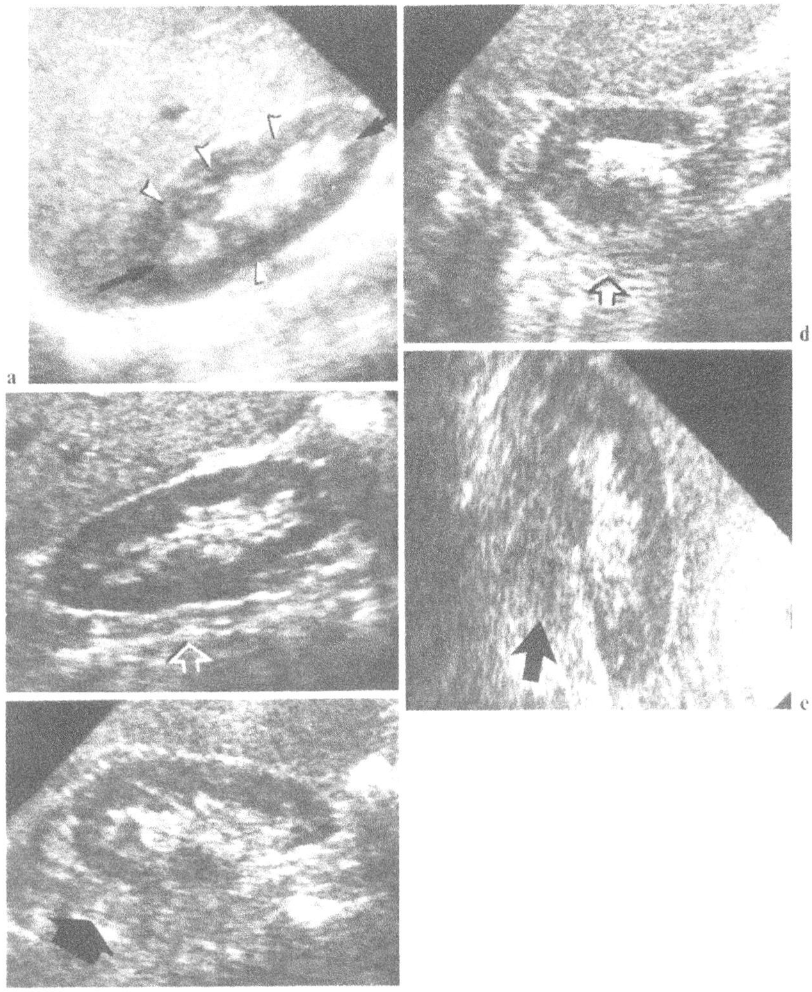

Fig. 1.2 a–e. Sections of the right kidney. **a** Sagittal sections. *Arrowheads* mark the pyramids, which are more sonotransparent than the columns; between the pyramids *arrows* point to the central zone. **b–e** Four sections of the right kidney. **b** Sagittal section; **c** oblique section; **d** transverse section; **e** coronal section. Note (*open arrows* in **b, d**) section of the musculus quadratus lumborum and, in **c** and **e**, the section of the psoas muscle

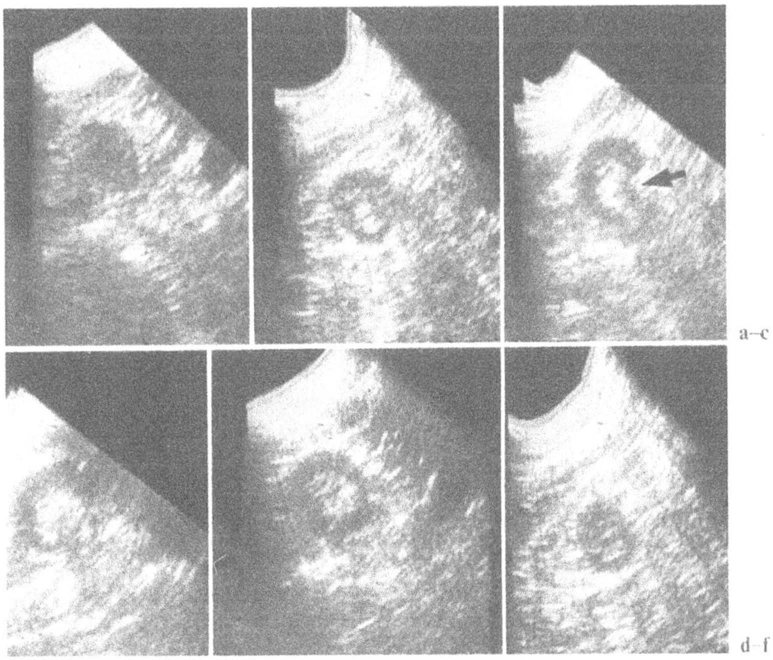

Fig. 1.3 a–f. Successive parallel transverse sections of left kidney (dorsal scanning, patient in prone position). Note the variations in diameter between upper pole (**a, b**), middle part of the kidney (**c–e**) and lower pole (**f**). Note also hilar identation (*arrow*) in **c**

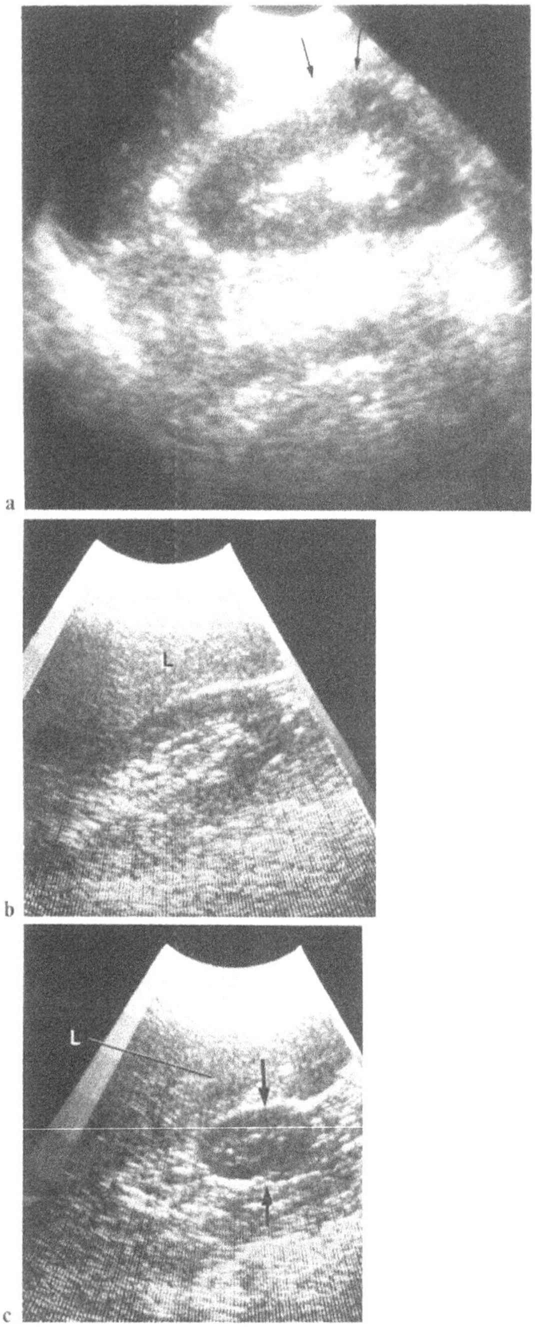

Fig. 1.4. a Dromedary hump: cortical hump (*arrows*) appear on coronal scan. **b, c** Pseudotumor: hypertrophy of sinus margin. **b** Right intercostal scan of normal kidney. **c** Parallel, more internal scan. Oval sonolucent area (*arrows*) corresponds to upper margin of renal sinus. This pattern is not pathologic. *L*, liver

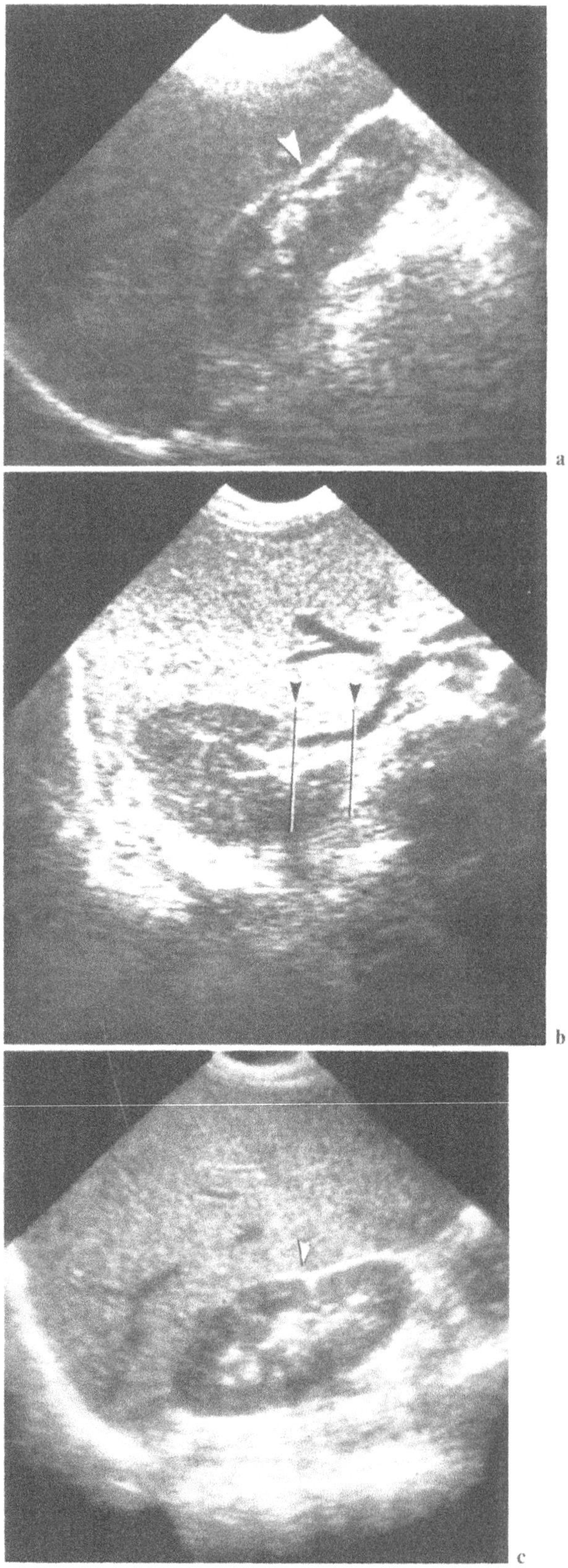

Fig. 1.5 a–c. Anterior aperture of the renal sinus. **a** Coronal ► section shows anterior cortical depression (*arrowhead*). **b** The depression pattern is explained by transverse section: posterior sinusal margin extends further internally than anterior margin, as shown by linear landmarks. Sagittal section passing between the lines deals with anterior sinusal apperture. **c** Another example

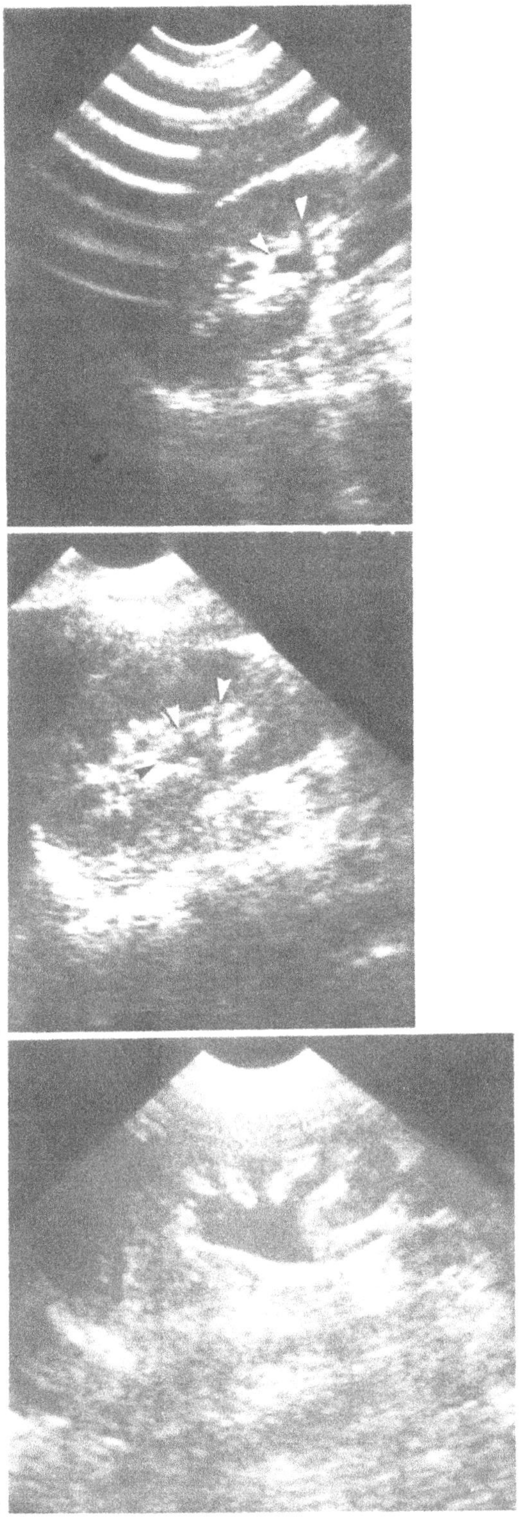

Fig. 1.6. a, b Coronal section of left collecting system (*arrowheads*). **c** Slightly distended collecting system (left coronal section)

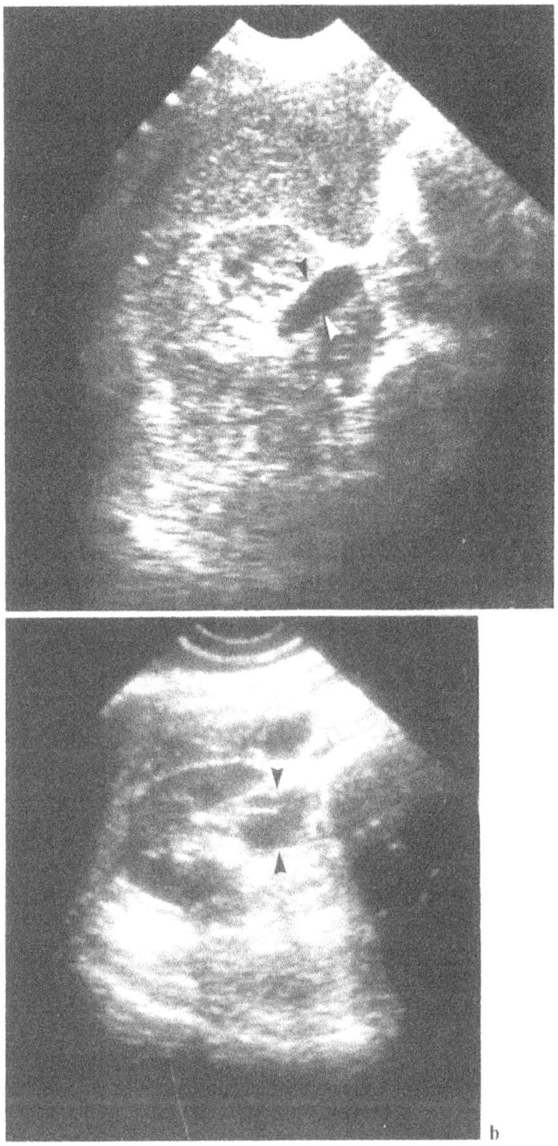

Fig. 1.7 a, b. Transverse sections of renal pelvis (*arrowheads*). **a** Intrasinusal pelvis; **b** extrasinusal pelvis

can be due to large columns (Fig. 1.8). We shall look at the usual pattern of *columnar hypertrophy* later.

Sinusal lipomatosis has several appearances. The first appearance is considered by most authors as the only true pattern of sinusal lipomatosis. It consists of a widening of the central zone, whose echogenic echotexture extends peripherally (Fig. 1.9 a, b).

Another pattern has been described by YEH (1977). It corresponds to multiple central cystic areas (see Fig. 4.13 p. 66); for a long time we considered such an appearance as rather typical of sinusal lipomatosis. However, the fatty nature of this pattern has been brought into discussion by other authors for theoretical and objective reasons.

In our opinion the theoretical objection does not hold, since it relies on the argument that fat is never sonotransparent. But fat within the abdominal wall is always transparent. We shall see later on that fat can be rather transparent in the juxtarenal compartments. In some patients liver scans show a sonotransparent hilar fat pad.

The objective arguments are much more relevant. CRONAN et al. (1982) punctured the central cystic areas and proved their true cystic nature in all cases. That pattern definitely corresponds then to juxtapyelic cysts and not to sinusal lipomatosis.

But, on the other hand, we believe that sinusal lipomatosis can indeed be transparent: a sonotransparent pattern can be encountered, less transparent, however, than that of cysts and with less regular contours (Fig. 1.10 a).

Correlation of computed tomography (CT) with densitometry is quite convincing in such cases (Fig. 1.10 b), even taking into account the possibility of partial volume artifacts. In a similar case, Cronan (personal communication) has found a magnetic resonance imaging (MRI) correlation in favor of fluid. A larger series of MRI correlative studies is, however, required.

Finally, we consider that there are two patterns in sinusal lipomatoses: (a) a widening of the echogenic central zone and (b) a sonotransparent central zone (sonotransparent, but not cystic).

Renal Parenchyma

In average imaging conditions (low attenuation, excellent image resolution), ultrasound scans disclose the pattern of the pyramids, columns, and cortex. A linear reflection may even show the arcuate arteries (Cook et al. 1977), (Fig. 1.11). An exceptionally sharp delineation of the pyramids is encountered in the transplanted kidney rejection process (see Fig. 8.14, p. 135).

Under good technical conditions and in a well-hydrated patient, minor calices may also be visualized. They appear as small, well-delineated echo-free areas, in direct relation with the distal part of the pyramids (Fig. 1.12). This corresponds to the lobar architecture of the kidney. However, if the image quality is lower, the pyramids are not as sharply individualized. The renal parenchyma appears then as a homogeneous area between the PCA and the renal contour; it is less echogenic than the liver. Exactly as on conventional intravenous urogram (IVU) images, its width does not vary abruptly.

Abnormal lobulations may be outlined within the parenchyma (Fig. 1.13). Their sonolucent pattern constitutes another kind of pseudotumor in the normal kidney, along with the nonpathological marginal bulges mentioned above. Oblique sections of the pyramids may appear as pseudolobulations (Fig. 1.14, see also Fig. 1.1 a). We have already referred to a pattern of division of the PCA due to *columnar hypertrophy* (Fig. 1.8 a, b). Columnar hypertrophy also gives rise to sonolucent, isoreflective nodules adjacent to the central area, which they can depress (Figs. 1.8 c, 1.15). Columnar hypertrophy has the same level of echogenicity as the surrounding parenchyma. It does not have its own boundary, and it does not bulge out of the renal contour (Fig. 1.8 d).

In Table 1.1 we have summarized the steps in ultrasound evaluation of the kidney. Table 1.2 lists the different kinds of *pseudotumor*.

Table 1.1. Ultrasound evaluation of the kidney

Shape and size (comparative)
Regularity of contours
Width of parenchyma
Homogeneity of parenchyma (taking into account whenever possible individualization of pyramids and minor calices)
Echogenicity of parenchyma
Shape and size of pyelovascular central area; diameter of pelvis
Doppler

Table 1.2. Pseudotumors in normal kidney

Sinus lipomatosis
Marginal fetal lobulation
Marginal infrasplenic hump (dromedary hump)
Intraparenchymal lobulation
Pseudolobulation due to pyramids
Columnar hypertrophy
Hypertrophy of margin of hilus

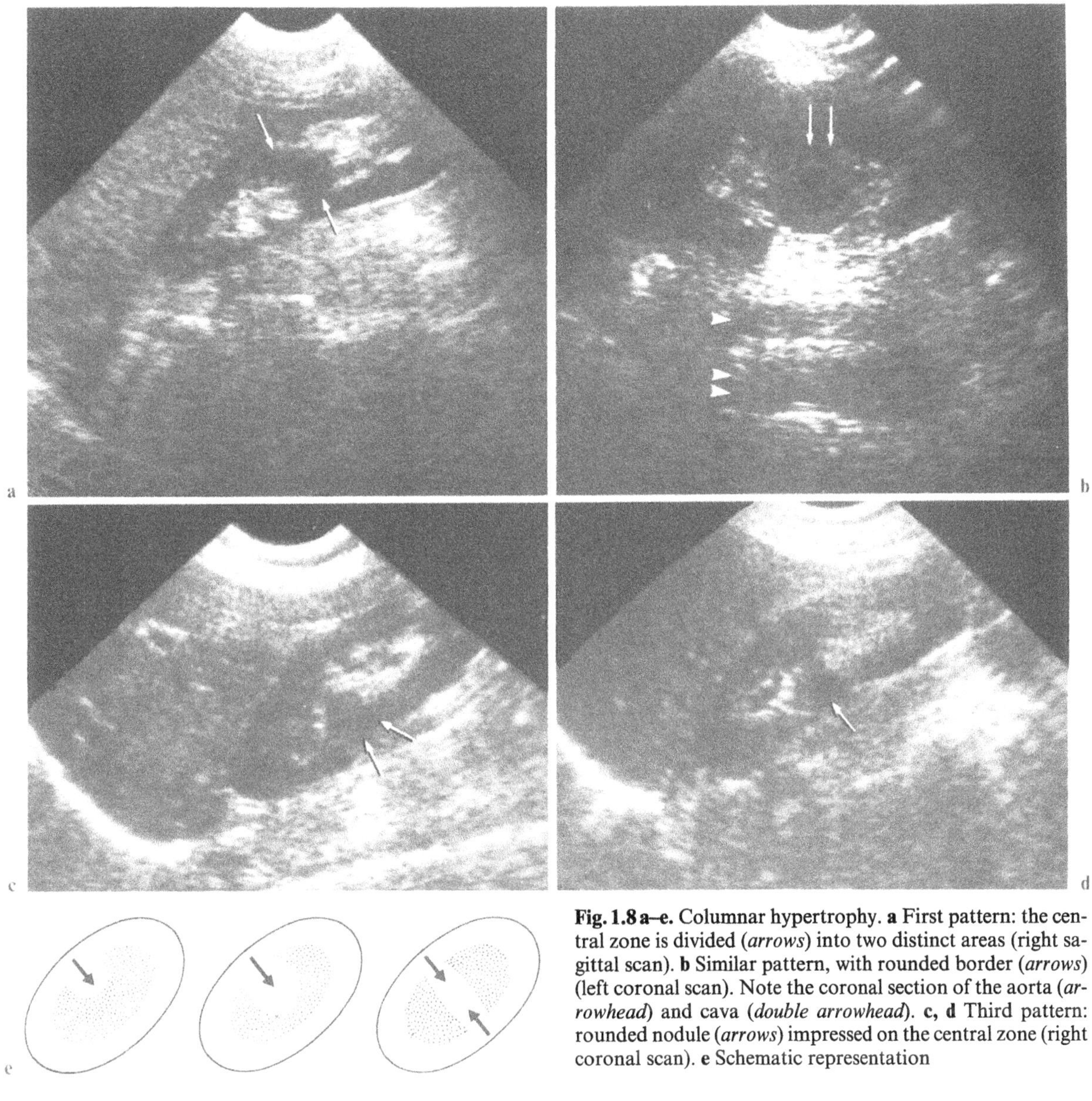

Fig. 1.8 a–e. Columnar hypertrophy. **a** First pattern: the central zone is divided (*arrows*) into two distinct areas (right sagittal scan). **b** Similar pattern, with rounded border (*arrows*) (left coronal scan). Note the coronal section of the aorta (*arrowhead*) and cava (*double arrowhead*). **c, d** Third pattern: rounded nodule (*arrows*) impressed on the central zone (right coronal scan). **e** Schematic representation

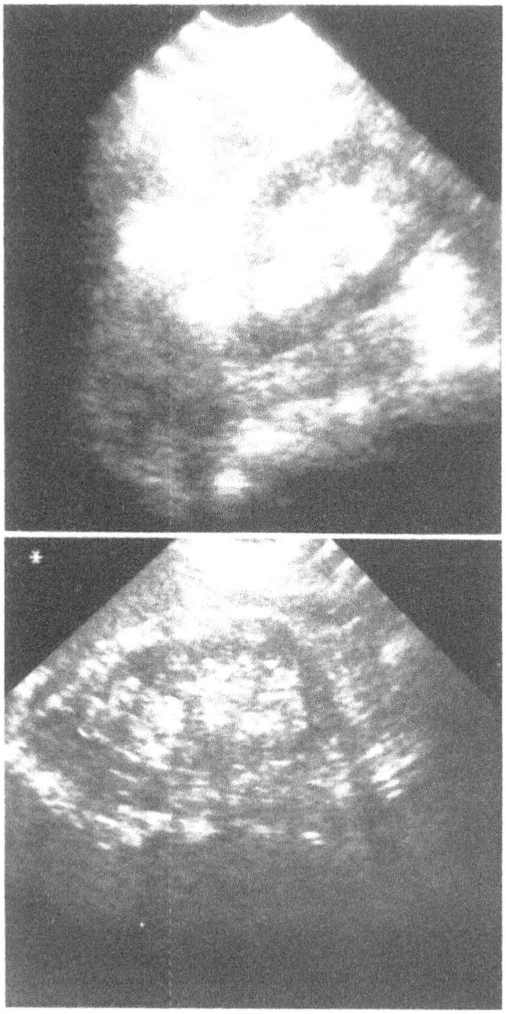

Fig. 1.9 a, b. Sinusal lipomatosis: widening of the central echogenic zone

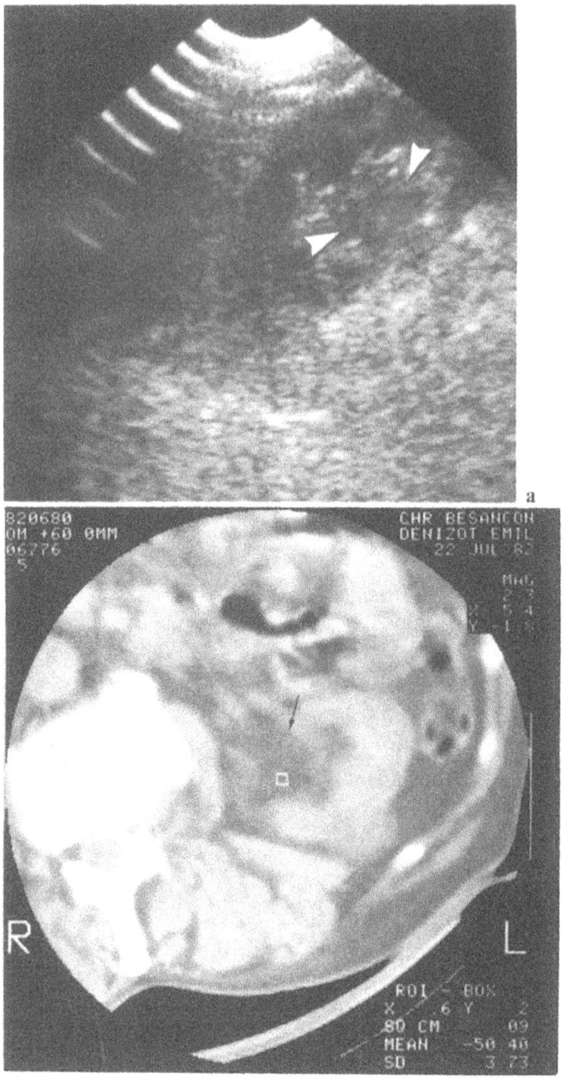

Fig. 1.10 a, b. Sinusal lipomatosis: **a** Sonotransparent area (*arrowheads*) in the central zone. **b** Noncontrasted CT. The sinus (*arrowbox*) shows a density of −50 HU

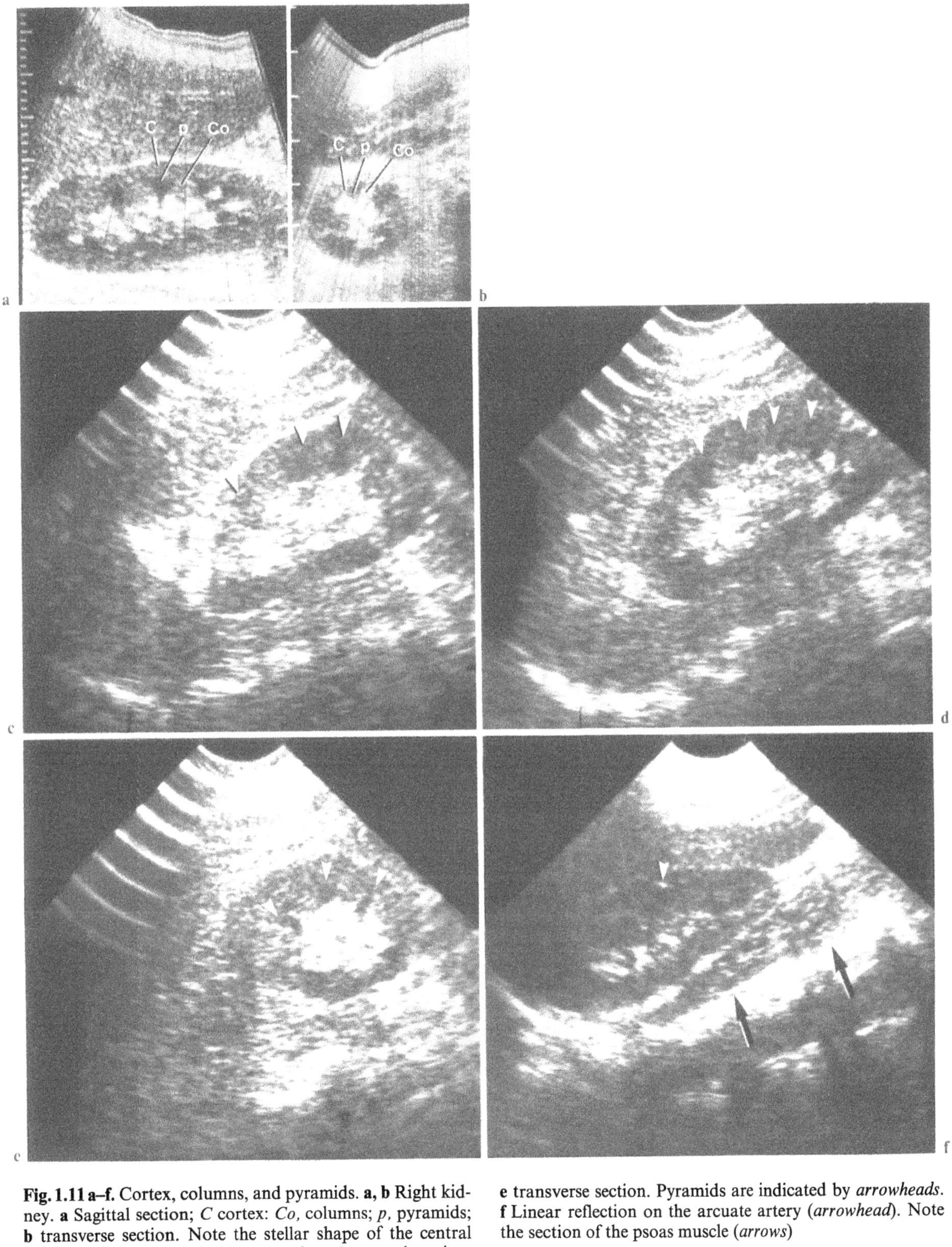

Fig. 1.11 a–f. Cortex, columns, and pyramids. **a, b** Right kidney. **a** Sagittal section; *C* cortex: *Co*, columns; *p*, pyramids; **b** transverse section. Note the stellar shape of the central zone; **c–e** left kidney; **c** oblique section; **d** coronal section; **e** transverse section. Pyramids are indicated by *arrowheads*. **f** Linear reflection on the arcuate artery (*arrowhead*). Note the section of the psoas muscle (*arrows*)

Fig. 1.12. Minor calyces (*black arrowheads*) adjacent to pyramids (*white arrowheads*) ►

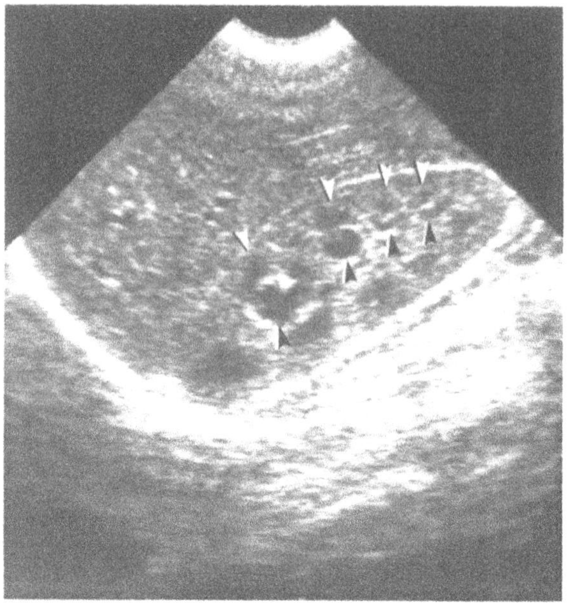

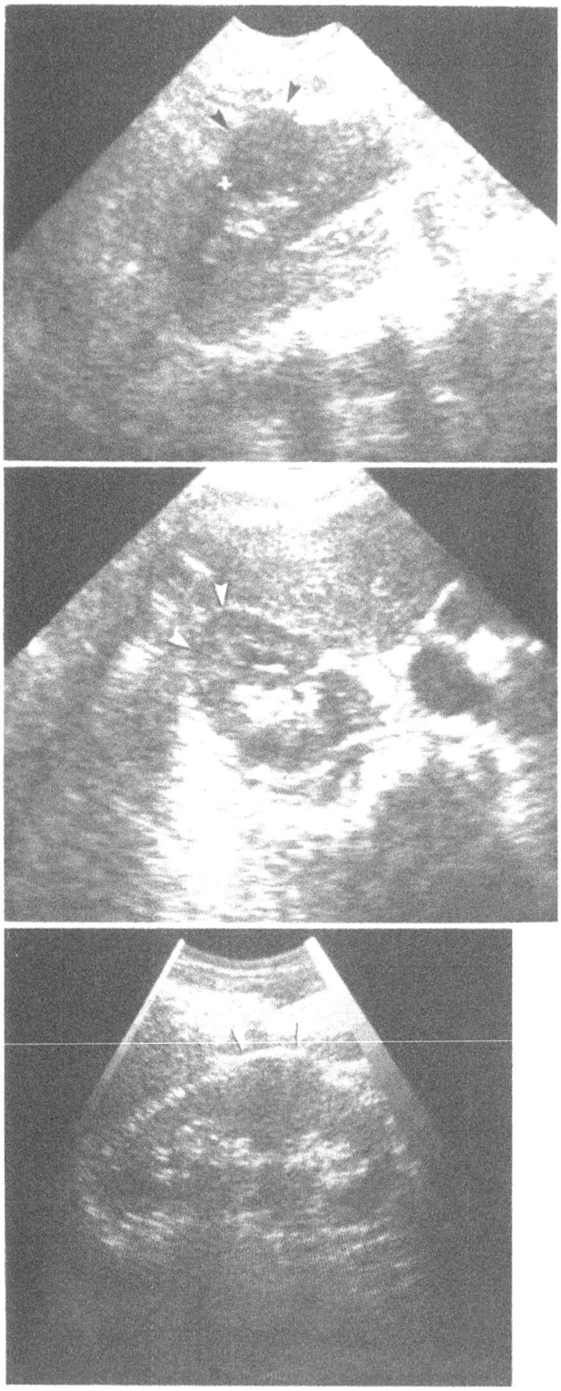

a

b

c

Fig. 1.13a–c. Fetal lobulation. **a, b** First case. **a** Coronal cut shows superficial nodule (*arrowheads*), with impression on the central zone. **b** Transverse cut shows merely external bulging. Contrast-enhanced CT confirms absence of tumoral process. **c** Another case, also evaluated by CT in a further step

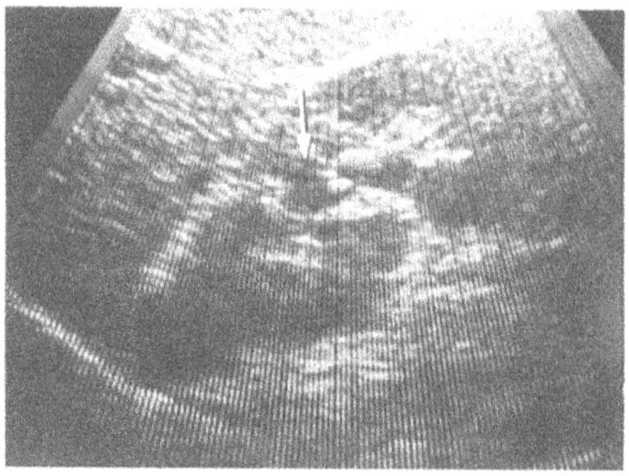

Fig. 1.14. Pseudolobulation due to obliquely cut pyramid (*arrow*) (see also Fig. 1.1 a, b)

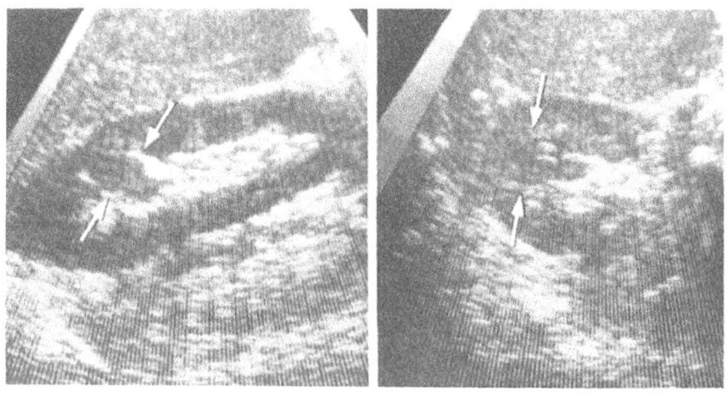

a

Fig. 1.15a, b. Nodular pattern of columnar hypertrophy (*arrow*). **a** Sagittal section, **b** transverse section (real time)

1.2 The Kidney as a Part of the Retroperitoneal Compartment

Juxtarenal Compartments

The analysis of juxtarenal fluid collections requires a precise knowledge of the anatomy of the juxtarenal compartments, a region which was thoroughly studied by MEIERS (1977). The particular architecture of that region is based on the perirenal fascia (Zuckerkandl's fascia anteriorly, Gerota's fascia posteriorly) (Fig. 1.16a).

The perirenal compartment extends form the renal capsule to the perirenal fascia, the anterior and posterior pararenal compartments surrounding the perirenal fascia and compartment. The perirenal fascia is continuous cranially, but open caudally: the three compartments merge in the lower part of the retroperitoneal space. The posterior peritoneum constitutes the anterior limit of the anterior pararenal compartment, within which the pancreas is located. This explains the migration of fluid of pancreatic origin to the perirenal compartment, or even to the kidney, within its capsule. The anterior pararenal compartment also contains the retroperitoneal segments of the colon, which represent a classical anatomical relation of the kidney.

The architecture of the juxtarenal compartments is rather ill defined on anatomical specimens (Fig. 1.16b). But it is readily displayed on CT scans, because of the particular radiological transparence of fat (Fig. 1.16c). On sonograms the juxtarenal compartments are not visualized in lean patients (Fig. 1.17). But they are clearly displayed in fat subjects (Fig. 1.18). The echogenic pattern of the juxtarenal fat, due to its richness in connective fibers, is a classical feature. However, the echogenity of fat is extremely variable. Juxtarenal fat is, in fact, sonotransparent when abundant. In such conditions the fascias and compartments are easily identified (Fig. 1.18a, b). Even the lateroconal fascia can be visualized (Fig. 1.18c). Recently, KUNIN (1986) described bridging septa within the perirenal compartment, whereas RASTOPOULOS et al. (1980) demonstrated that the anterior pararenal space extended posteriorly within two sheets of the posterior renal fascia.

The kidney and the surrounding fatty layer move according to the respiratory cycle (Fig. 1.19). This classical effect is particularly well demonstrated in real time.

Due to the high reflectivity gradient existing between the perirenal fat and the renal cortex, the specific role of the renal capsule in delineating the limits of the kidney's image remains unclear. In fact, the capsule proper is not sharply delineated in images of transplanted kidneys, in which the absence of perirenal fat should bring about a better individualization of this element. But the capsule becomes apparent in case of perirenal or subcapsular hematoma (see Chap. 10).

Bone and Muscle

Because of the intense reflection of ultrasound upon bone, skeletal elements do not figure in this chapter, except that we should recall that they are liable to cast acoustic shadows (Fig. 1.20). The section through the psoas muscles is well delineated between the kidneys and the spine. This muscular pattern must be kept in mind to avert confusion with pathological masses (Fig. 1.21). The quadratus lumborum and paraspinal muscles are also readily identified.

Vessels

The pattern of the *aorta* and of the *vena cava,* in both sagittal and transverse sections, is classical (Fig. 1.22). The aorta and vena cava can also be displayed on coronal scans. Their image is then rather similar to that in an angiogram (Fig. 1.23). The coronal approach is particularly efficient in Doppler studies (DUBBINS 1986).

Caval kinetics are visibly influenced by respiration (WEILL 1973): the vena cava expands during expiration and collapses during inspiration.

Arteries and veins possess specific ultrasonic patterns: high-resolution scans show the thick pulsating wall of arteries. The arterial lumen, probably because of intense, rapid turbulence, is not absolutely echo-free (Fig. 1.22). These morphological features are displayed both in the aorta and in its branches. Veins, on the other hand, have thin walls. As mentioned above, they expand during expiration. Transmitted pulsations may be observed, in association with respiratory kinetic changes. The venous lumen is echo-free, typically liquid, with one exception: in real time examination (sonoscopy) a few fugitive intraluminal echoes are often seen moving with the blood flow. These momentary echoes are particularly clear in the caval lumen, proximal to the confluence of the renal or hepatic veins (Fig. 1.24).

Proper scanning planes, mainly in real time, make it possible to visualize the renal vessels. The *right renal artery* is retrocaval (Figs. 1.24, 1.25). It must not be confused, on transverse sections, with

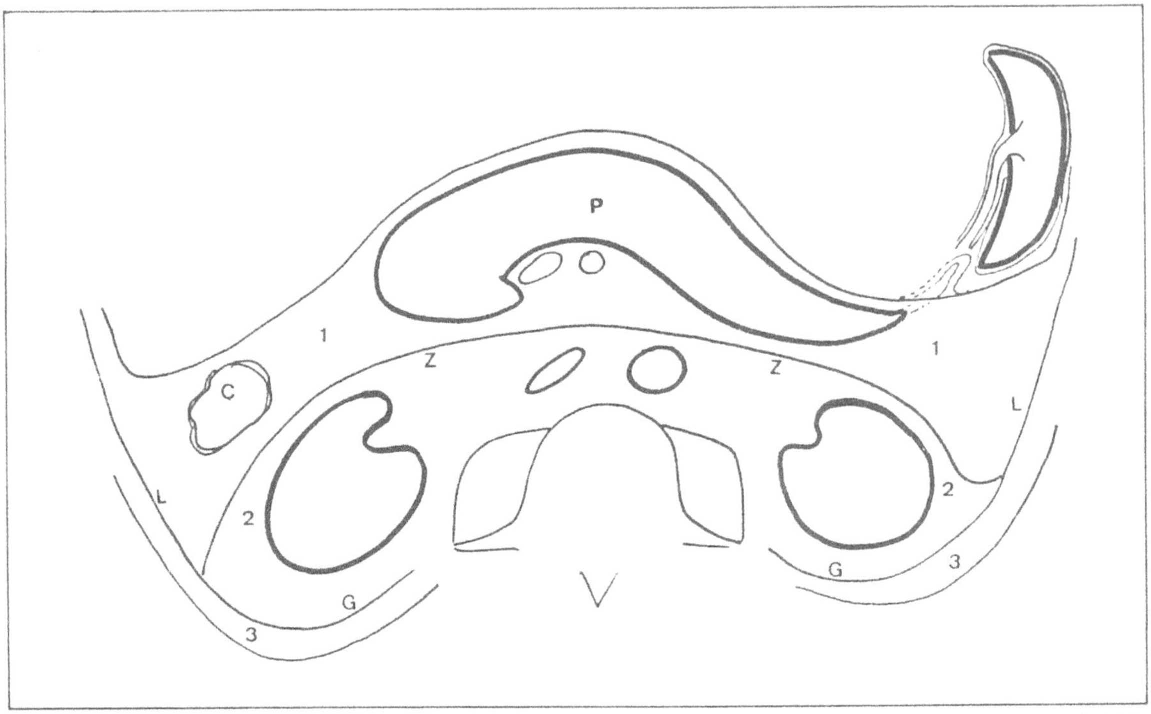

a

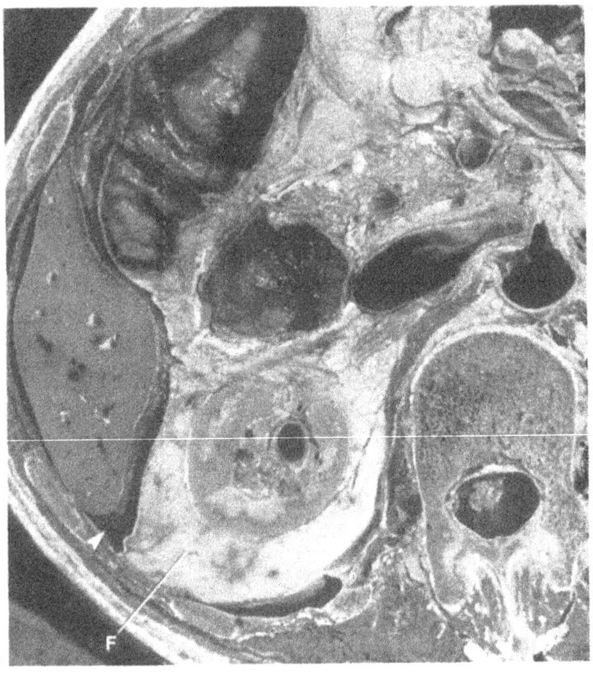

b

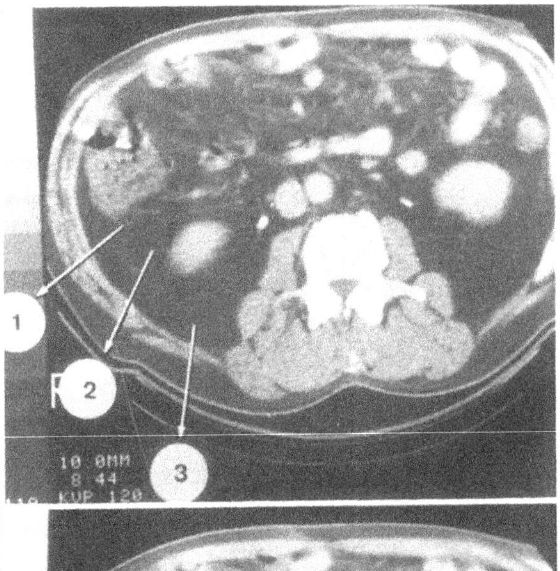

c

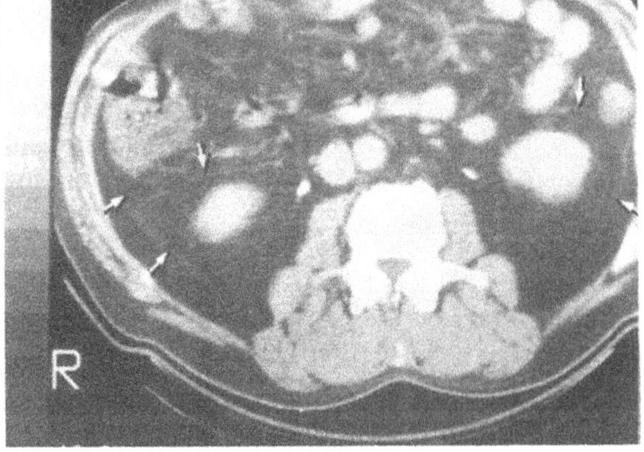

d

Fig. 1.16. a Scheme of retroperitoneal compartment. *1*, anterior pararenal compartment, with pancreas (*P*) and colon (*C*); *2*, perirenal compartment; *3*, posterior pararenal compartment; *Z* and *G*: Zuckerkandl and Gerota's fascias (perirenal fascia). *L*, lateroconal fascia. **b** Anatomical specimen. Perirenal and pararenal fat (*F*) appear continuous. Note Morison's pouch between the posterior peritoneum and the liver (*arrowhead*). **c, d** CT display of the retroperitoneum. The perirenal fascia is indicated by *arrows*. *1, 2, 3*, identify the different compartments

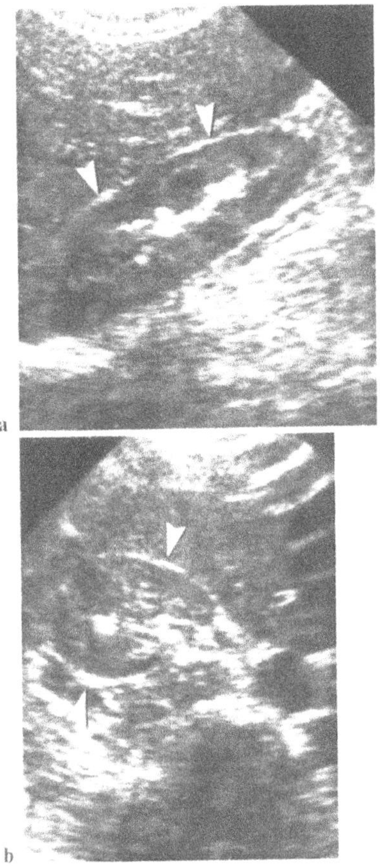

a

b

Fig. 1.17 a, b. Juxtarenal fat (*arrowheads*) in a lean patient. **a** Sagittal scan; **b** transverse scan

the right crus of the diaphragm (CALLEN et al. 1979) (Fig. 1.26). The *left renal artery* usually originates from the anterolateral aspect of the aorta (Fig. 1.27). The *right renal vein* is short and oblique (Fig. 1.28). The *left renal vein* runs more horizontally, curling around the anterior wall of the aorta (Fig. 1.29). A Valsalva maneuver may contribute to a better display of the renal veins.

Normal lymph nodes may appear on transverse scans, proximal to the large vessels (Fig. 1.29). Their maximum diameter is 15 mm (see Chapt. 6).

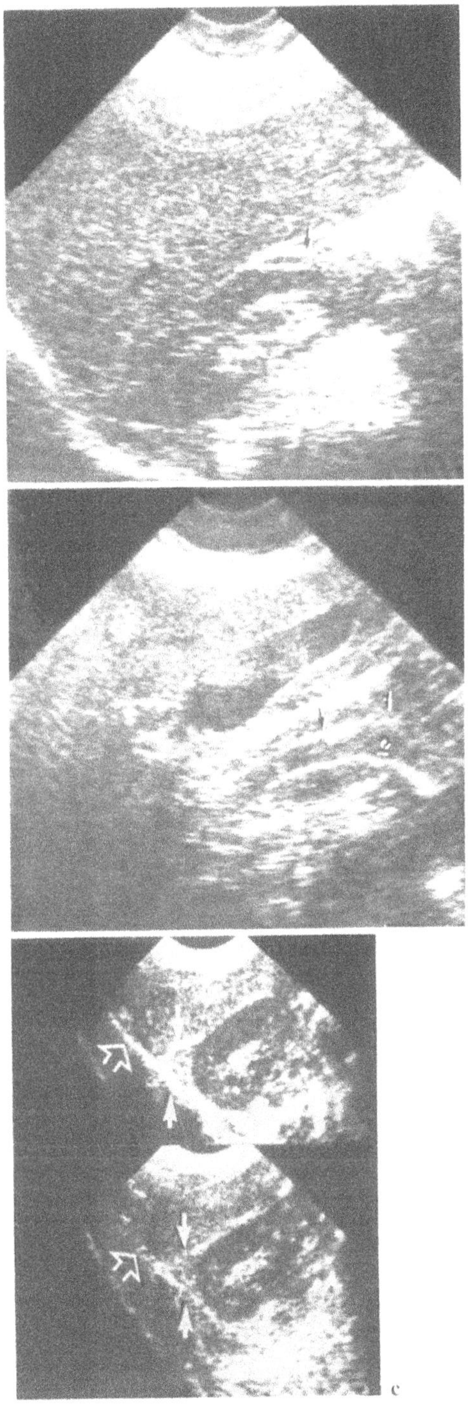

a

b

c

Fig. 1.18 a–c. Juxtarenal compartments: ultrasonic study in fatter subjects. **a** Sagittal section in first subject: perirenal fascia (*arrow*) is visualized between sonotransparent fatty layers of perirenal and anterior pararenal compartments. **b** Sagittal section in other subjects. *Arrows* indicate the perirenal fascia. Note the sonotransparency of fat. **c** Perirenal (*arrows*) and lateroconal (*open arrow*) fascias

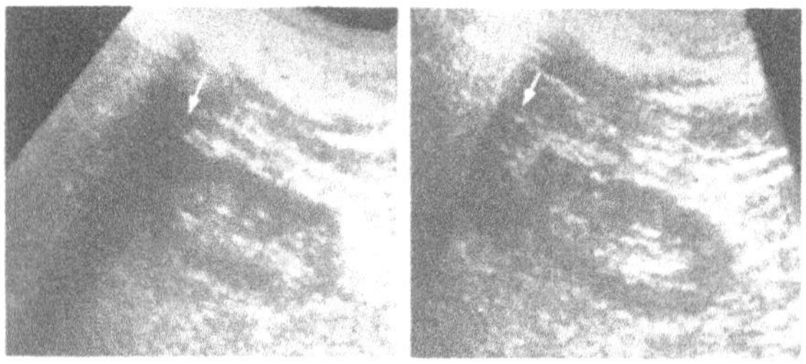

a, b

Fig. 1.19 a, b. Respiratory mobility of the kidney. **a** Sagittal cut (prone position), in neutral apnea. Lowest rib is shadowing (*arrow*) renal upper pole. **b** Deep suspended inspiration: upper pole has moved caudally, below shadow

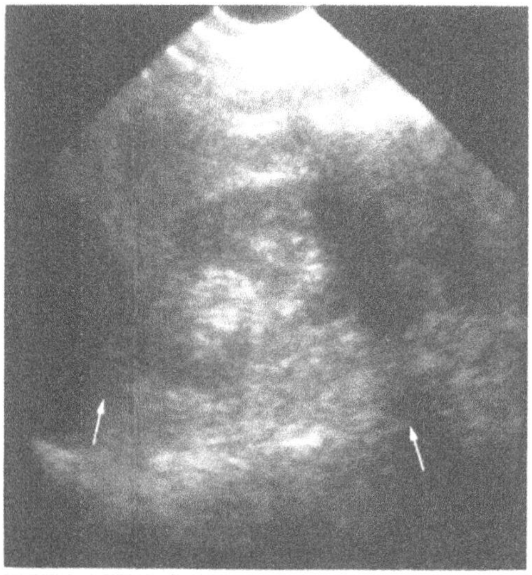

1.20 a

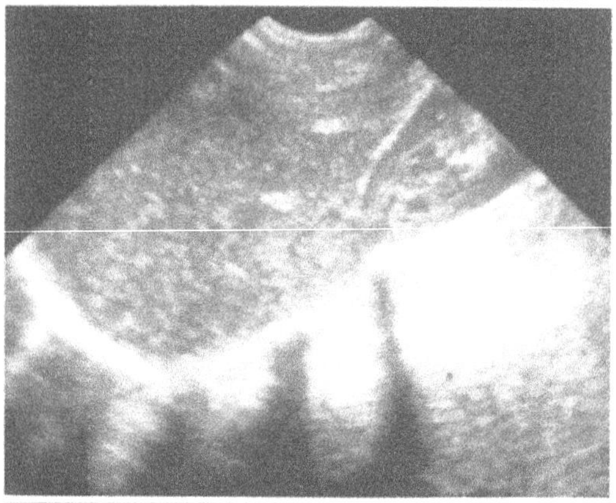

1.20 b

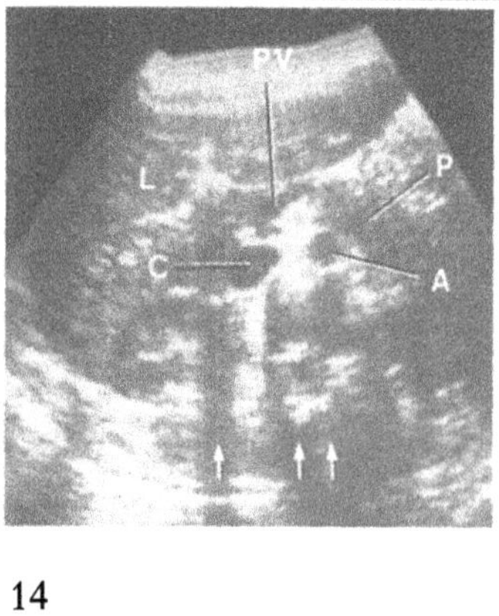

1.20 c

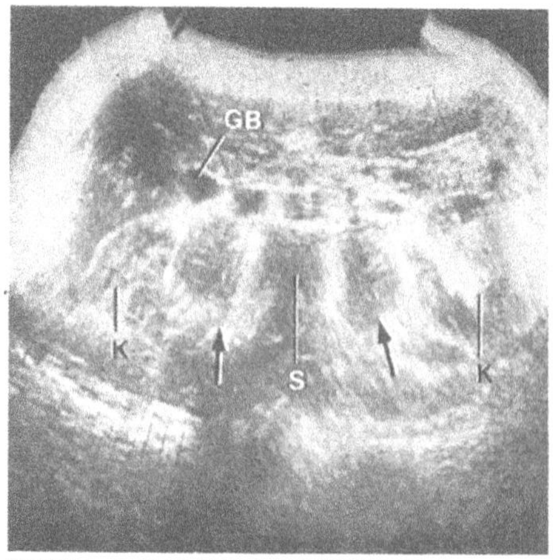

1.21 a

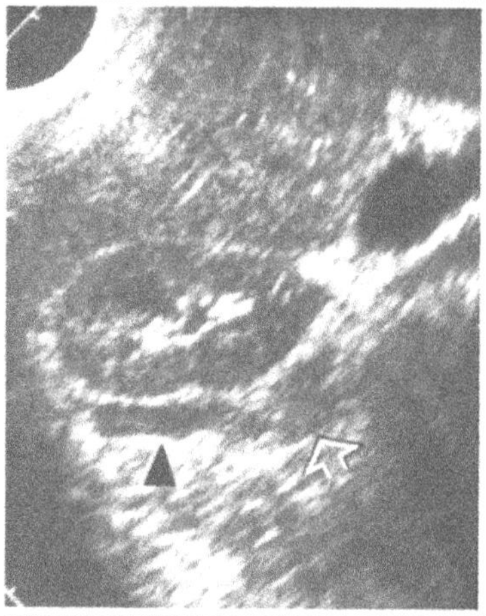

1.21 b

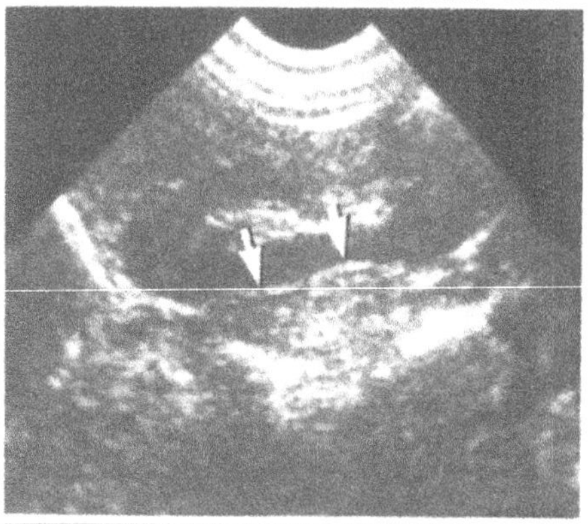

1.21 c

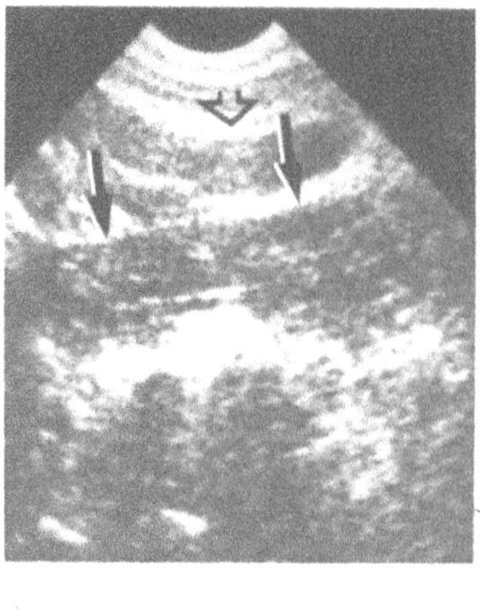

1.21 d

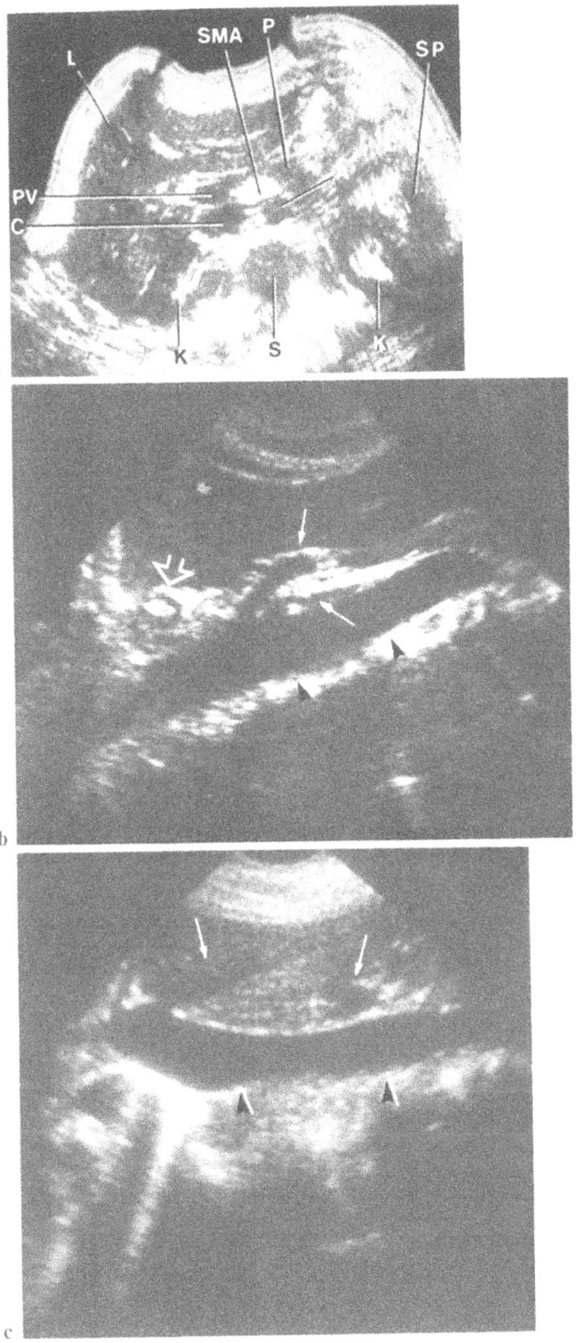

a

b

c

◂ **Fig. 1.22 a–c.** Aorta and vena cava. **a** Transverse section (*A*, aorta; *C*, vena cava; *SMA*, superior mesenteric artery; *PV*, portal vein; *L*, liver; *S*, spleen; *P*, pancreas; *K*, kidneys). **b** Sagittal section of aorta (*arrowheads*). *Arrows* point to SMA and inferior mesenteric artery (IMA) origins. Note esophagogastric junction (*open arrow*). **c** Sagittal section of inferior vena cava (IVC) (*arrowheads*), hepatic vein, and portal vein (*arrows*)

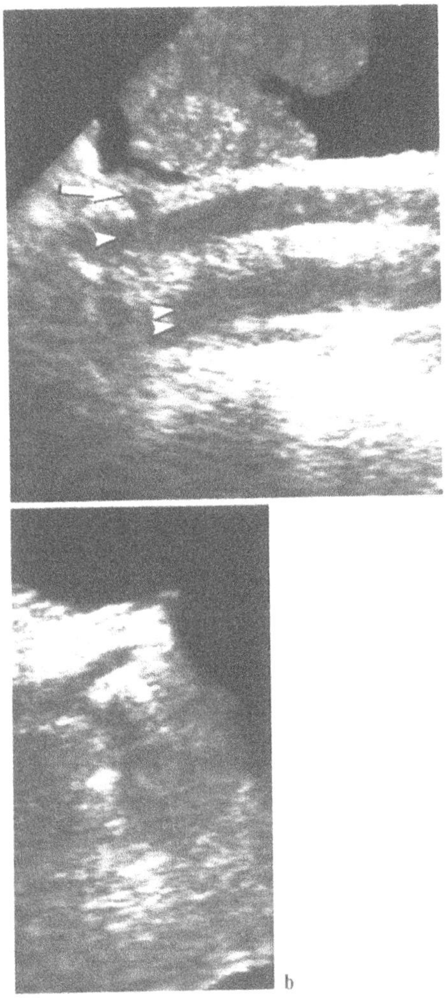

a

b

Fig. 1.23 a, b. Coronal section of aorta (*arrowheads*) and cava (*double arrowhead*). Note left renal artery (*arrows*) and origin of the iliac arteries

◂◂ **Fig. 1.20. a** Shadows of ribs (*arrows*). **b** Shadows of ribs and transverse apophyses (*arrowheads*). **c** Transverse section: shadows of duodenal gas (*single arrow*) and of spine (*double arrow*). *PV*, portal vein; *A*, aorta; *C*, cava; *P*, pancreas; *L*, liver

◂ **Fig. 1.21. a** Psoas muscle. Transverse section (*GB*, gallbladder; *K*, kidneys; *S*, spine). **b** Transverse section shows right kidney in contact with muscle quadratus lumborum (*arrowhead*), and adjacent internally to psoas muscle (*open arrow*). **c, d** Coronal sections of psoas muscle (*arrows*). *Arrowhead* in **d** points to the colon

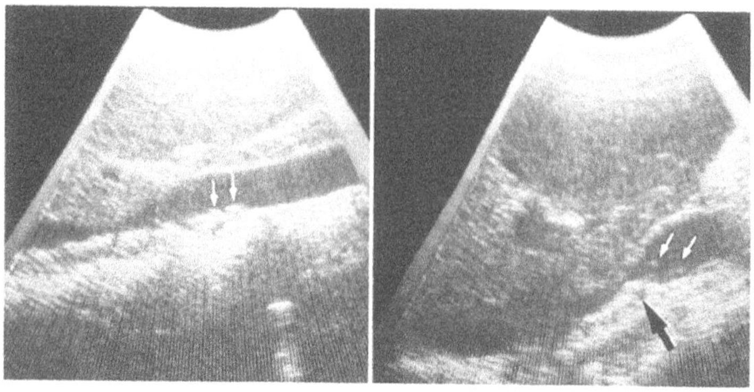

a b

Fig. 1.24 a, b. Caval intraluminal turbulences displayed on sagittal real time sections. Note, in **b**, the anterior bulging of the right renal artery, particularly marked during inspiration (*arrow*). In **a** retrocaval sonolucent line corresponds to the right crus of the diaphragm

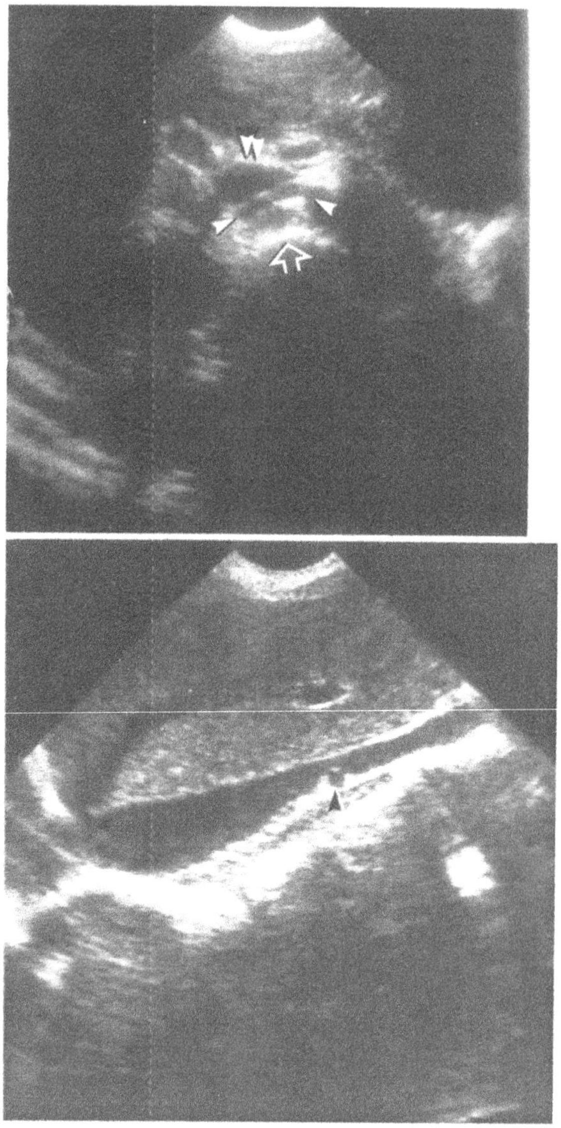

a b

Fig. 1.25 a, b. Right renal artery. **a** Transverse section: the artery (*arrowheads*) runs posterior to IVC (*double arrowhead*), anterior to normal lymph node (*open arrow*). **b** Sagittal section of artery (*arrowhead*) behind the IVC

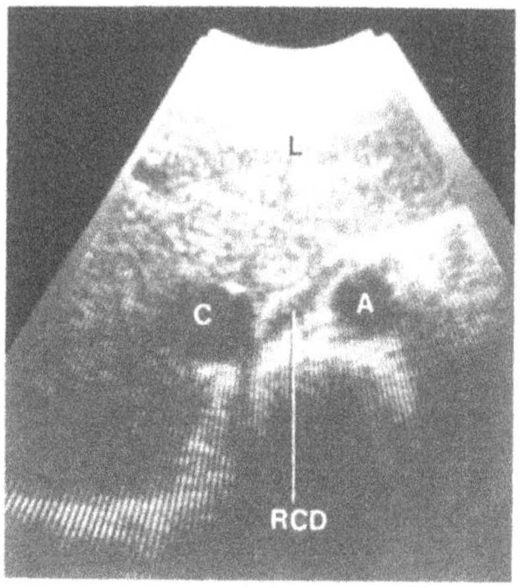

Fig. 1.26. Right crus of the diaphragm (RCD) displayed on a real time transverse scan. *L*, liver; *A*, aorta; *C*, vena cava

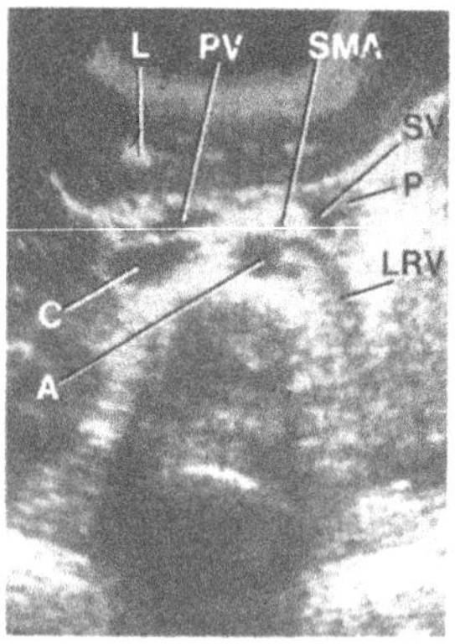

Fig. 1.27. The left renal artery is seen proximal to the aorta (transverse section). *L*, liver; *P*, pancreas; *PV*, portal vein; *SV*, splenic vein; *SMA*, superior mesenteric artery; *C*, IVC; *A*, aorta; *LRV*, left renal vein

Fig. 1.28 a, b. Right renal vein (*black arrowheads*) **a, b** two adjacent oblique sections. Note how splenoportal confluence is close to IVC (*white arrowheads*). Both vessels are separated by the virtual space of Winslow's foramen. Note image of normal lymph node (*open arrow*)

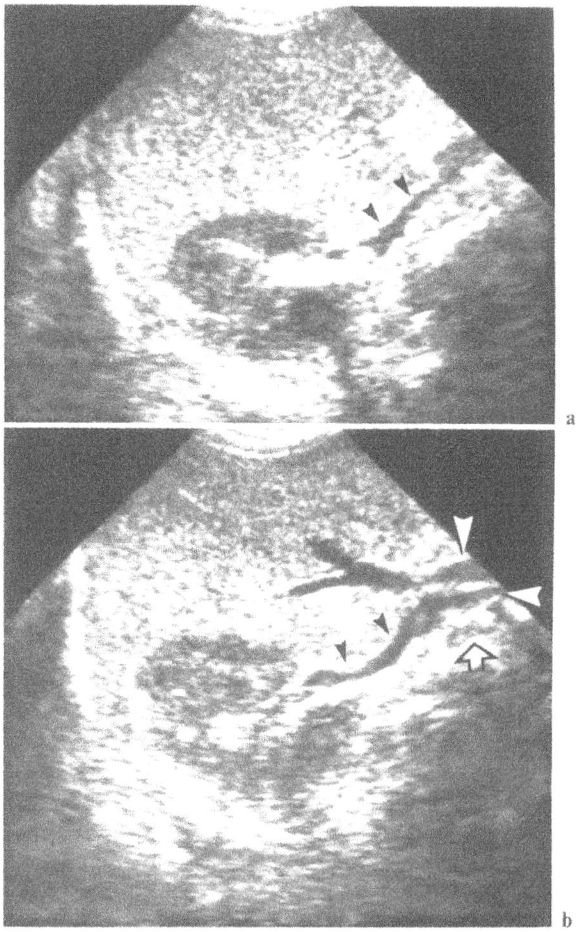

Fig. 1.29 a–d. Left renal vein. **a, b** Preaortic course of the vein. Transverse section. The left renal vein (*LRV*) curls around the aorta (*A*). *C*, IVC; *SV*, splenic vein, *arrowhead*, SMA; *P*, pancreas. **b** Another example. *P*, portal vein; *M*, SMA; *V*, left renal vein; *C*, IVC; *A*, aorta and origin of the left renal artery; *R*, right kidney; *LN*, normal lymph node. **c, d** Initial course of the vein (*small arrowheads*). Note again the vicinity of the pancreas (*broad arrowheads*)

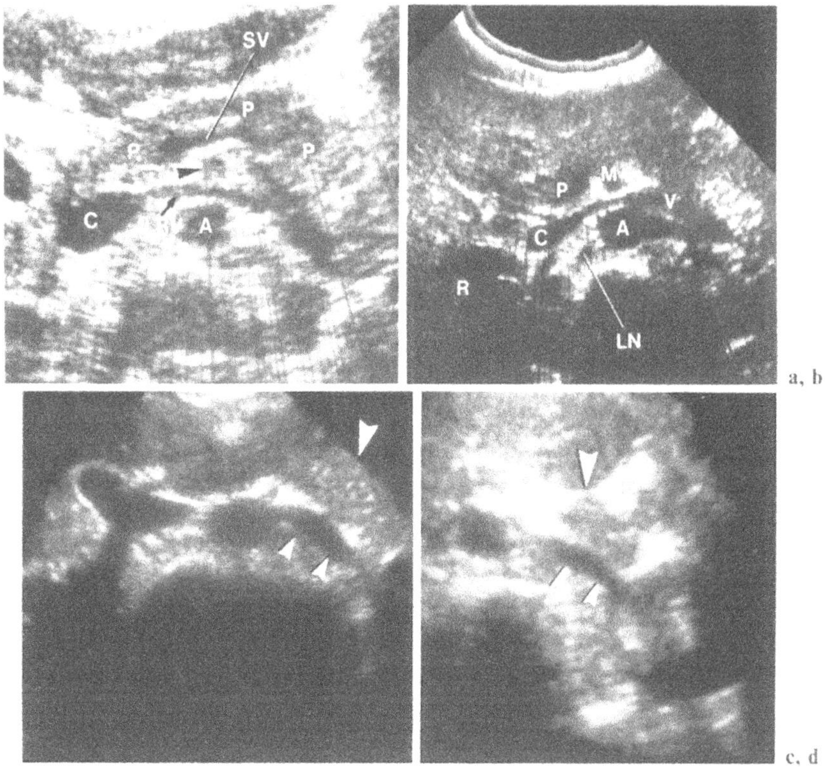

Adrenal Gland

The suprarenal area is displaced on frontal scans, or slightly oblique scans, as a strongly echogenic, triangular area. It lies between kidney, aorta, and spleen on the left side, and between kidney, liver, and vena cava on the right side. In fact the right adrenal is partly retrocaval, whereas the left gland is prerenal.

In good acoustic conditions the adrenal can be fully visualized with its particular shape. On the right side its retrocaval segment is commonly displayed. But in most subjects sonograms show only an echogenic triangle of suprarenal fat. We shall study the ultrasonic appearance of the normal adrenal in more detail in Chap. 11.

Retrocaval Kidney

A retrocaval position of the right adrenal is classical. We have also encountered a retrocaval right kidney (Fig. 1.30) in 0.2% of patients. This unusual situation is immediately recognized on a transverse section. But on a sagittal section the image produced by a retrocaval kidney will suggest a tumoral mass – until a succession of sweeping real time scans show it is simply a matter of morphological and topographic variation (WEILL et al. 1979), due to hypertrophy of the upper margin of the renal hilus.

Pancreas

The right kidney is not directly adjacent to the pancreas (Fig. 1.31). Even if it was adjacent to the pancreas, the right kidney is separated from it by the perirenal fascia. We have stated already that the fascia does not constitute a solid barrier to fluid migrations of pancreatic origin, which can involve the kidney. The close relationship of the pancreas to the left renal vessels must be emphasized.

This fact does not seem widely recognized: many sonologists advocated an oblique scanning direction for examining the pancreas, on the grounds that the left part of the pancreas is in contact with the upper third of the kidney (MEIRE 1979). This would mean that the left part of the pancreas is located above the level of the renal hilus. We studied the pancreas of 100 normal subjects in real time, with the subjects standing. A direct relationship between the left renal vessels and the pancreas was found in 62%. This ultrasound study was supplemented by that of 17 anatomical preparations (16 dissections and 1 transverse scan of frozen cadavers) (WEILL et al. 1980). The relationship between the renal vessels and the pancreas was found in 9 of these 17 preparations – a result which should be no surprise, since it has already been given in the classical textbook, *Gray's Anatomy* and since precisely that relationship makes it possible to achieve splenorenal anastomoses. As shown by retrograde pancreatography, it is the tail of the pancreas only which ascends frankly in the direction of the splenic hilus, above the level of the renal vessels.

1.3 Less Direct Renal Relationships

Right Side

The right lobe of the *liver* could be said to be directly related to the kidney, even though the two organs are separated by the virtual space of Morison's pouch (hepatorenal peritoneal recess) (Fig. 1.16b). Depending on the development of the right lobe of the liver, this relationship may extend along the entire anterior and lateral aspect of the kidney, or may cover a smaller area only.

Liver tissue is usually more echogenic than renal parenchyma. Sagittal sections of the liver often show a posterior bulge (infrarenal hump) just below the kidney's lower pole (WEILL 1978) (Fig. 1.11a).

As mentioned above, the relationship between the liver and right kidney strictly speaking is not direct, since two peritoneal membranes separate the organs. Morison's pouch is, in normal conditions, only a virtual, invisible space, but it can also contain fluid (ascites, blood, pus, liquid resulting from peritoneal inflammation or from acute pancreatic autodigestion). When it contains fluid, ultrasonic scans will display a thin sonolucent strip between liver and perirenal fat; we term this the "crescent moon sign" (WEILL 1978, 1980) (Fig. 1.32).

The *gallbladder*, though also separated by the peritoneal membranes, is often in close relation to the anterior aspect of the right kidney (Fig. 1.33, see also Figs. 1.30b).

When the right kidney is not entirely covered by the right lobe of the liver, the *right colonic flexure* lies proximal to it. In anterior scanning, gas in the colon may cast an acoustic shadow on the kidney. The ascending colon, which is located in the anterior pararenal space, may extend up to the renal lower pole.

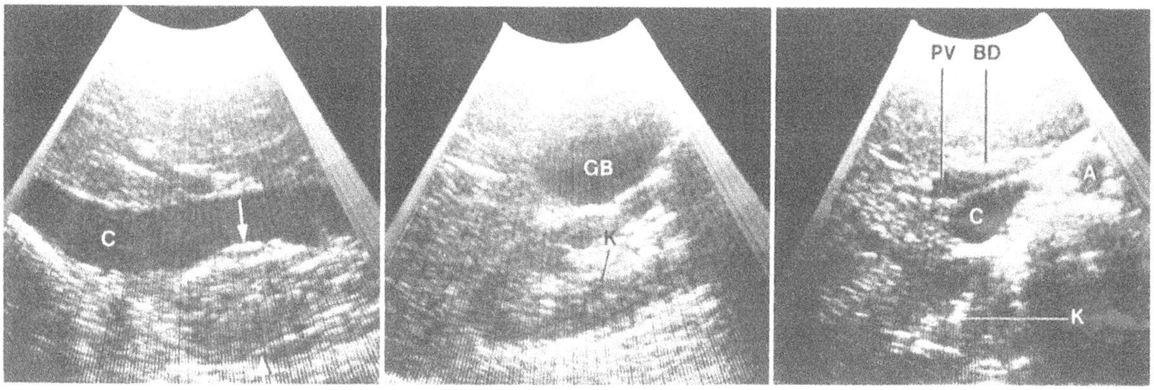

Fig. 1.30 a–c. Pseudoretrocaval mass. **a** Sagittal caval scan displays an oval mass (*arrows*) posterior to vessel, with slight forward bulging into vascular lumen. *C*, IVC. **b** Parallel, more external section shows right kidney (*K*). In fact, multiple sections during sweeping movement of real time head confirms the continuity of "mass" and right kidney (*K*). *GB*, gallbladder. **c** Transverse section clearly shows kidney in the retrocaval situation. *PV*, portal vein; *BD*, bile duct; *C*, IVC; *A*, aorta; *K*, right kidney. Note in **a** retrocaval sonolucent oval element adjacent to the upper limit of the kidney. It could correspond to the right adrenal

a

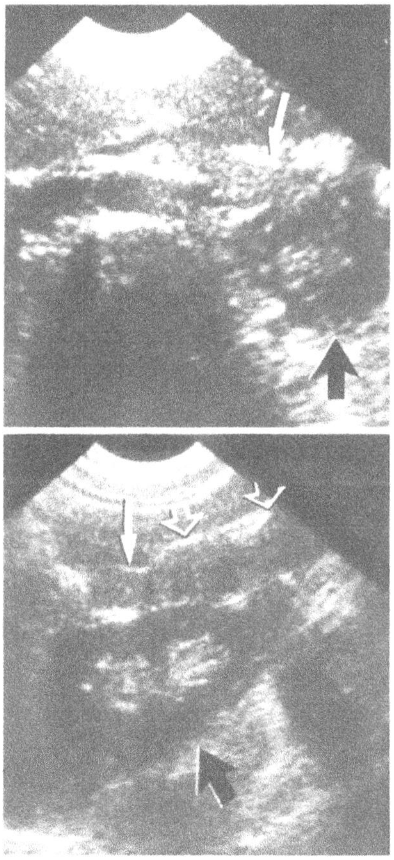

b

Fig. 1.31 a, b. Relation of the pancreatic tail (*white arrows*) to the left kidney (*black arrows*). **a** Transverse section; **b** sagittal section (*open arrows* points to the colon, close to the kidney within the anterior pararenal compartment)

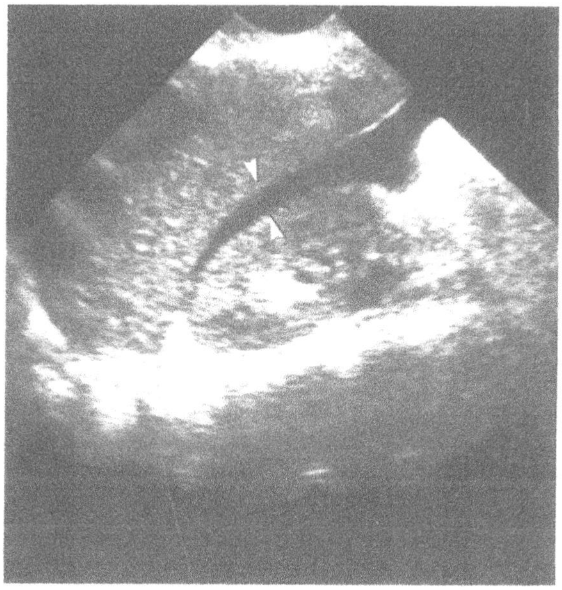

Fig. 1.32. Fluid (*arrowheads*) in Morison's pouch

a 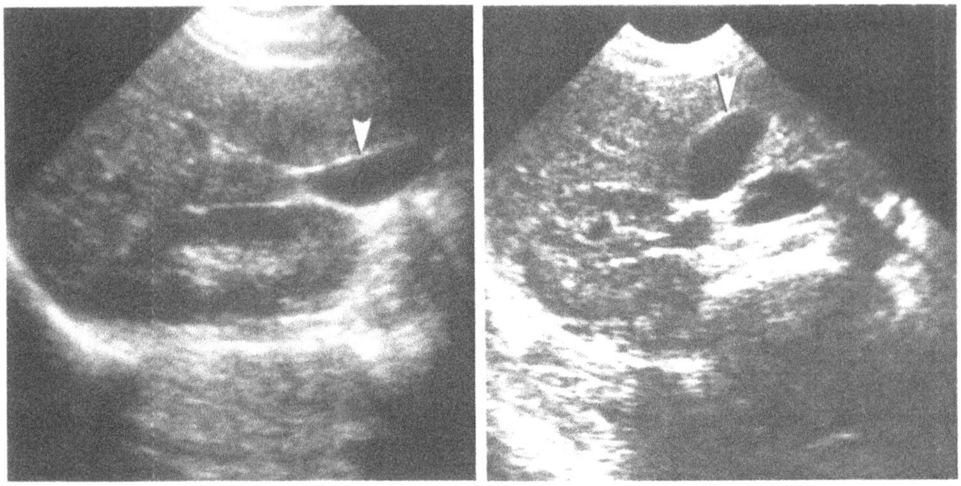 b

Fig. 1.33 a, b. Relation of kidney to gallbladder (*arrowhead*). **a** Sagittal section; **b** transverse section

a 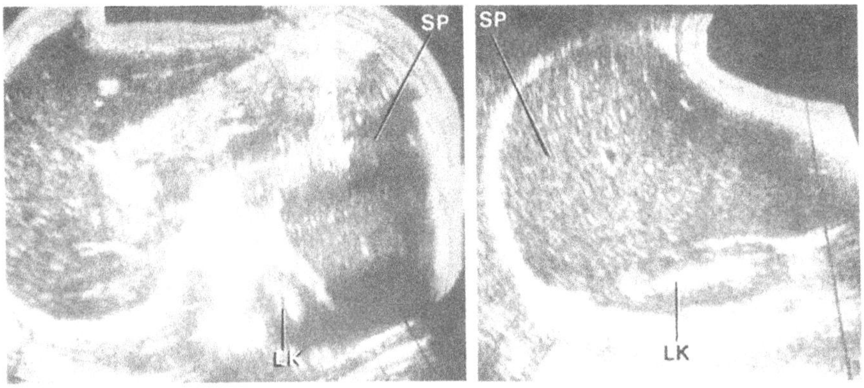 b

Fig. 1.34 a, b. Relationship between the left kidney (*LK*) and massively enlarged spleen (*SP*). **a** Transverse section; **b** sagittal section of left upper quadrant

a–c 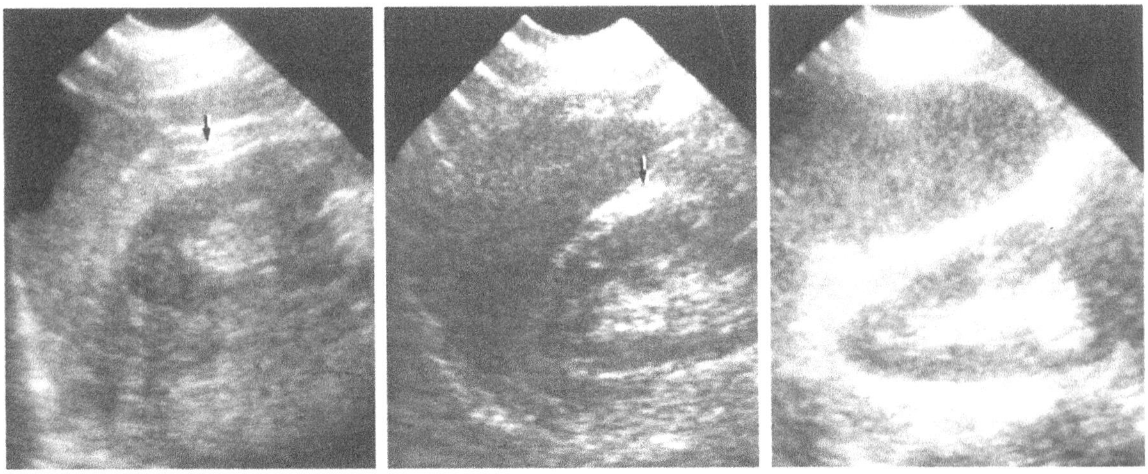

Fig. 1.35 a–c. Relation of the left kidney to normal-sized spleen (coronal sections). Note in **a** and **b** (*arrows*) the perirenal fascia

Left Side

The left kidney's upper and lateral aspects are in close relationship to the spleen. A massively enlarged spleen will entirely cover the left kidney, mimicking the relationship of the liver with the right kidney (Fig. 1.34). But in normal conditions the area of contact is limited to the renal upper pole and to the upper half (or third) of the lateral cortex. As on the right side between the liver and right kidney, there is a peritoneal recess between the spleen and left kidney. It is smaller than Morison's pouch, owing to the presence of the phrenicocolonic ligament, but a crescent moon sign may still be observed here when intraperitoneal fluid is present.

Intercostal or frontal scans visualize very clearly the vascular elements of the splenic hilus, in the vicinity of the upper third of the kidney's outer contour (Fig. 1.35).

The *descending colon* is located in the anterior pararenal space, in direct relationship to the anterior aspect of the left kidney. Acoustic shadows caused by gas in the descending colon often make it difficult to display the left kidney in anterior scans. Conversely, posterior scans of the prone patient usually show the descending colon in front of the kidney (Fig. 1.36).

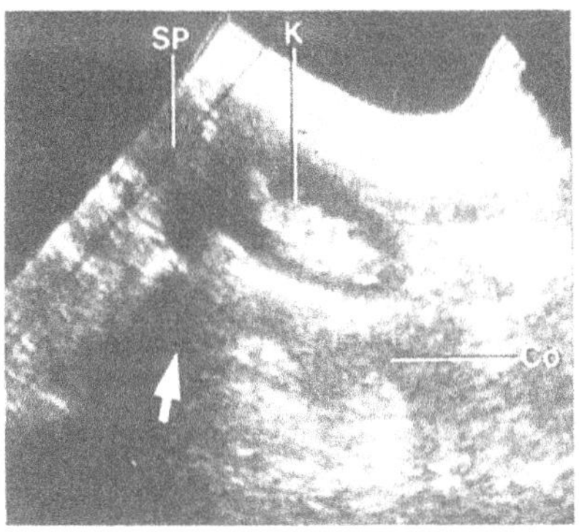

Fig. 1.36. Vicinity of the left kidney (*K*) and descending colon (*Co*). Note acoustic shadow due to colonic gas. *SP*, spleen. Sagittal scan in prone position

1.4 Basic Tissue Echopatterns: Pitfalls and Artifacts

Tissue Echopatterns

The differentiation between solid tissue and fluid collections is now classical and does not deserve detailed study. A fluid collection is sonotransparent and shows posterior enhancement (Fig. 1.37) (see also ascitis, Fig. 1.32, and the gallbladder, Fig. 1.33). Conversely, solid tissues are characterized by multiple echoes, whose pattern corresponds to normal and pathological architectures. The pattern of some fluid collections is less specific due to attenuating fluid, such as pus.

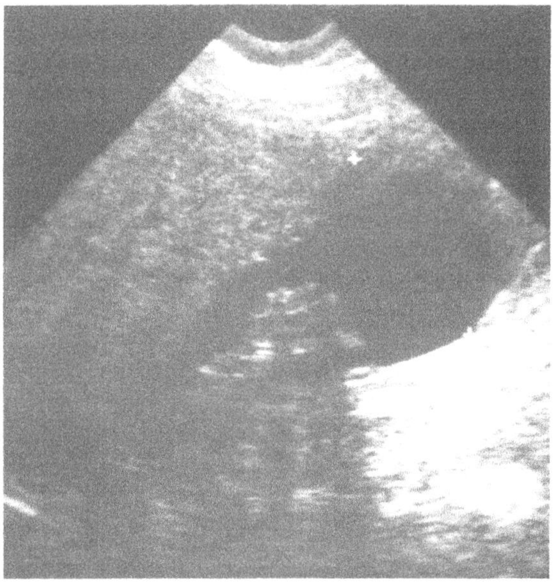

Fig. 1.37. Typical liquid pattern of benign cyst. Note posterior enhancement

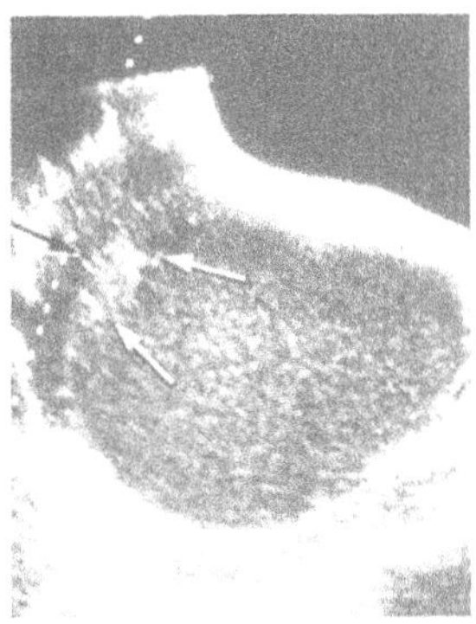

Fig. 1.38. Pseudosolid pattern of blood-filled cavity in a case of necrotized carcinoma: sagittal cut shows typical heterogeneous area (*arrow*). Rounded area filled with homogeneous echoes corresponds to almost pure blood disclosed by puncture: level of density at CT was 70 Hounsfield units

Some scattered echoes can then appear, whereas posterior enhancement is less marked or even absent. A similar pattern is encountered in slightly attenuating tissues, in edema for instance ("semisolid" pattern). Thus, some ultrasonic patterns are quire unspecific before puncture. However, the density resolution of present machines has rendered such situations much rarer.

On the other hand, the pattern of thick fluid, of blood, or of pus with debris or gas bubbles can be quite similar to that of solid tissues (Fig. 1.38). In such cases CT densitometry will show a lower density, and puncture will definitely demonstrate the presence of fluid. In some collections an echogenic component can accumulate in a dependent position, creating a fluid-fluid level (see Fig. 4.7, p. 63).

The gallbladder, the renal pelvis, and the vessels (see Figs. 1.22–1.25, 1.33, 1.37) display wall images. Gerota's fascia (Figs. 1.18, 1.35) is an example of what we term an image of septation. However, if such images indicate the existence of an interface, they do not necessarily correspond to an anatomical entity. This is particularly in the case of multiple layers of tissue, as in the gastric wall or in the wall of the urinary bladder. Some interfaces may correspond to artifacts.

Artifacts

Shadowing

We have already encountered acoustic shadows behind bone (Fig. 1.20). Calcifications, such as lithiases and, on the other hand, gas bubbles also give rise to acoustic shadows (Fig. 1.39). But all shadows are not caused by focal reverberation. The tangential distortion of the ultrasonic beam by cystic or solid elements gives rise to a linear shadowing called refraction artifact (Figs. 1.40, 1.41). Within the normal kidney such shadows can arise from vessels or major calices and also from the renal margin (Fig. 1.41). Pathological processes can also give rise to such shadows.

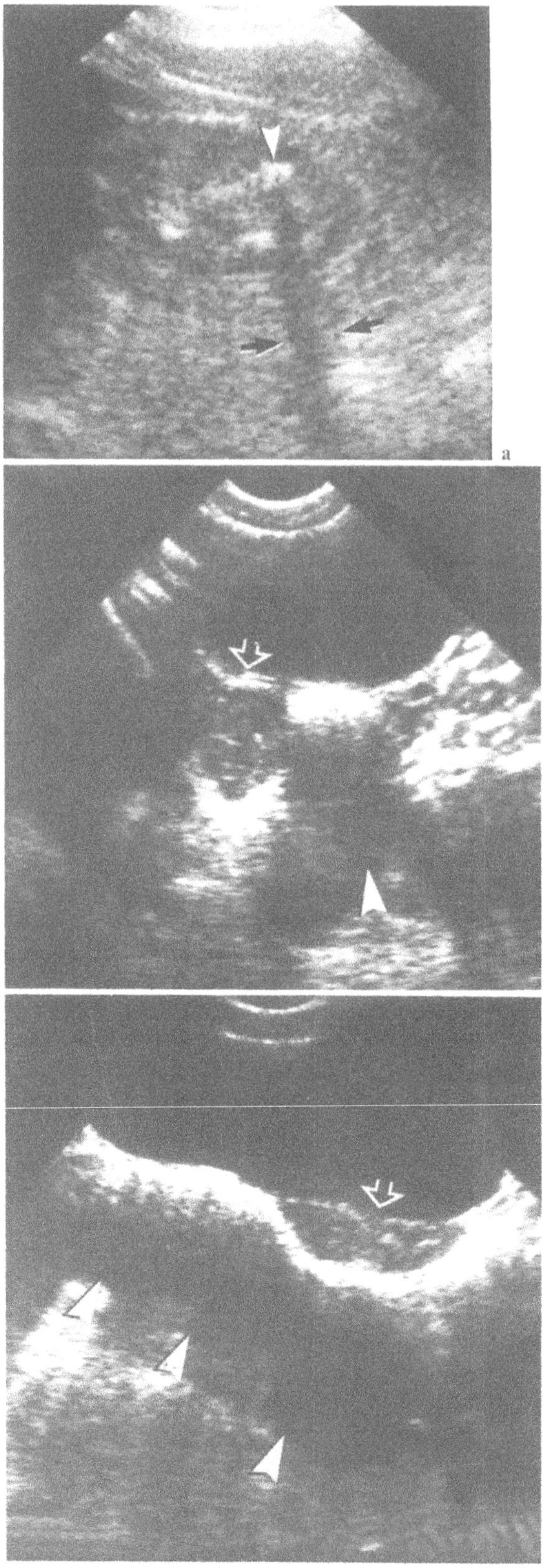

Fig. 1.39. a Shadows (*arrows*) of caliceal stone (*arrowhead*). ► **b, c** Shadows of intestinal gas (*arrowheads*). **b** Transverse section of urinary bladder and of hemorrhagic cyst in right ovary (*open arrow*). The shadow posterior to the bladder is due to gas-filled colonic loop (*arrowhead*). **c** Sagittal section of bladder and uterus (*open arrow*). Shadows are due to gas-filled colon and rectum (*arrowheads*)

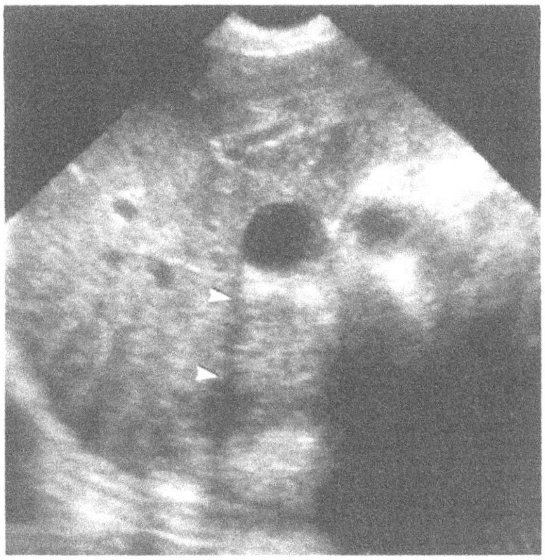

Fig. 1.40. Refractive shadow (*arrowheads*) arising from the margin of the vena cava, running through the right kidney

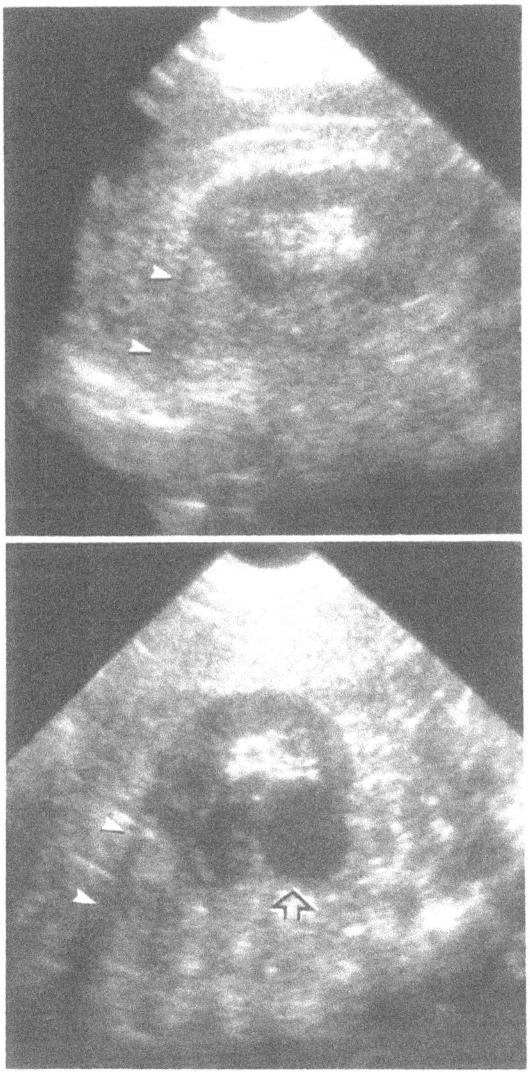

a

b

Margin Artifacts

The ultrasonic beam, even when focused, is far from being an ideal line. Even in the area of optimal focusing, its sectional diameter reaches several millimeters. It can thus deal with the lateral part of a fluid collection and with adjacent tissue simultaneously. The latter appears then within the liquid pattern, mimicking a sediment (Figs. 1.42, 1.43).

Mirror Artifacts

Mirror artifacts arise when a first interface A is located a short distance from a curved and strongly reverberating interface B. The ultrasonic beam first traverses A; reflected by B, it follows a new course and encounters B a second time (Fig. 1.44) before coming back along the same course. The display of an echo on the screen is related to the calibration of the machine, which converts a duration (the time required by the sound pulse to come back from B to A) into a distance, related to the sound's velocity. Thus, the machine converts the time of propagation ABB into a new signal, posterior to the interface B. This gives rise to a symmetrical, mirror-like pseudoimage of A (Fig. 1.45).

The third echogenic line which is often encountered along the diaphragm (Fig. 1.45 a) is a mirror artifact: the line proximal to the liver corresponds to the diaphragm. The medial line, classically depicted as the diaphragmatic image, corresponds to the pleura. The third line is a mirror artifact of the first line (WINSBERG 1983).

Comet-tail Artifacts

Intense reverberation can occur between the adjacent surfaces of a metallic clip or of a small stone, giving rise to adjacent harmonics. Once again the machine transforms a duration into a spatial signal. Thus the successive delays separating successive reverberations are displayed as multiple signals along the *y*-axis, giving rise to an echogenic strip made of adjacent echoes (Fig. 1.46). Similar artifacts, due to resonance phenomena, appear posterior to gas bubbles.

◄ **Fig. 1.41 a, b.** Refractive shadow (*arrowheads*) arising from the kidney margin: **a** Sagittal section; **b** transverse section. Note, in **b**, large juxtapyelic cyst (*open arrow*)

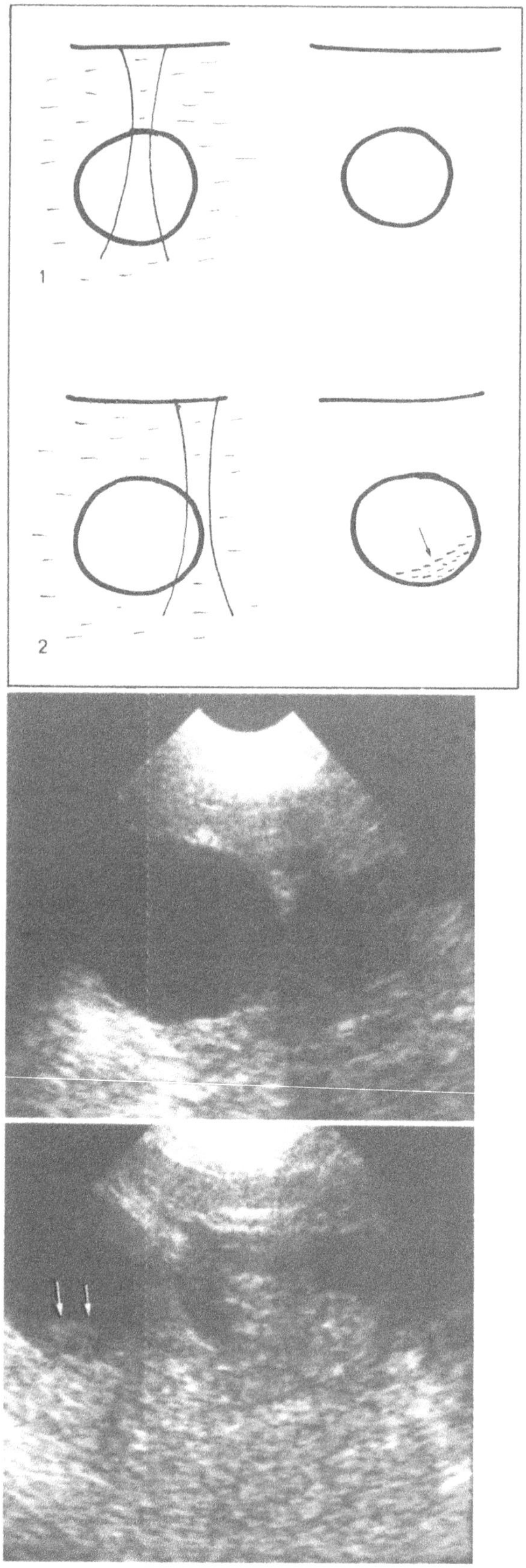

a b c

◀ **Fig. 1.42 a–c.** Margin artifact. **a** Scheme: *1*, ultrasonic beam passes through cyst; image of cyst is clearly outlined; *2*, course of beam is more lateral; it deals with cyst and neighboring tissue. Pseudosediment (*arrows*) is displayed. **b** Juxtarenal hepatic cyst displayed in conditions of **A***1*. **c** Pseudosediment (*arrows*) appears: conditions of scanning are those of **A***2*. Note, in **c**, refractive shadow

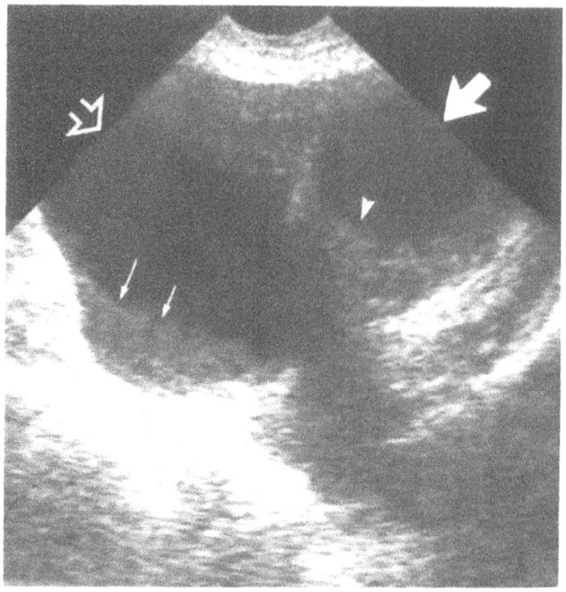

Fig. 1.43. Margin artifact: two similar images of different meaning. Transverse suprapubic scan shows an ovarian cyst (*broad arrow*), adjacent to urinary bladder (*open arrow*). The posterior echogenic area within the cyst corresponds to solid tissue (*arrowhead*). Similar pattern within the bladder (*arrows*) corresponds to margin artifact

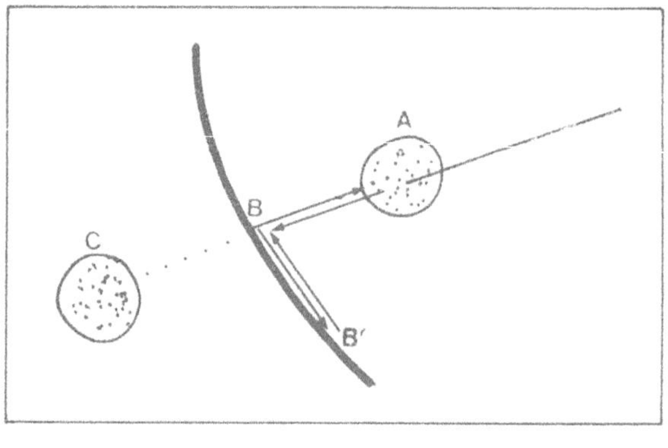

Fig. 1.44. Mirror artifact: the duration of the course *BB′* is converted into a distance and induces the image of a pseudo-object *C* (*BB′* = *CB*)

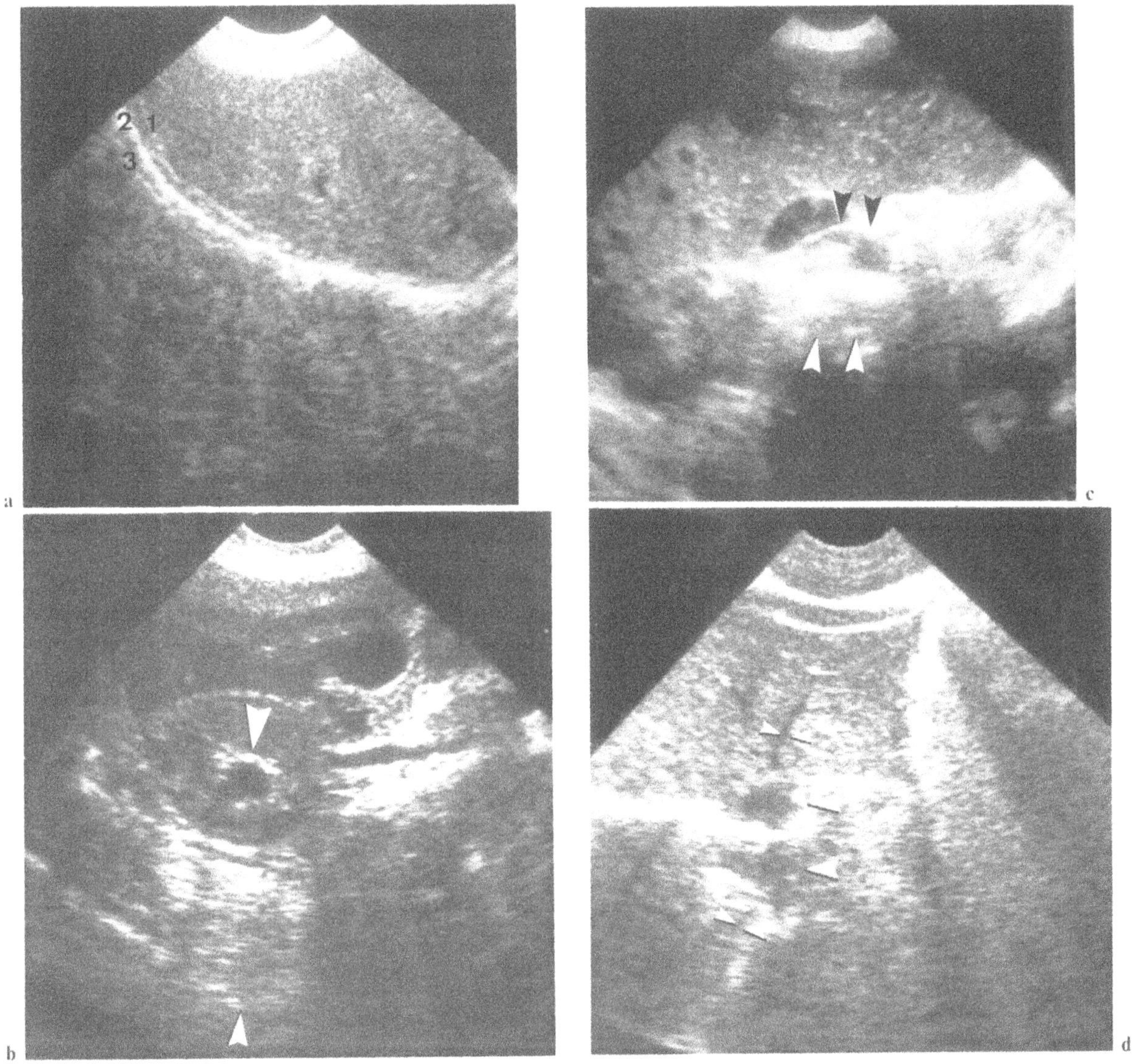

Fig. 1.45 a–d. Examples of mirror artifacts. **a** The three diaphragmatic lines: *1*, diaphragm; *2*, pleura; *3*, mirror of line *2*. **b** Transverse section of right kidney: mirror artifact (*small arrowhead*) of pelvis (*broad arrowhead*). **c** Transverse section of aorta and right renal artery (*black arrowhead*) with their mirror image (*white arrowheads*). **d** Mirror image of hepatic vein (*small arrowheads*) and vena cava (*broad arrowheads*)

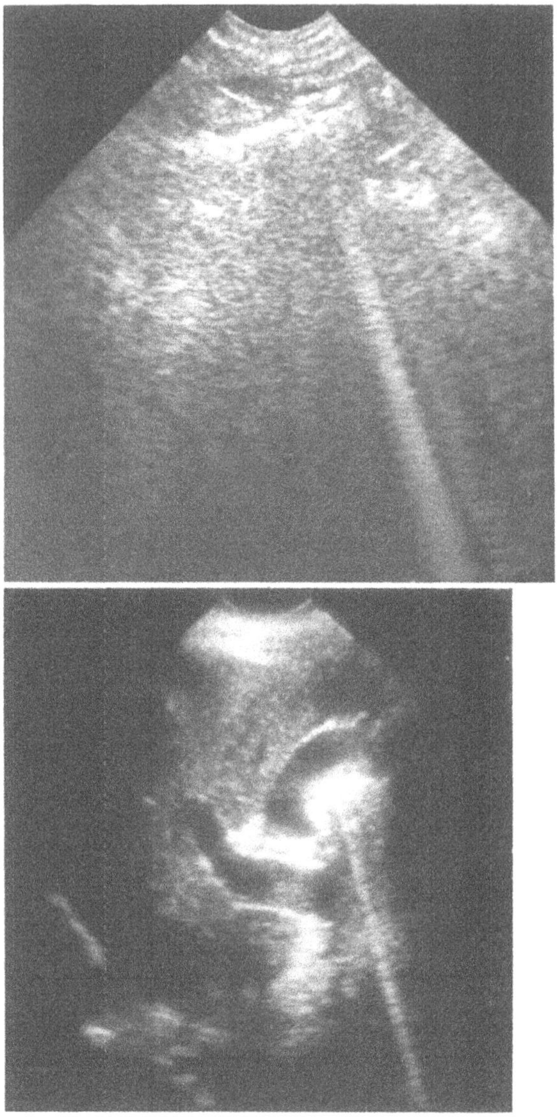

a

b

Fig. 1.46 a, b. Comet-tail-like artifacts arising from air bubbles within the digestive tract

Velocity Artifacts

Ultrasound progressing through fluid is decelerated, whereas it is accelerated through solid elastic tissue. Once again the display of the signal on the screen represents the time required by the sound propagation at average velocity. Changes in velocity induce changes in the location of the signal (FILLY 1982).

The phenomenon of velocity artifacts explains the flattened appearance of large biliary or renal stones. It also explains why while puncturing large cysts or large masses the tip echo does not always appear where expected.

The study of so many artifacts must not induce the feeling that sonography is a constant succession of pitfalls. The display of an artifact means that a local interaction between sound and a particular interface is occurring. This also means that the artifact will be modified or will disappear if that interaction is modified, that is, if the direction of the beam is altered. Such changes in the direction of sound are absolutely constant during a real time examination. And real time has become, as we shall see in Chap. 2, practically the only procedure utilized in daily routine. In real time, artifacts are *fugacious;* they are erased immediately under echoscopic monitoring. They must be kept in mind in order to be identified, and then suppressed, thanks to a dynamic technique of examination – thus avoiding, for instance, the diagnosis of stones whenever a shadow is outlined. But artifacts are also useful clues to existing interfaces.

2 Examination Techniques

The scanning planes used in renal examinations will be logically inferred from the successive steps of the previous anatomical study; we shall first scan the kidneys along their longer axis, using sagittal and coronal sections (Fig. 2.1). To these two longitudinal scanning directions, we shall add oblique scans, corresponding to intercostal scanning. And, of course, we shall eventually scan the kidneys across, using transverse sections.

To proceed from mere organ sections to incidences in the patient, it is still necessary to specify the different scanning directions with reference to superficial anatomical landmarks and to describe the patients' positioning.

Classically, the kidney is examined with the help of posterior scans carried out on the prone patient. Anterior scanning with the patient supine is advocated for the right kidney, using the liver window. In fact, thanks to the high-resolution real time now available, the successive steps of ultrasonic renal examinations have been fundamentally modified: as we shall see later on, most examinations are now carried out in decubitus and in the standing position. We shall study incidences and section planes in more detail later on.

2.1 Technical Data

This study will in fact be very short: we do not intend to deal in detail with ultrasonic technology, since this book is primarily focused on clinical applications. Details can be found in another book by one of us (Weill 1982).

There are two main methods of creating an ultrasonic (echographic) image: real time and contact scanning.

Contact Scanning

In this mode, a transducer is moved across the skin of the examined area, in a given geometrical plane (Fig. 2.2).

The summation of the different echoes, created at the interfaces encountered by the moving ultrasonic beam, builds up a laminagraphic image. Image construction in contact scanning needs a rather long time, from a few tenths of a second when using single-sweep scanning to a few seconds in the case of compound scanning. Contact scans are sequential; they are carried out following a previously chosen scanning direction, using parallel sections every 5, 10, or 15 mm.

In contact scanning machines, it is very easy to change transducers, and therefore the frequency and beam focusing. On machines of the latest generation, the echo display is digital, with a large dynamic range of gray shades.[1]

Real Time

In real time, the image is continuous, dynamic, and fluoroscopic. In fact, real time imaging corresponds to a rapid succession of images. The summation effect is achieved by retinal retention. In mechanical devices the transducer(s), instead of being manually displaced, constantly revolve automatically in a fluid-filled enclosure which is applied to the skin (Fig. 2.3). In some real time heads the transducer is static. The linear movement of the ultrasonic beam results from reflection on an oscillating mirror.

The frequency of the successive section images, which are displayed on a cathode ray tube, is high enough (15–30 revolutions/s) to obtain, as said before, a retinal summation. Mechanical devices give rise to sectorial fields. The image is digitized and can be frozen into a single frame, which is photographed. The real time images in this book were obtained with this type of machine.[2]

---

[1] The machine used for the illustrations in this book is a Phosonic (Searle).

[2] Combison 100 (Kretztechnik), Diasonics DS1 and DRF 1.

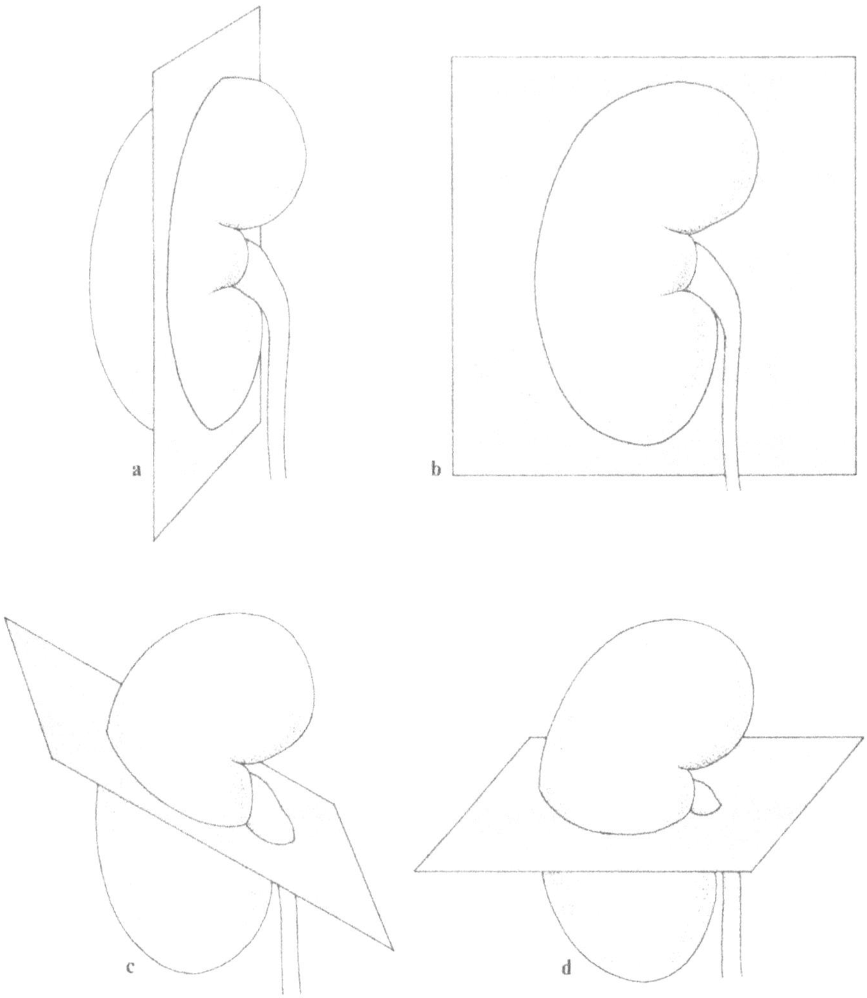

Fig. 2.1 a–d. Scanning directions used in renal examination. **a** Sagittal sections. **b** Coronal sections. **c** Oblique sections. **d** Transverse sections

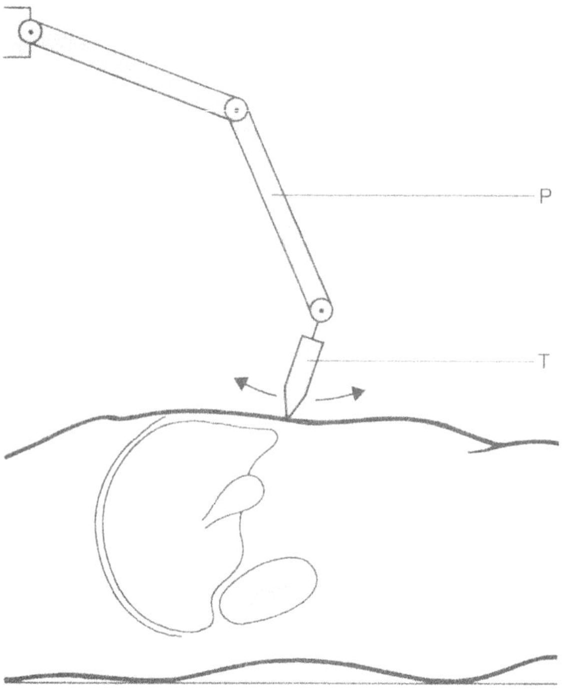

Fig. 2.2. Contact scanning: the transducer (*T*) and its pantographic attachment (*P*)

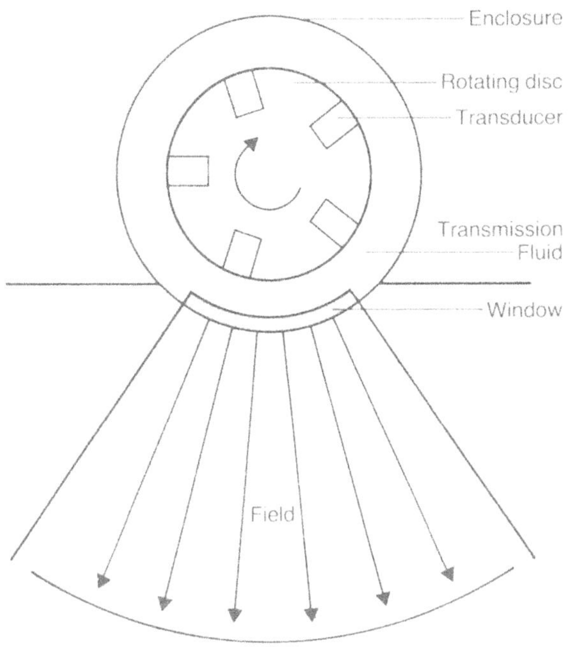

Fig. 2.3. Schematic diagram to illustrate the principle of a mechanical real time device

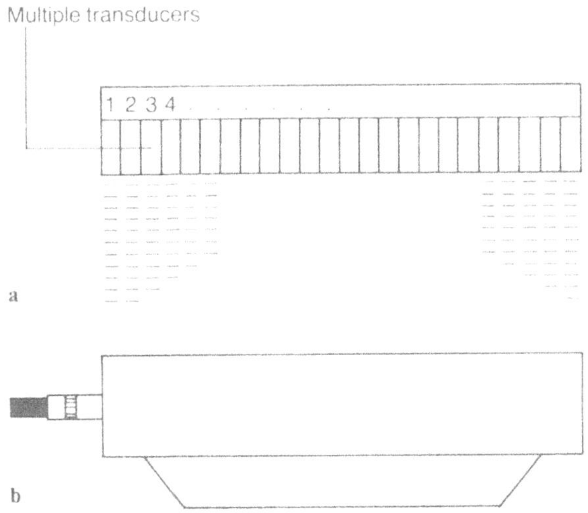

Fig. 2.4 a, b. Principle of an electronic array. **a** The multiple adjacent transducers: according to triggering phases, the wave front is oblique, transverse, or convergent. **b** External appearance of array

Other real time machines have arrays (Fig. 2.4) of numerous small transducers (60, 120, 240, or 480). The successive dephased triggering of these transducers gives rise to the equivalent of a mechanical displacement of the ultrasonic beam. Different triggering modalities (switched arrays, phased arrays) result in different kinds of fields (parallel scans, sector scans). They also make beam focusing and even dynamic focusing possible. These electronic devices possess a higher image frequency than mechanical devices.[3] Curved linear arrays are now also available. With rare exceptions, phased arrays do not yield ideal results in abdominal examinations, but they have built-in Doppler capabilities.

In real time machines, it is necessary, in order to change frequency, to change the whole real time "head," whether this is a mechanical rotating device or an electronic array.

Real time permits great flexibility of method, with constant information feedback. Since the image is continuously displayed on the monitor screen, the direction of scanning can be immediately modified and adapted, according to the shape, size, or orientation of the anatomical structure under examination.

On the other hand, thanks to the continuous display, an infinite number of close parallel scans in different directions can be obtained if sweeping movements are communicated to the real time head. The sequential steps of the contact scanning technique are therefore replaced by a continuous examination process. There is no "blind space" left out by the different sections. The whole organ volume is scanned across. Such a multidirectional sweeping scanning eventually enables one to achieve an effortless, natural three-dimensional cerebrovisual reconstruction.

Another advantage of real time is its flexibility in intercostal scanning.

It is our current experience that with high-resolution real time, small renal lesions (0.5 cm in diameter) (Fig. 4.2 a) are displayed which were not visualized with conventional, sequential contact scanning. On the other hand, contact scanning was able in selected cases, thanks to larger fields, to provide invaluable information. Currently we use only large field, high-resolution real time.

[3] The image frequency could be easily increased. However, 30 to 40 is an upper limit: with higher frequencies the sound pulse would not have time enough for its course down to the deeper interfaces and back.

Peroperative Sonography

Ultrasound has entered the operative theater (SIGEL 1982). Peroperative sonography enables the surgeon to localize at once renal stones or small renal tumors, thus markedly shortening the duration of surgery. A small renal time head, of high frequency, set within a sterile glove, is directly applied on the renal capsule, without coupling gel. Sectorial heads or small arrays are utilized.

2.2 Technological Prospects

A completely automatic examination mode is possible thanks to special machines using a water bed (KOSSOFF 1974). The patient lies in the prone position, in contact with a flexible membrane which is deeply depressed; the body is almost surrounded by fluid. Several transducers, moving synchronously, scan across the water window.

However, automatic scanning has not met the expectations, while high-resolution real time has become widely diffused.

Transmission imaging, which brings about a summation image, instead of a section, was announced as clinically and commercially available by GREEN in 1978. But it was never produced out of research laboratories.

Digitization makes possible the pre- and post-processing of the signal. It should also make possible its quantified analysis, which would represent an important step toward tissue characterization. But quantified analysis of attenuation has not yet (1985) achieved really specific results. We shall mention research based on the analysis of diffracted ultrasound frequencies, on the one hand, and on measurements of sound velocity on the other hand. Permanent bidimensional monitoring enables one to now propose duplex Doppler for evaluating the renal blood flow – not without difficulties due to the deep location of the renal vessels. This obstacle disappears when dealing with the transplanted kidney.

2.3 Technical Factors of Image Quality

Suppression of Kinetic Blurring

In contact scanning, rapid single sweeps reduce the time taken for image construction and therefore lessen the risk of kinetic blur. This risk does not exist in real time.

Axial and Lateral Spatial Resolution

Axial resolution, i.e., resolution along the axis of the ultrasonic beam, is related to its frequency. Lateral resolution (i.e., resolution along an axis perpendicular to the beam) is related to focusing: both parameters are transducer dependent.

Frequency. It would seem logical to increase the frequency of the beam in order to increase the spatial resolution. But as the frequency is increased, attenuation also increases. A compromise frequency of 3.5 MHz is used; a frequency of 2.5 MHz may be necessary in a large patient (the more so since the thick posterior abdominal muscles attenuate much more than the thinner anterior muscles).

Unfortunately, most companies abandoned the low frequency despite its evident advantages in stout patients. A frequency of 5 MHz will be chosen for studying lean patients or children, and also for evaluating fluid collections, in cases of hydronephrosis or cysts for instance.

Focusing. The depth of focusing is 5–10 cm (5 cm for children). Some real time sector scanners operating with several revolving transducers have multiple different focusing depths.[4] On the other hand, some electronic arrays have dynamic focusing. So do sectorial scanners operating with an oscillating mirror and an annular array.

[4] So does the machine used in this book.

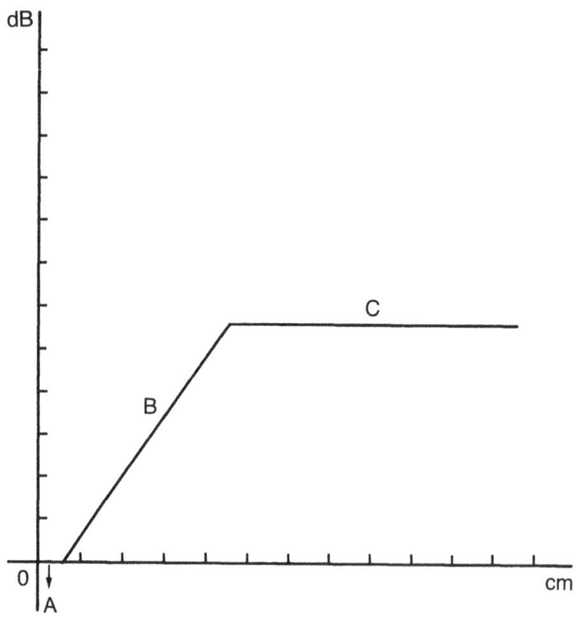

Fig. 2.5. TGC curve. *A*, delay; *B*, slope; *C*, maximal far gain

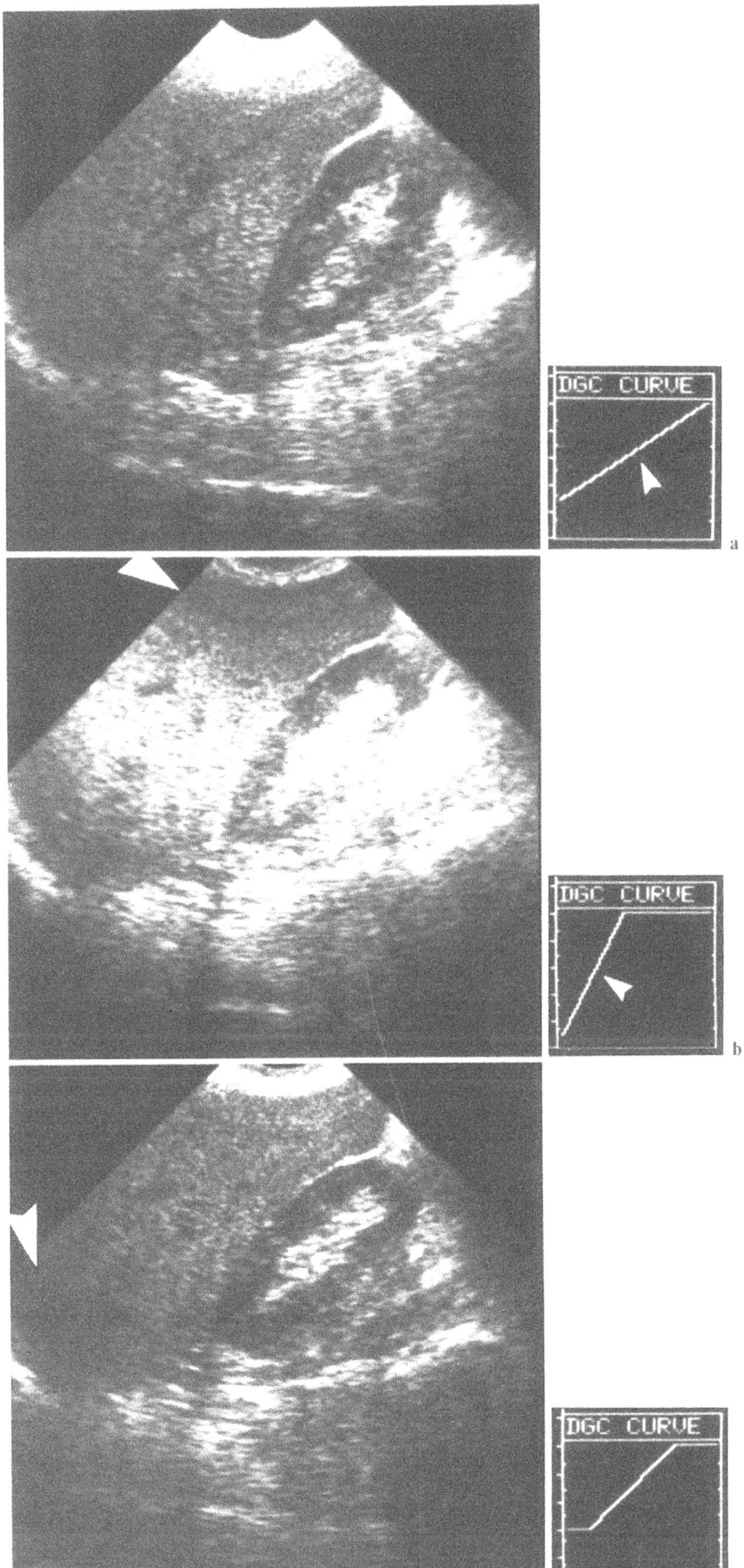

Fig. 2.6 a–c. Effect of TGC setting on image quality. **a** Satisfactory adjustment. Echo amplitude is similar in superficial areas and depth. The curve is displayed on the right. **b** Slope is steeper (*small arrowhead*). The image is imbalanced with too intense amplification in depth and too poor enhancement in superficial layers (*broad arrowhead*). **c** Now the slope is flatter (*small arrowhead*). Echo amplitude at depth is insufficient (*broad arrowhead*)

Total Gain and Time Gain Compensation Settings

Total Gain. This setting is easy to adjust immediately if the echo intensity is too low or too high. In fact an average setting is usually convenient for most patients.

Time Gain Compensation (TGC). The progressive attenuation of the ultrasonic beam in the deeper tissues is an unavoidable physical phenomenon. In order to obtain a good balance of the echo intensity from surface down to depth, it is necessary to amplify selectively the deeper echoes. The depth of the interfaces and of their echoes is evaluated by the machine, since the latter is able to measure the time needed by ultrasonic waves to travel from the transducer down to the interface and back. This evaluation makes it possible to set a TGC curve in relation to depth (Fig. 2.5).

An average setting is suitable for most patients (Fig. 2.5, 2.6a). Bad adjustments bring about important image defects and artifacts (Fig. 2.6b, c). Small adjustments are sometimes necessary, on the spot, during examinations: a permanent display of the TGC curve is absolutely mandatory. A proper TGC setting is mandatory when changing from a child to a large adult patient, from a heavily attenuating patient to a weakly attenuating one, or even from the supine to the prone position. A new setting is also necessary when changing frequency, attenuation being directly related to frequency.

The different parameters we have just examined are summarized in Table 2.1.

Table 2.1. Image quality parameters

Intrinsic to the transducer or real time head:
Frequency
Focusing
Adjustable by the user:
Total gain
Time gain compensation
Pre- and postprocessing

2.4 Positioning and Scanning Directions

Real Time

Right Kidney. The patient assumes the supine position. The real time head is applied sagittally on the right upper quadrant, immediately below the costal edge. The patient is asked to breathe deeply in and hold the breath. The real time head is then moved from left to right and from right to left, in order to carry out a succession of parallel sagittal scans through the liver window (Fig. 2.7). If the kidney is in a high position, the real time head will be angled cephalad, so as to scan across the whole organ, upper pole included. A few successive suspended inspirations will be enough for the required single-frame images to be obtained. Intercostal scans are then carried out with normal respiration, before coronal scans in deep suspended respiration are performed.

The patient is then positioned in left lateral decubitus. A series of intercostal scans (Fig. 2.8) are first carried out, in neutral apnea, followed by coronal scans (Fig. 2.9). The lateral positioning helps to bring the liver clear of the costal edge, especially in deep suspended inspiration. This increases the area of the liver window. Transhepatic sagittal cuts are then repeated. A series of transverse scans are then performed with a sweeping movement of the real time head along the anterior and lateral wall of the right upper quadrant (Fig. 2.10).

Left Kidney. The patient is placed in the supine position, or in an incomplete left anterior oblique position. The real time head is vertically applied on the axillary line, under the last rib, with a cephalad angulation, in order to scan across the kidney along a frontal (coronal) plane (Fig. 2.11). The patient is asked to take a deep breath and hold it. A sweeping succession of parallel frontal scans is then carried out.

The orientation of the real time head is then adapted to that of the intercostal spaces, in order to carry out a series of intercostal scans (Fig. 2.12). Intercostal scanning is easier in the left lateral decubitus position.

Thanks to a sweeping movement of the real time head from the lateral thoracic wall to the posterior wall of the lumbar fossa, intercostal scans are transformed into oblique and posterior sagittal scans which also show the aorta and branches. The scanning phases are thus multiplied, ensuring a thorough and complete study of the renal volume. In some patients the gas-filled left colon impedes the lateral approach. Posterior scans are then invaluable.

On the left side, intraintestinal gas is liable to interrupt the propagation of the ultrasonic beam in anterior scanning: sagittal scans are therefore only rarely possible by anterior approach. Sagittal scans are more successful by posterior approach; this is possible, in real time, using the same position of lateral decubitus.

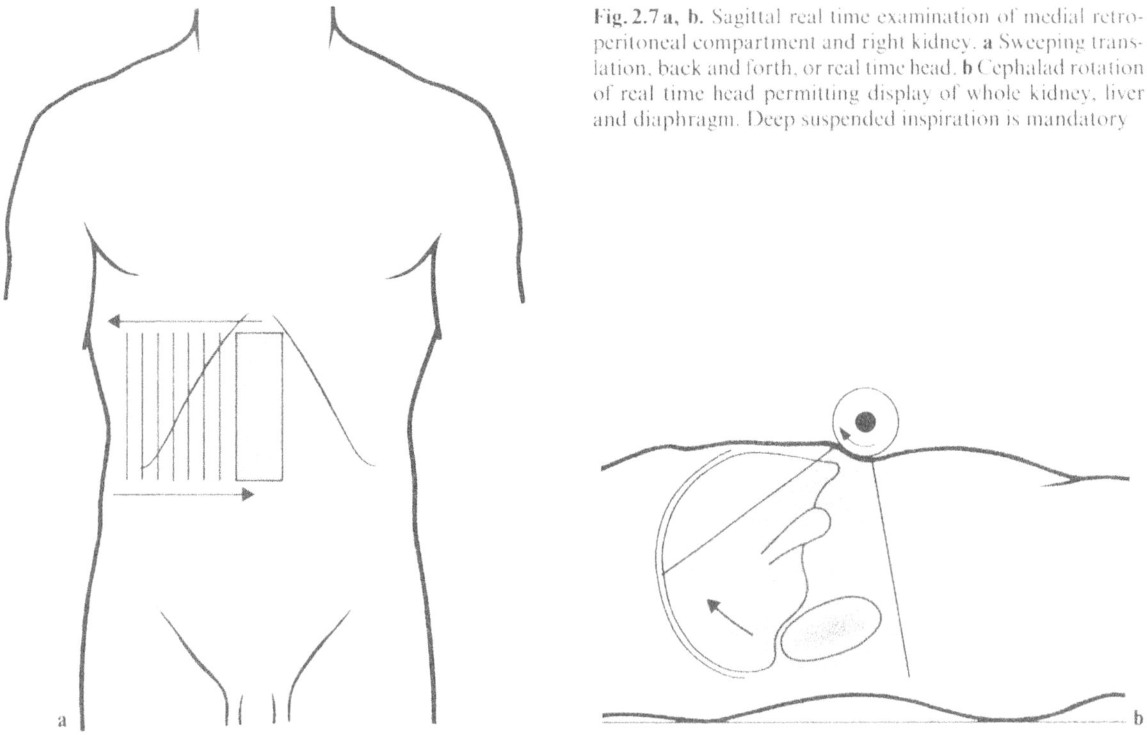

Fig. 2.7 a, b. Sagittal real time examination of medial retroperitoneal compartment and right kidney. **a** Sweeping translation, back and forth, or real time head. **b** Cephalad rotation of real time head permitting display of whole kidney, liver and diaphragm. Deep suspended inspiration is mandatory

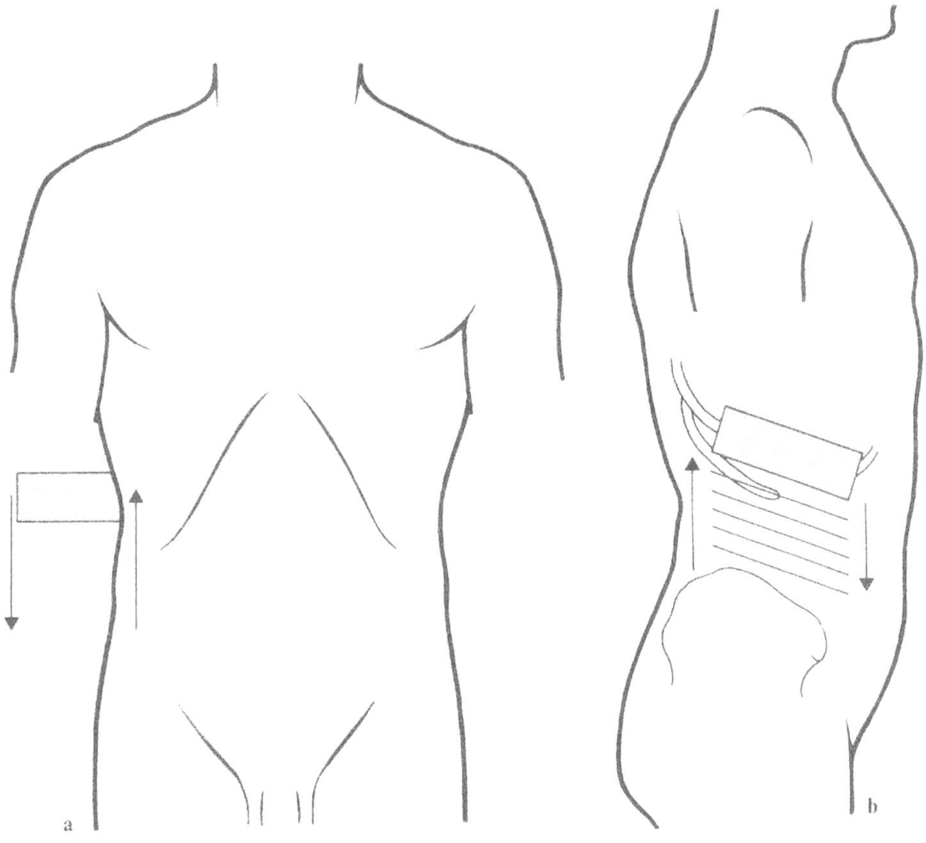

Fig. 2.8 a, b. Patient positioning and scanning direction during right intercostal examination: respiration is neutral

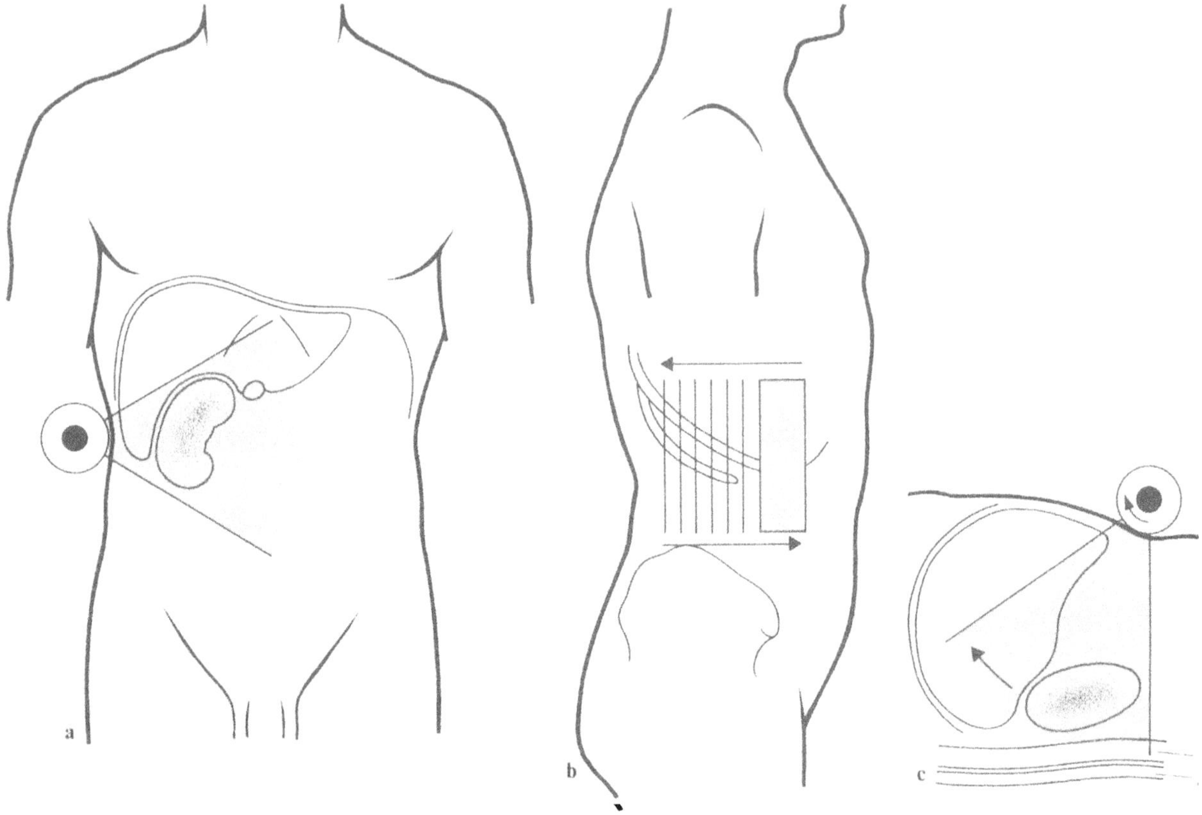

Fig. 2.9 a–c. Right lateral axillary scanning. **a** Positioning of patient. **b** Scanning direction. **c** Coronal display of kidney, suprarenal area and liver thanks to cephalad rotation of real time head. Deep suspended inspiration is again necessary

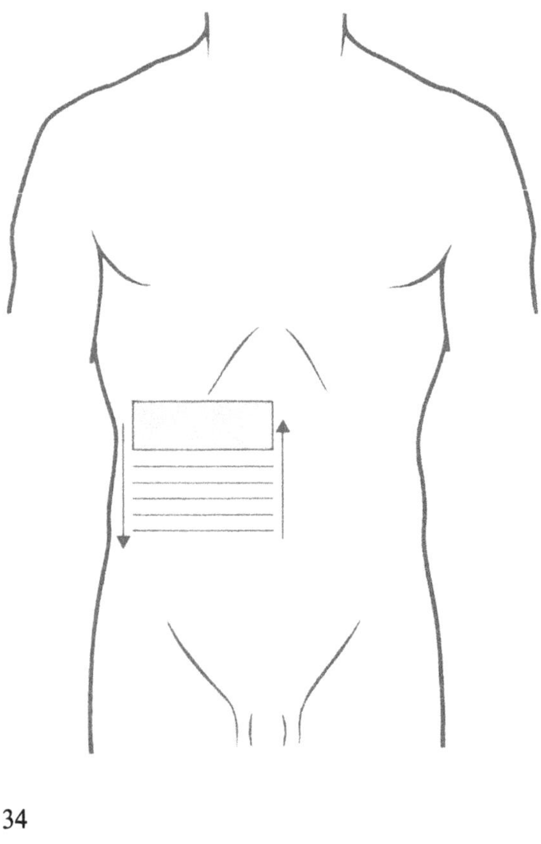

Fig. 2.10. Transverse real time examination of right kidney. Patient lies in supine position. A better positioning is achieved by left lateral decubitus, or, failing this, left posterior oblique position. Deep suspended inspiration is necessary

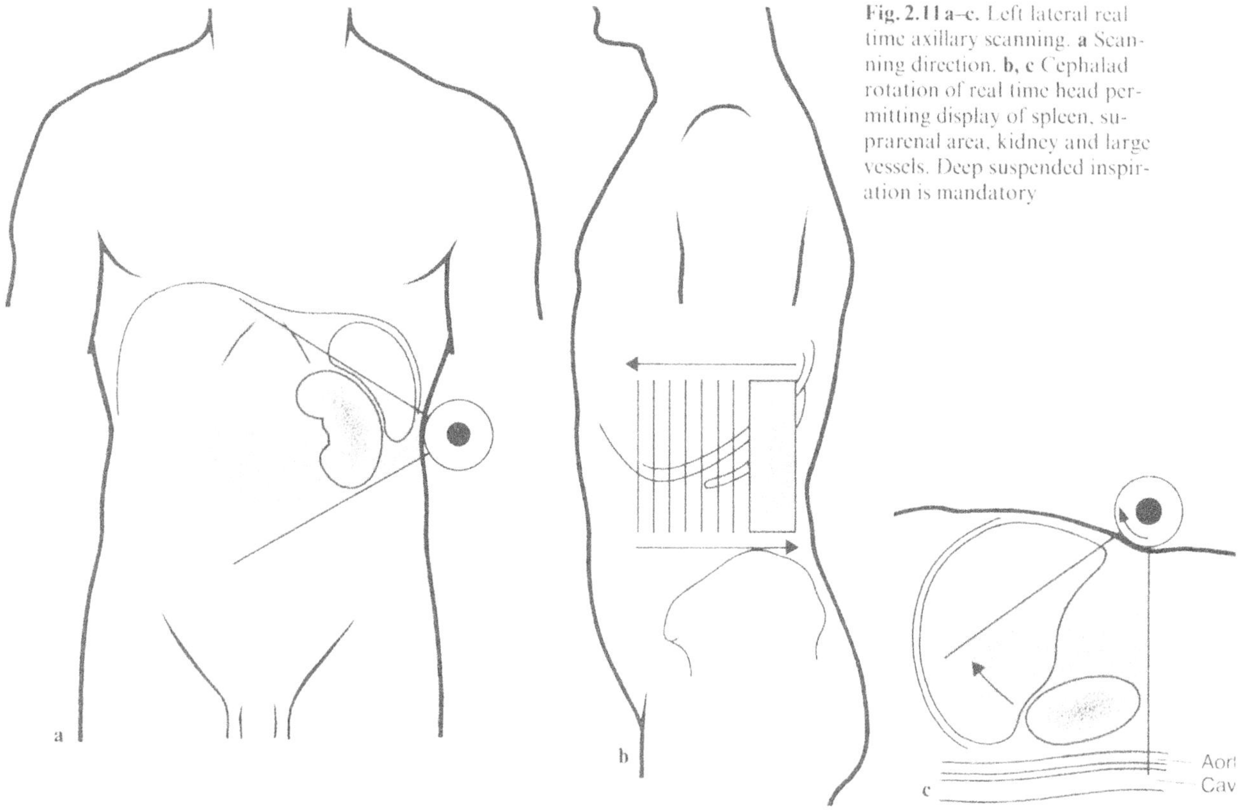

Fig. 2.11 a–c. Left lateral real time axillary scanning. **a** Scanning direction. **b, c** Cephalad rotation of real time head permitting display of spleen, suprarenal area, kidney and large vessels. Deep suspended inspiration is mandatory

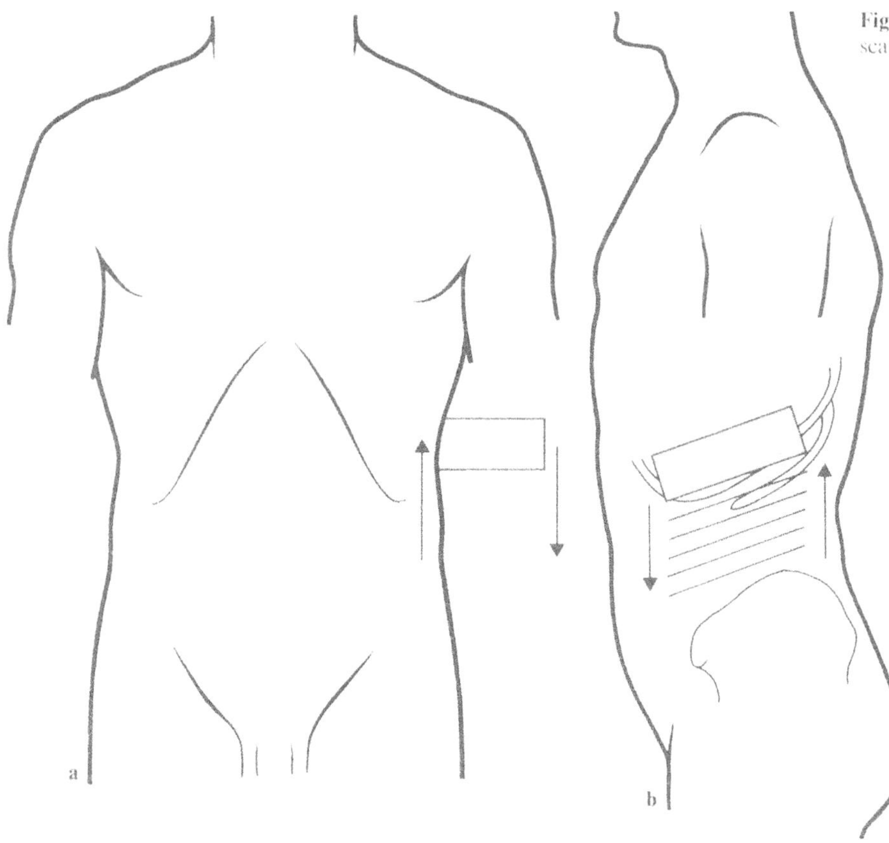

Fig. 2.12 a, b. Left intercostal scanning

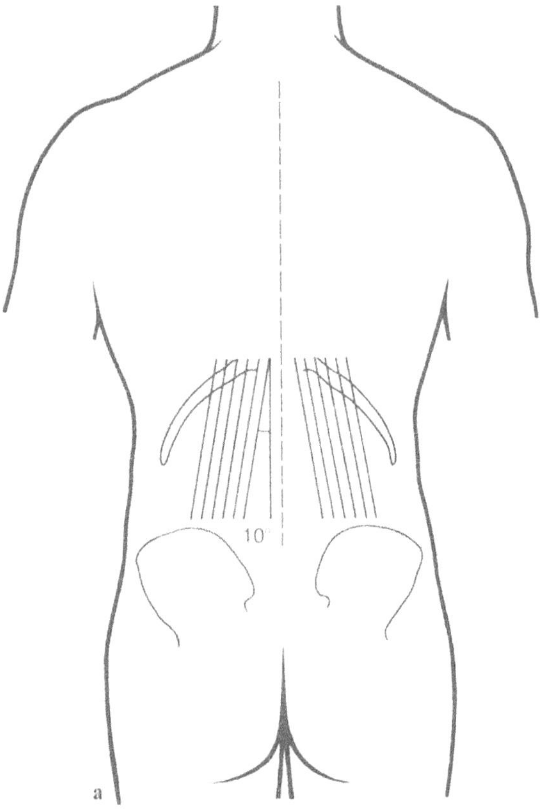

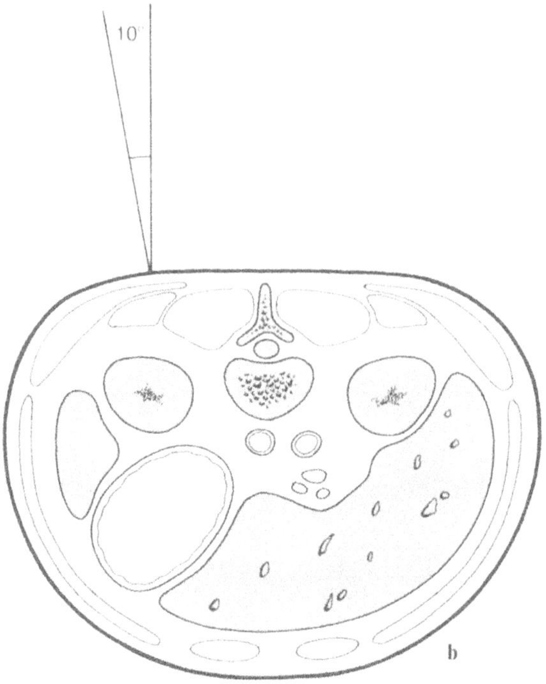

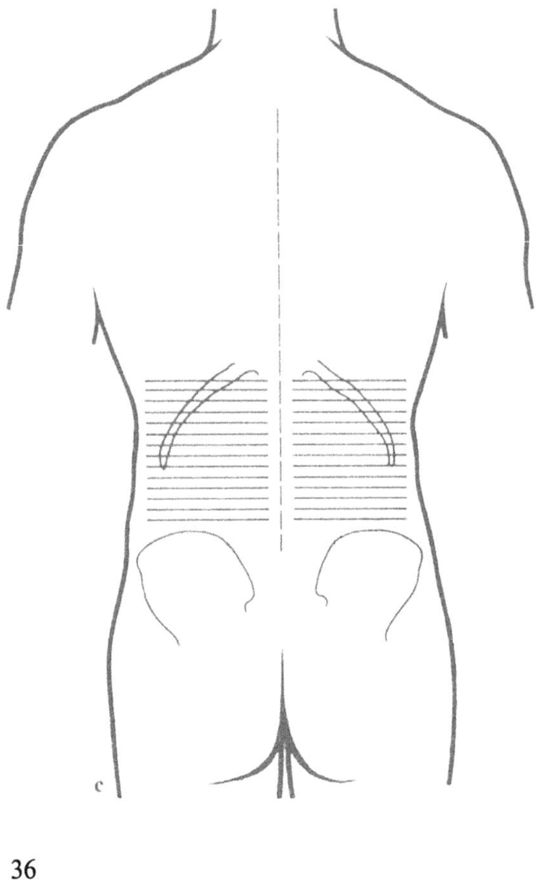

Fig. 2.13 a–c. Posterior scanning. **a** Sagittal scanning: note slight angulation. **b** Transverse representation of scanning direction during sagittal examination. Note slight angulation. **c** Transverse scanning

When the spleen is small, the left kidney may lie in a high position. It can then be useful to have the patient standing. With the help of a deep suspended inspiration, the kidney will then be brought more effectively clear of the costal edge. In fact, we now use scanning with the patient in the upright position systematically at the end of the procedure.

These successive phases of real time examination show, in addition to the kidneys, the retroperitoneal compartment, the liver, and the spleen: an ultrasonic examination must always be a comprehensive radiological and clinical examination, as we shall again emphasize later. Even carried out as a complete upper abdomen examination, a real time renal examination only lasts a few minutes in a normal subject. Screening examination of the lower urinary tract (see Chap. 12), in complement, only takes a few seconds.

Ureter. On both sides, lateroposterior scanning yields images of the upper half of the abdominal ureter.

Contact Scanning

All the positions and scanning directions just detailed for real time scanning were also be used in contact scanning. We used to carry out contact scans only for large lesions, whose diameter is frankly superior to the field covered by wide-angle sector scanning. We then used, on the right side, anterior transhepatic sagittal scans, performed in decubitus. We also used, on both sides, classical posterior scans, the patient lying in the prone position. Posterior scanning includes bilateral transverse scans and sagittal scans (Fig. 2.13).

In view of the orientation of the kidney, sagittal scans should in fact be slightly oblique (Fig. 2.13 a); the scanning plane should also have an axial angulation of 10° (Fig. 2.13 b).

2.5 Particular Problems

Critically Ill Patients; Recently Operated Patients; Traumatized Patients

It is impossible, in such patients, to use the prone position. The anterior and lateral approach, so easy with small real time heads, is then especially suitable. To scan a recently operated area, it is advisable, after removing the dressing, to fix on the skin a sterile adhesive mylar sheet, of the kind surgeons use to prepare the operative field (A. Eisenscher 1977, personal communication). The ultrasonic beam passes very easily across such a thin plastic membrane if less than 5 MHz.

Newborn and Infant

Here again real time is particularly useful since it enables one to avoid kinetic blurring. A frequency of 5–7 MHz, with superficial focusing and water-delay, is particularly convenient. The main requirement is adapting the focusing to the area of interest. Even without a special transducer, excellent images can be obtained at 3.5 MHz, provided that focusing is brought from a depth of 7–10 cm to a depth of 3–5 cm. This can be achieved by interposition of a water delay, the simplest being a perfusion bag of saline. However, with such a water delay, harmonics are displayed at a depth equivalent to the course of ultrasound in water. The best intermediate medium currently available is a thick block of flexible plastic.[5]

When examining infants (and, more rarely, very lean adults) in the prone position, it may be helpful to lie them on a pillow, so as to correct the lumbar lordosis.

Puncture Techniques

Ultrasonically guided puncture (Holm et al. 1975) will remain an essential complement to mere imaging in many cases, until reliable noninvasive tissue characterization methods become available. Puncture under ultrasonic guidance can also be carried out in order to position a renal or vesical catheter either for infusion of contrast medium or for drainage. That technique also permits the nonoperative extraction of renal stones. Puncture was first carried out with B scanners (Fig. 2.14). It relies now on real time, which permits one to monitor the needle's progression on the screen.

Guided puncture may be carried out with real time and contact scanning. Contact scanning guided puncture relies on a special transducer (Fig. 2.14) through which a central canal permits the passage of a sterile needle. The puncture itself is blind, but the puncture direction and depth are evaluated on the organ section image, displayed on the monitor screen.

In real time there are different technical modalities. A steerable tunnel-shaped guide may be fixed

[5] Kitecho – 3M –

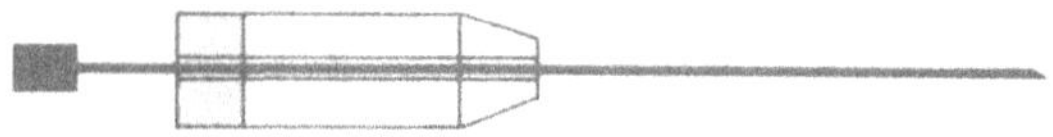

Fig. 2.14. Special contact scanning transducer for guided puncture

on the side of a real time head (HOLM 1975) (Fig. 2.15a). There are also (SAITOH et al. 1979a, b) special hollow real time arrays (Fig. 2.15b), through which the puncture needle passes. Free puncture, without direct coupling to the real time head, is also possible. With these real time devices it is possible to monitor on the screen the progress of the needle. This enhances the precision of the procedure. We perform puncture under real time guidance, with a linear array, but without any particular steering device.

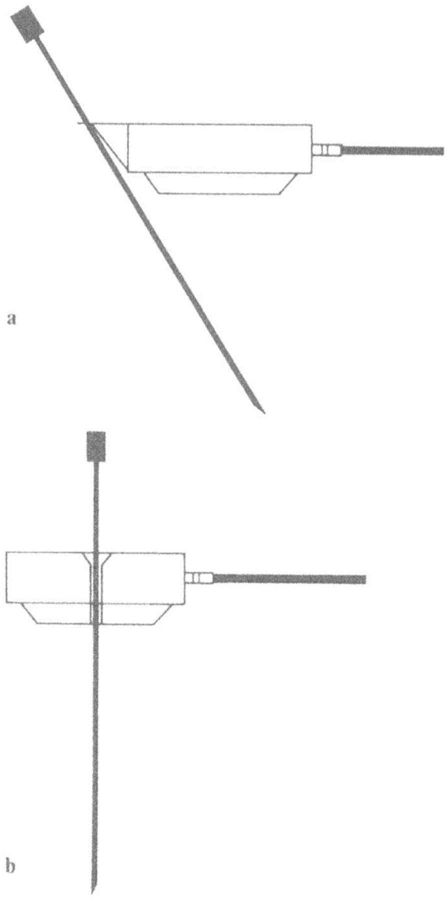

Fig. 2.15a, b. Devices used for real time guided puncture. **a** Lateral guide (Holm). **b** Central channel through real time head (Saitoh)

2.6 General Management of Ultrasonic Examinations

A simple renal ultrasonic checkup can be carried out on the nonprepared patient. Some preparation is nevertheless advisable for a comprehensive abdominal examination: as we stated before, a correct examination must be comprehensive: the discovery of a renal tumor will be followed by the evaluation of the retroperitoneal space and of the liver. The discovery of a pelvic dilatation associated with the presence of liver metastases will lead to the search for a pelvic mass. In the presence of cystic renal lesions, hepatic scans are mandatory. These are only a few examples: like any radiological examination, sonography is a clinical procedure which would be artificial and fruitless if limited to the particular organ initially suspected to be abnormal.

The best preparation, in our opinion, does not rely on complete fasting. Conversely the patient is advised to drink freely, since gastric and intestinal repletion enables a better examination to be made of the central part of the retroperitoneum, whereas bladder filling ensures a correct analysis of the lower urinary tract. Ingesting sweetened fluid provides some calories and renders waiting less unpleasant, particularly for older people.

Thus, our patients replace full breakfast by sweetened tea or coffee for a morning examination. For an afternoon examination, breakfast is allowed, whereas lunch is replaced by tea or coffee. During the procedure a complementary gastric filling is obtained whenever colonic gas impedes correct visualization of the retroperitoneum. Ingestion of 300 ml at least is required. The patient is then examined in the following positions: decubitus, right and left lateral decubitus, and upright position.

In the majority of cases, renal ultrasonic examinations are considered in a few standard clinical conditions only:

1. Presence of a palpable mass
2. Abdominal pain, with or without accompanying hyperthermia
3. Hematuria
4. Unexplained fever
5. Discovery of liver, bone, or lung metastases
6. Abnormalities disclosed by an intravenous urogram (IVU): a nonsecreting kidney, presence of a "urographic" renal mass, etc.

A particular item is the frequency with which renal abnormalities are disclosed by comprehensive upper abdomen examinations carried out for nonrenal purposes: in the course of a digestive ultrasonic screening examination; the right kidney is scanned across while the liver is evaluated, and the left kidney while the pancreas and the spleen are examined.

3 Hydronephrosis

Ultrasonic images of hydronephrosis are encountered in the following clinical conditions:
- Abdominal pain, with or without fever
- Presence of a palpable mass
- Complementary ultrasound after discovery of a nonsecreting kidney on an IVU
- Evaluation of anuria or renal insufficiency
- Evaluation of the lower urinary tract and pelvis
- Systematic complementary renal evaluation during an obstetrical ultrasonic examination
- Abdominal screening

3.1 Beginning Hydronephrosis

Beginning hydronephrosis will be evaluated at the level of the renal pelvis on the one hand, and at the level of calices on the other.

Pelvis Dilatation. In Chap. 1 we gave the maximum anteroposterior diameter of the normal renal pelvis as 3 cm. A dilated pelvis may appear with two different patterns. One is that of an intrarenal pouch, giving rise to an echo-free pattern inside the reflective central area, with convex limits (Fig. 3.1). The other is that of a pouch in the renal sinus, internal to the kidney rather than intrarenal (Fig. 3.2). In both patterns the dilatation gives rise to a convexity of contours – intercostal, coronal and poserolateral scans make possible a precise analysis of the ureteric junction.

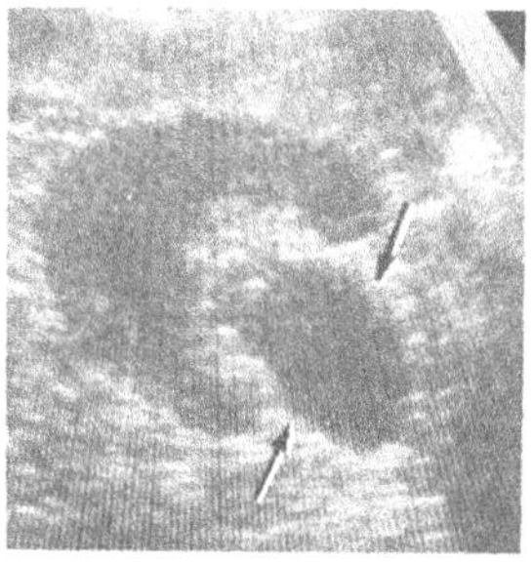

Fig. 3.2. Extrasinusal dilated pelvis (*arrows*) (transverse cut)

Caliceal Dilatation. Infundibular dilatation gives rise to small fluid-filled peripheral pouches (Fig. 3.3). Fluid-filled areas will appear inside the reflective zone due to a dilatation of the major calices (Fig. 3.4). Multidirectional real time scans will display the confluence of the different parts of the dilated collecting system. Intercostal scans show at best the general architecture of the dilated collecting system (Fig. 3.5).

There may be a discrepancy between the sizes of the calices and the pelvis. Ultrasonic scans may display a widely dilated pelvis while calices are only moderately dilated or even of normal size (Fig. 3.6). In such cases, the pelvis seems to act for a while as a valve, particularly after the rapid onset of an obstruction.

As we mentioned in Chap. 1, according to Morin and Baker (1979) the amount of water intake and the degree of bladder repletion must both be considered when evaluating the size of the col-

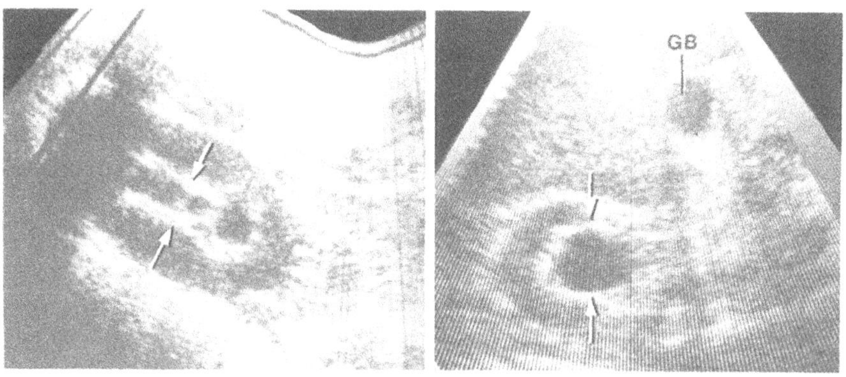

a, b

Fig. 3.1 a, b. Beginning dilatation of intrasinusal pelvis. **a** Sagittal scan of left kidney in prone position shows enlarged pelvis (*arrows*). **b** Oblique cut of right kidney. Diameter of rounded, dilated pelvis (*arrows*) is 3.5 cm. Shadowing posterior to gall bladder (*GB*) is due to sound bending lecting system in borderline cases: a moderate dilatation may only signify increased secretion and ureteral blockage due to urine retention in the bladder. In such cases the seemingly dilated collecting systems are symmetrical. A further examination when the patient is fasting and after vesical evacuation must then be considered, rather than carrying out immediately an excretory urogram. ROSENFIELD (1979a, b) advocates increasing the water intake to display borderline dilatations better. In the pregnant woman a moderate dilatation of the collecting system is normal (Fig. 3.6). In case of functional disorders (pain, signs of infection), dilatation of the affected side alone, or more pronounced on the affected side, is a relevant sign.

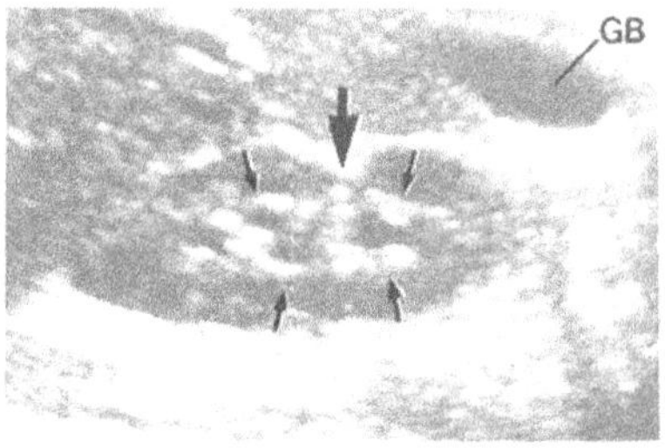

Fig. 3.3. Discrete caliceal dilatation (*arrows*)

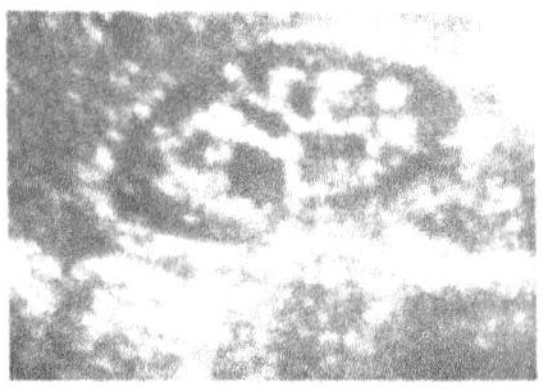

Fig. 3.4. Multilocular pattern due to dilatation of major calices. Similar pattern arise from multiple parapelvic cysts

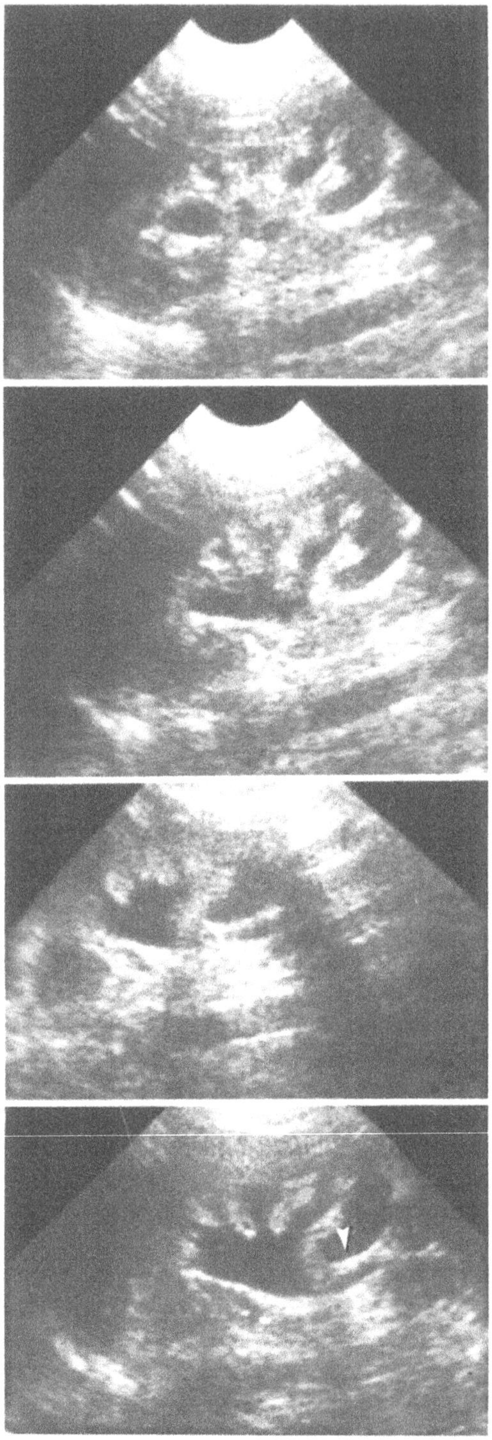

Fig. 3.5 a–d. Pelvicaliceal dilatation. Four parallel left posterolateral scans. Note, in **d**, junctional dilatation (*arrowhead*). Note also display of aorta

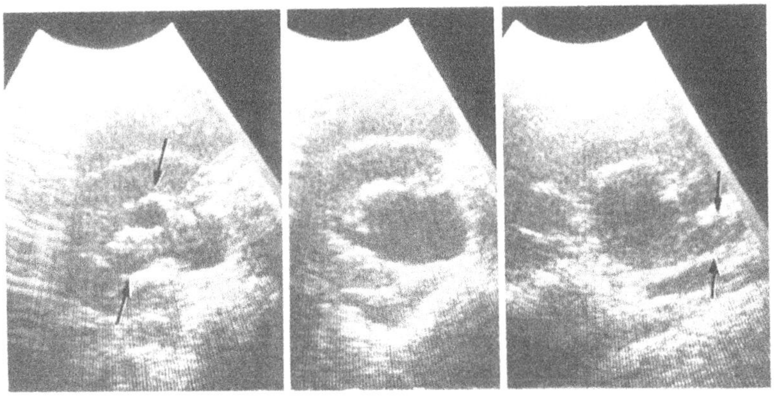

a–c

Fig. 3.6 a–c. Pelvicaliceal dilatation in 6 months pregnancy. **a** Dilated pelvis and calices (*arrows*). **b** Pelvis. **c** Pelvis and initial ureter (*arrows*)

3.2 Frank Hydronephrosis

We term frank hydronephrosis a condition in which a markedly dilated pelvis (over 5 cm in anteroposterior diameter) is associated with dilated infundibula and calices (Figs. 3.7, 3.8). Such images of dilatation affecting the entire collecting system are quite similar to those seen on a conventional X-ray urogram. The communications existing between the infundibula and the pelvis, and corresponding to the dilated calices themselves, are usually evident on most of the ultrasonic scans. If not, a multidirectional real time study of the collecting system will clearly display the confluences as defects, interrupting the infundibular and caliceal walls (Fig. 3.9). Pelvicalyceal confluences are usually well demonstrated on intercostal scans. The dilated calices outline then, above the pelvis, the "Mickey mouse" pattern (Figs. 3.6a, 3.7a, 3.8b, 3.9c). Cortical atrophy can be demonstrated (Figs. 3.8, 3.9).

Ultrasonic evaluation of hydronephrosis calls for a thourough analysis of the different territories of the kidney.

The discovery of a dilatation limited to only part of the collecting system has important etiological significance: a partial dilatation can be due to an inflammatory process, e.g., a renal tuberculosis, or to a pelvicaliceal urothelial tumor. In such cases sonography can only provide hypotheses, which will be checked by an IVU or by an instrumental opacification if necessary.

Partial hydronephrosis can also correspond to dilatation of one of the nephrons of a duplicated kidney (Fig. 3.11). In some cases, a bladder examination is then likely to display a ureterocele (Fig. 3.11). Acute dilatation may be complicated by a rupture, with developing urinoma ("uriniferous cyst") (see Chap. 10, Fig. 10.8).

Pelvic-Ureteric Junction. We have already stressed the interest in assessing the pelvic-ureteric junction. This particular segment is best visualized by intercostal, coronal and posterolateral sections. Such sections also readily show the first centimeters of a dilated ureter. It is therefore quite easy to differentiate a mere junctional syndrome from a uretero-hydronephrosis (Figs. 3.5d, 3.6c, 3.12–3.15).

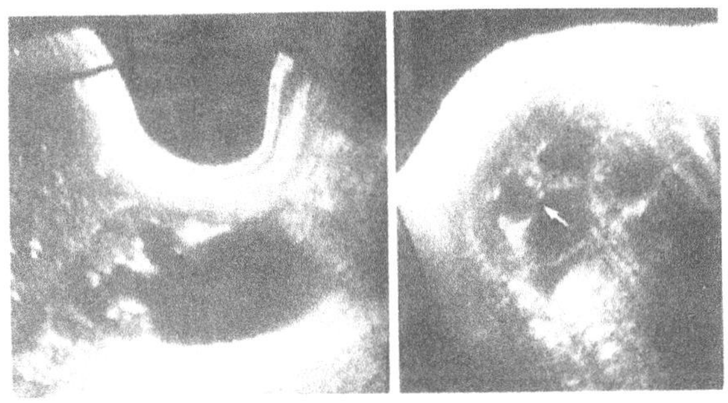

a, b

Fig. 3.7 a, b. Frank hydronephrosis. **a** Sagittal scan: pelvis diameter is 9 cm. Pelvicaliceal communications are readily demonstrated. **b** Transverse scan: pattern is multilocular but pelvicaliceal communication is displayed (*arrow*). Parenchymal thickness remains normal

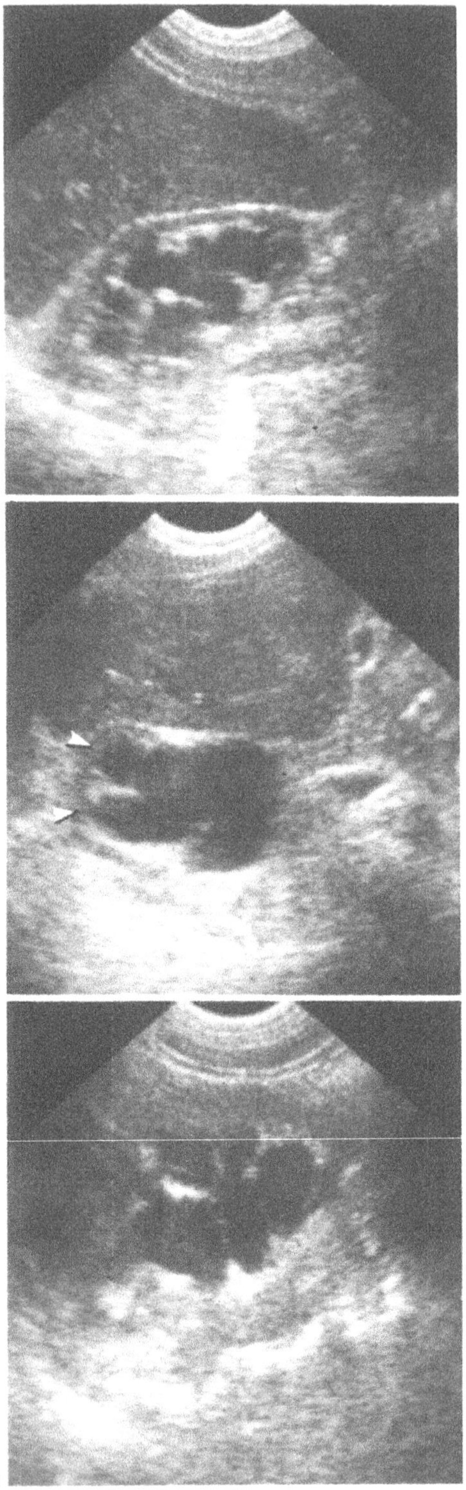

Fig. 3.8 a–c. Bilateral hydronephrosis. **a, b** Right kidney. **a** Sagittal scan: communicating multilocular pattern; parenchyma is thinned. **b** Intercostal scan shows "Mickey mouse" pattern (*arrowheads*). **c** Left kidney

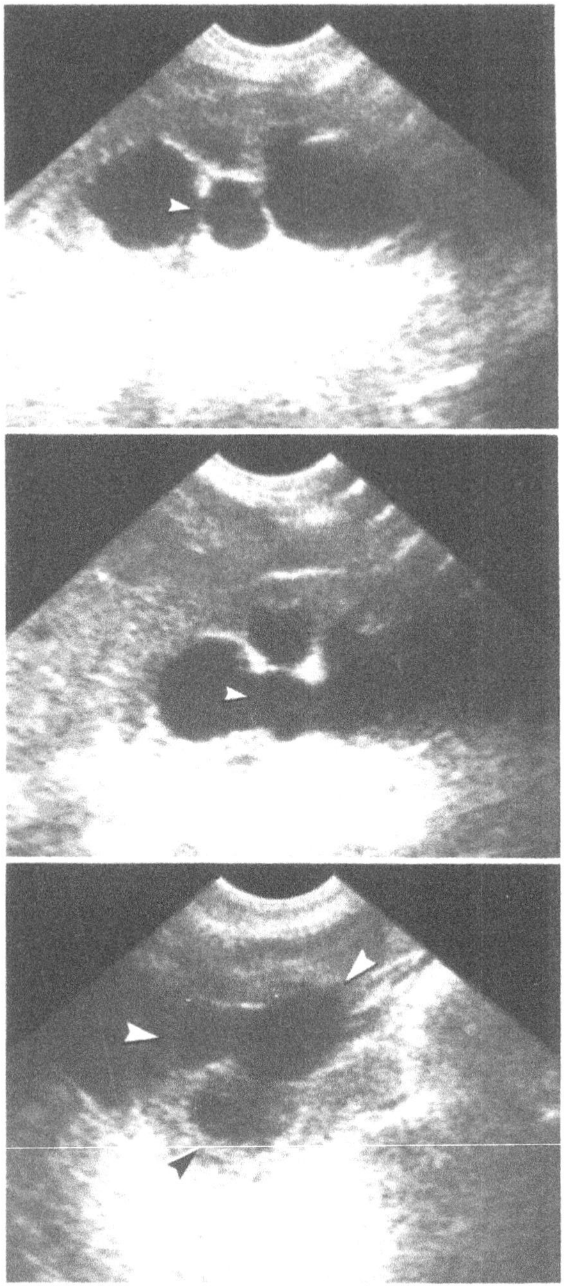

Fig. 3.9 a–c. Right hydronephrosis. **a, b** Sagittal scans. **c** Intercostal scan. Note, in **a** and **b,** interrupted septations (*arrowheads*). Note in **c** "Mickey mouse" pattern (*arrowheads*)

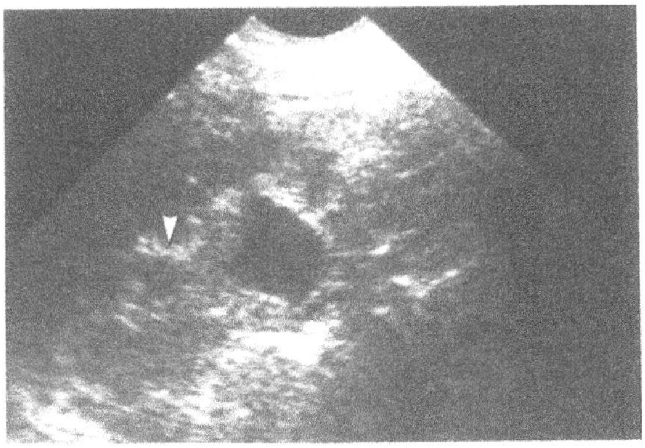

Fig. 3.10. Dilated lower nephron in duplicated kidney. Diameter of pelvis of upper nephron (*small arrowhead*) is normal. Dilatation is due to junction narrowing

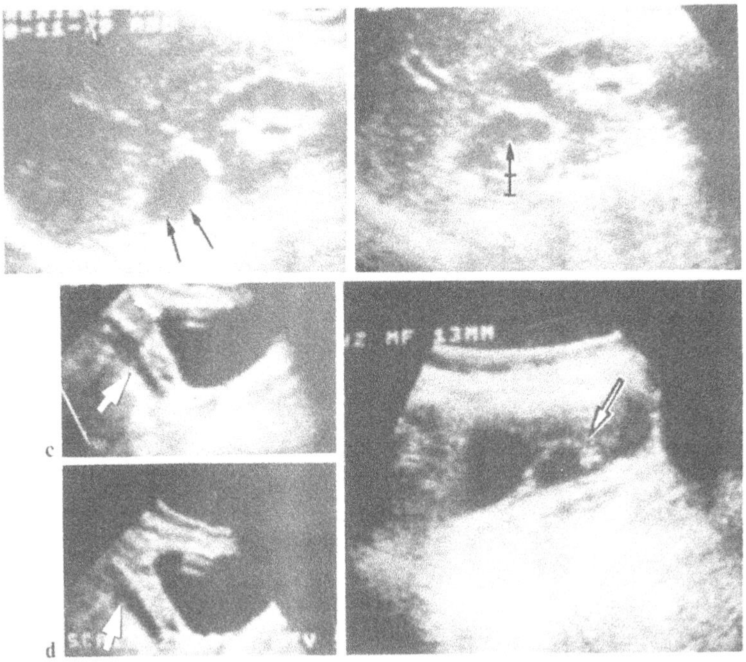

Fig. 3.11 a–e. Pseudocystic pattern. **a** Sagittal section shows cystic pattern in right upper pole (*arrows*). **b** Parallel scan shows irregular posterior wall (*arrow*): collection corresponds to hydronephrosis in the upper nephron of the duplicated kidney. **c, d** Oblique pelvic sections demonstrate the dilated ureter (*arrow*) behind the urinary bladder. **e** Transverse section of the bladder discloses septation proximal to the posterior wall (*arrow*), corresponding to wall of ureterocele. (Courtesy of M. Crevier, J. Y. Oueled, and J. Bourgeault, Montréal)

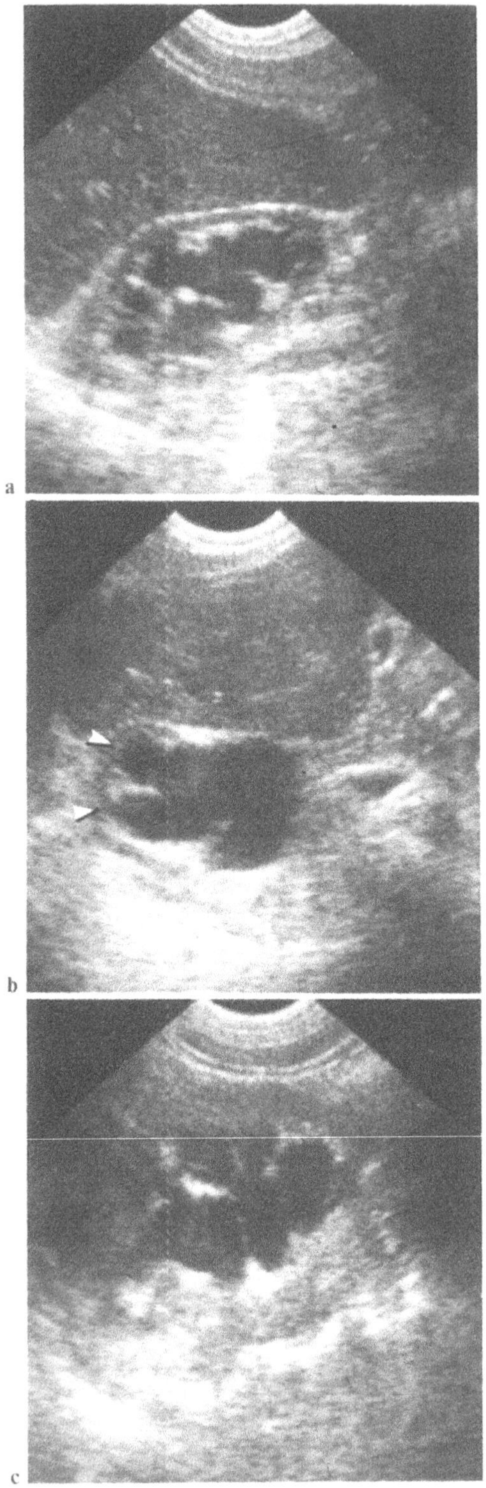

Fig. 3.8 a–c. Bilateral hydronephrosis. **a, b** Right kidney. **a** Sagittal scan: communicating multilocular pattern; parenchyma is thinned. **b** Intercostal scan shows "Mickey mouse" pattern (*arrowheads*). **c** Left kidney

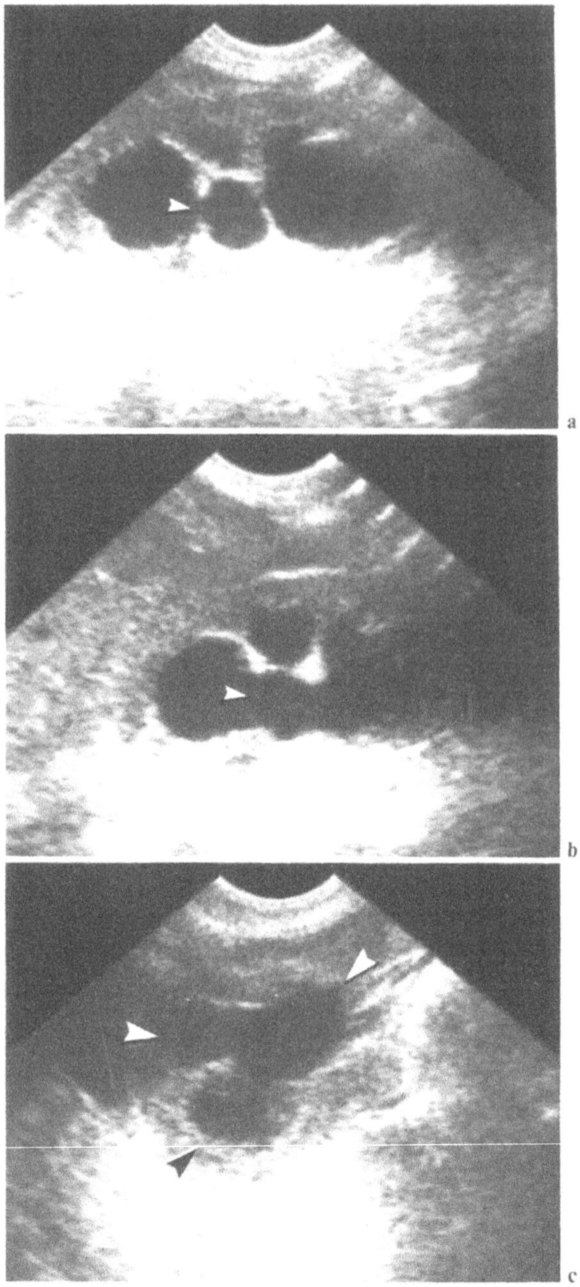

Fig. 3.9 a–c. Right hydronephrosis. **a, b** Sagittal scans. **c** Intercostal scan. Note, in **a** and **b**, interrupted septations (*arrowheads*). Note in **c** "Mickey mouse" pattern (*arrowheads*)

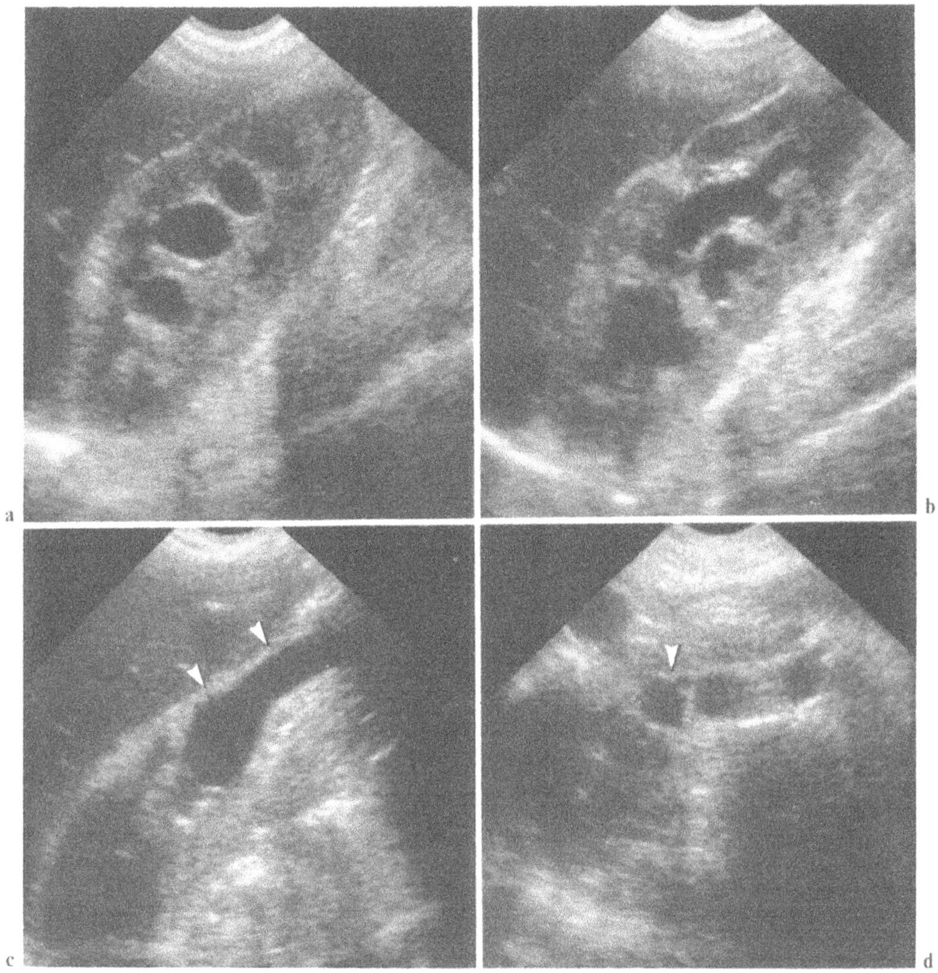

Fig. 3.13 a–d. Hydronephrosis with dilated ureter. **a, b** Coronal scans of the right kidney; **c** coronal scan of the dilated ureter (*arrowheads*); **d** transverse scan of the dilated ureter (*arrowhead*)

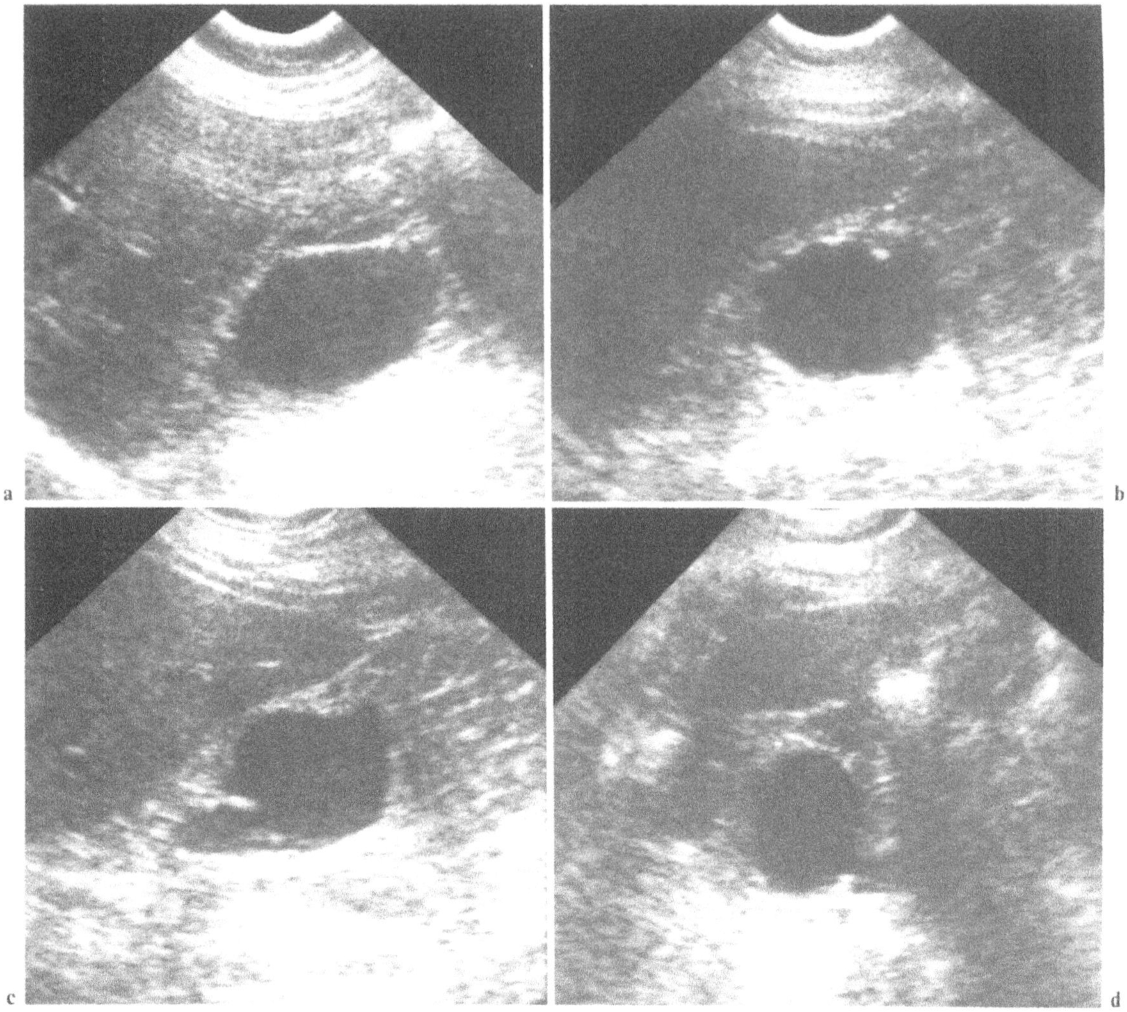

Fig. 3.14a–d. Junctional syndrome. **a–c** Three intercostal scans of the pelvis; **d** transverse scan. Ureter is not dilated

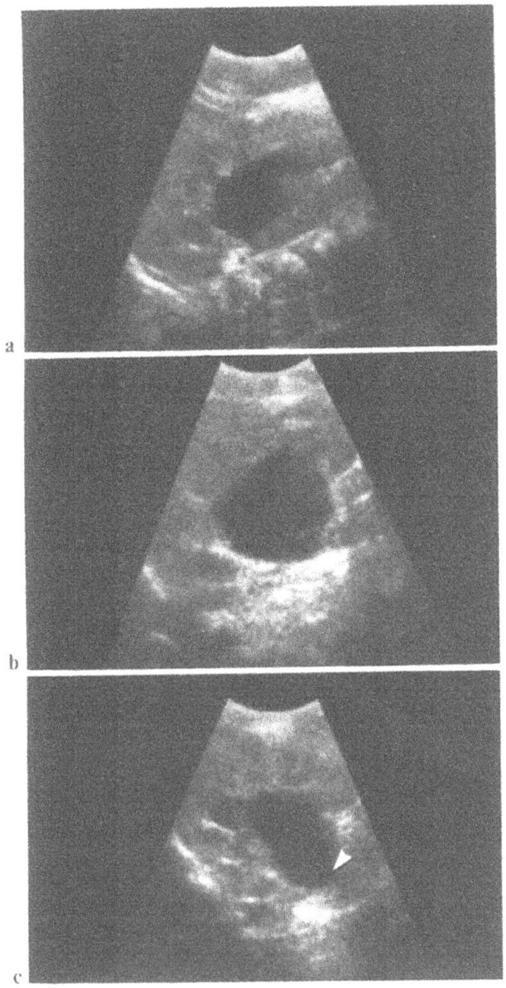

Fig. 3.15 a–c. Neonatal junctional syndrome. **a, b** Coronal scans; **c** intercostal scan; junction (*arrowhead*) is narrowed. Distal ureter is not dilated

3.3 Major Hydronephrosis

In major hydronephrosis a large abdominal mass is present. Ultrasonic scans disclose a *multilocular pattern* (Figs. 3.16–3.18), rather similar to that of multiple adjacent cysts. But there are communications between the different pouches, whose walls are discontinuous (Fig. 3.19). This constitutes a specific characteristic. It is not always possible, in such cases, to differentiate the dilated pelvis from hugely dilated calices.

The *thickness of the parenchyma* is markedly reduced (Fig. 3.16–3.19). The parenchyma may grow so thin as to possess the same pattern as a pelvis or intercaliceal wall (Fig. 3.15). In the presence of this kind of multilocular pattern, it is advisable to carry out high-frequency scans (5–7 MHz). Such scans will display, from time to time, scattered echoes, or a sediment layer, which indicate infection or hemorrhage (see Fig. 3.20). Pyonephrosis will be studied in Chap. 7.

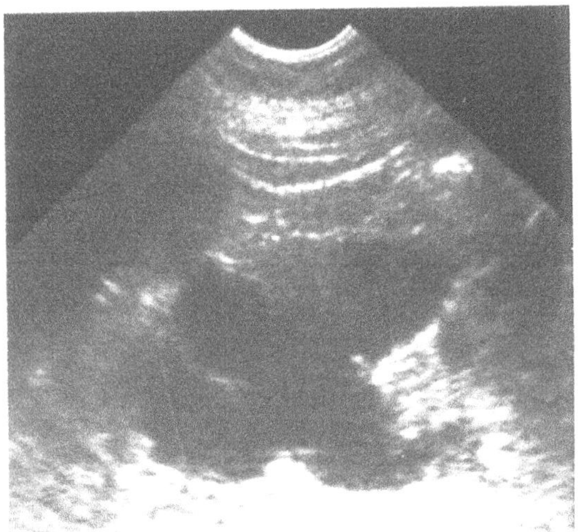

Fig. 3.16. Major hydronephrosis. This patient underwent ureteral ligation during removal of malignant pelvic tumor. Cortical atrophy is diffuse. Dilated ureter, pelvis, and calices are clearly demonstrated (left intercostal scan)

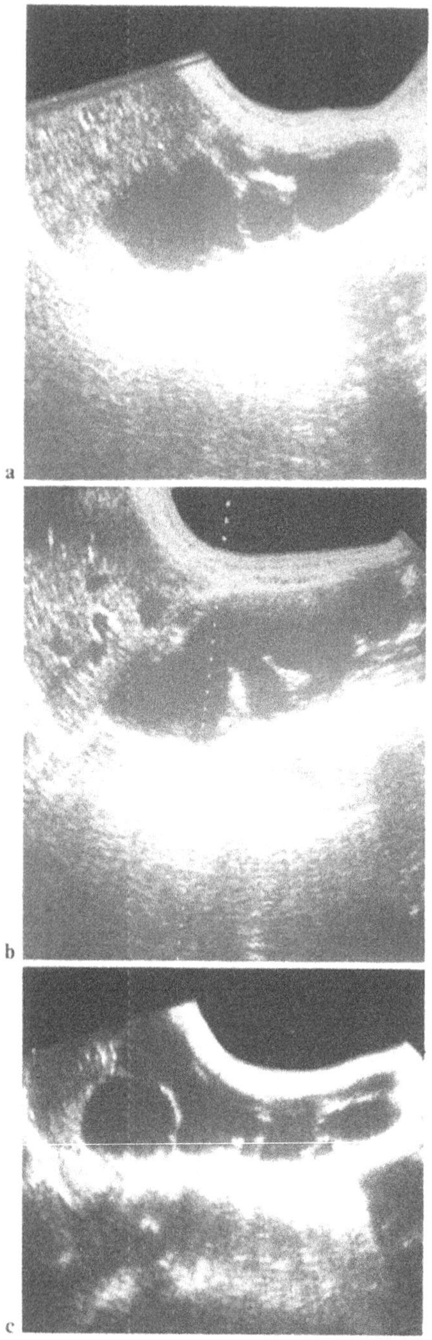

Fig. 3.17 a–c. Major hydronephrosis with pseudopolycystic pattern in hugely swollen kidney. **a, b** First case; **c** another case (three sagittal scans)

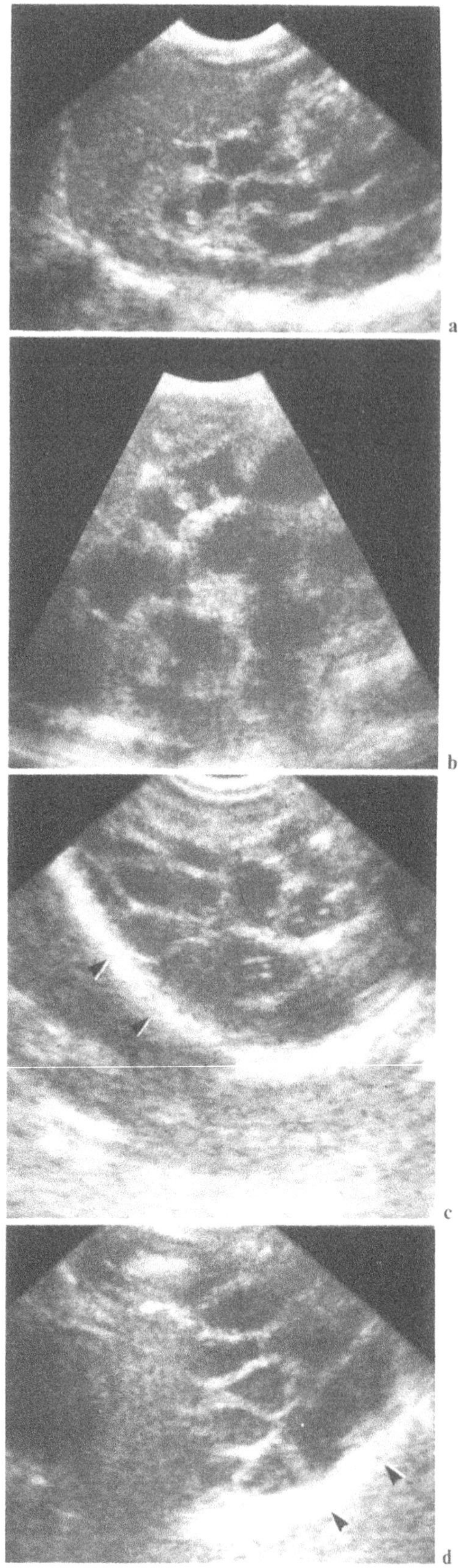

Fig. 3.18 a–d. Neonatal hydronephrosis (4-month-old infant) ▸ with pseudopolycystic pattern. **a** Right sagittal scan; **b** right transverse scan below the liver; **c** right transverse scan in the iliac fossa; **d** transverse scan of the left kidney in the iliac fossa; both kidneys come in contact. *Arrowheads* indicate the iliac bone

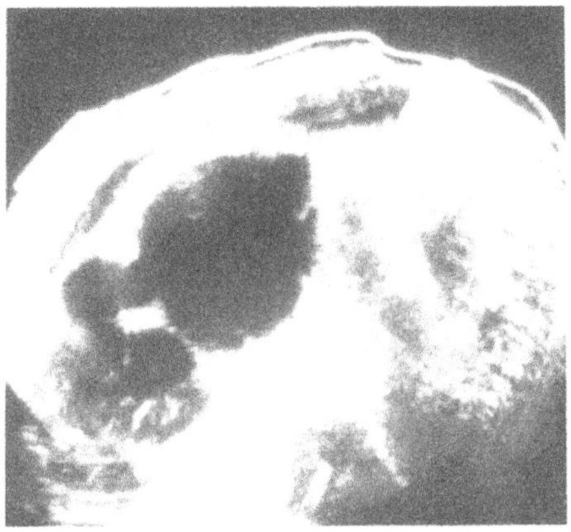

Fig. 3.19. Transverse abdominal scan shows massively enlarged extrasinusal pelvis. Dilated collecting system occupies entire right hemiabdomen

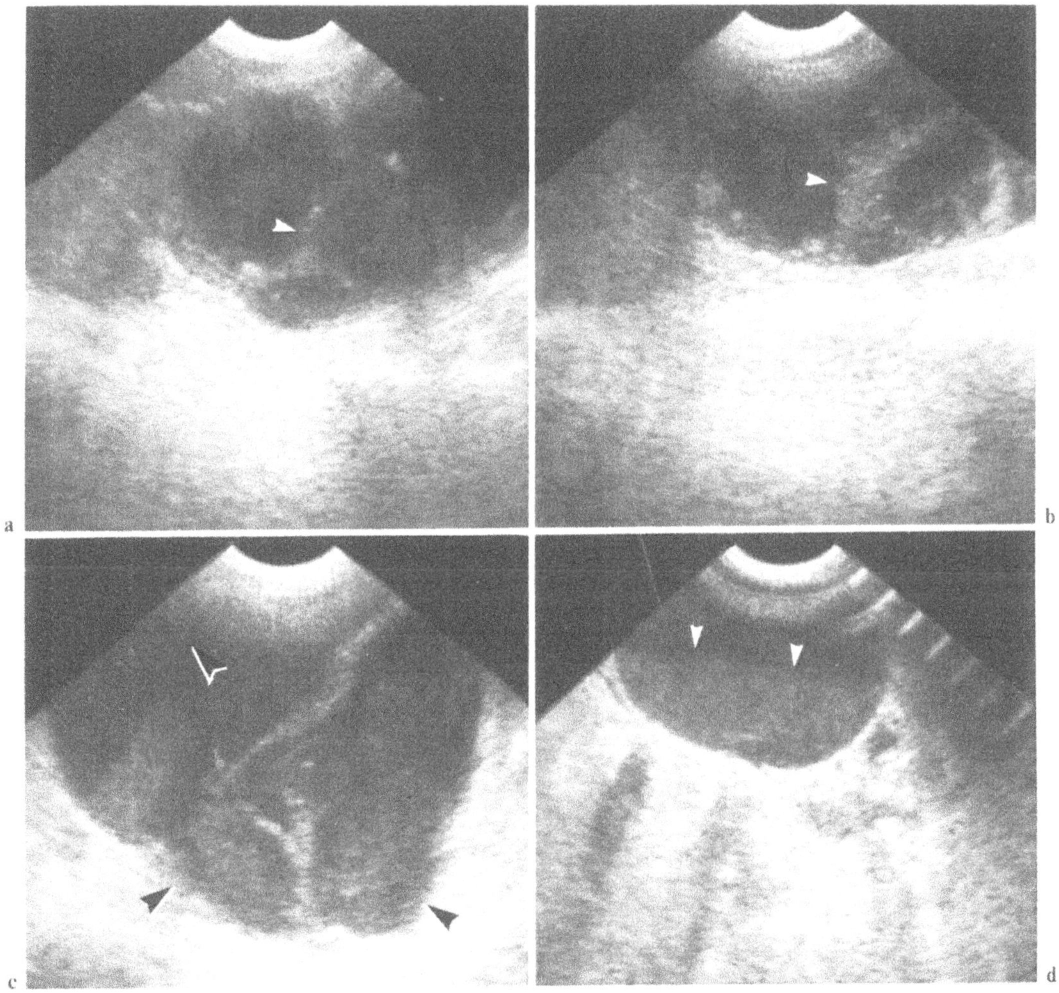

Fig. 3.20 a–d. Infected hydronephrosis. Four scans. Note, in **a** and **b**, thickened septations (*arrowheads*). Note, in **c** and **d**, dependent accumulation of infected urine (*arrowheads*) with, in **d**, "fluid-fluid" level (*arrowheads*)

3.4 Differential Diagnosis

Juxtapyelic cysts are often multiple. They develop within the echogenic pattern of the renal sinus. They can therefore mimick a beginning hydronephrosis (Fig. 3.21). But the pattern of interrupted septations, which characterizes hydronephrosis, is not present. And if finally the diagnosis remains unsettled, an intravenous pyelogram (IVP) will demonstrate the absence of pelvic dilatation. Another process can mimick early caliceal dilatation: in *papillary necrosis* the pyramids are replaced by cavities which communicate with the calices (HOFFMAN et al. 1982) (Fig. 3.21 d). Correct display of the arcuate artery enables one to identify the definite lobular architecture.

Other problems of differential diagnosis arise with large hydronephrotic fluid collections. The possibility of a *polycystic disease* will be discussed later. The true renal origin of the fluid collection should also be discussed. While a moderately dilated collecting system is clearly renal in origin, large multilocular collections may arise from *other tissues or organs* (septated ascites, mesenteric cysts, cystic mesenchymonas, cystic lymphangiomas, abdominal overian cysts, etc.). If the collection is renal, multiple scans in different scanning directions will show the abscence of a renal image, whether normal, distorted, or flattened.

Another reason why multiple scans must be carried out, even if the diagnosis of hydronephrosis is patent, is the possibility of associated other renal lesions. We shall examine that possibility later.

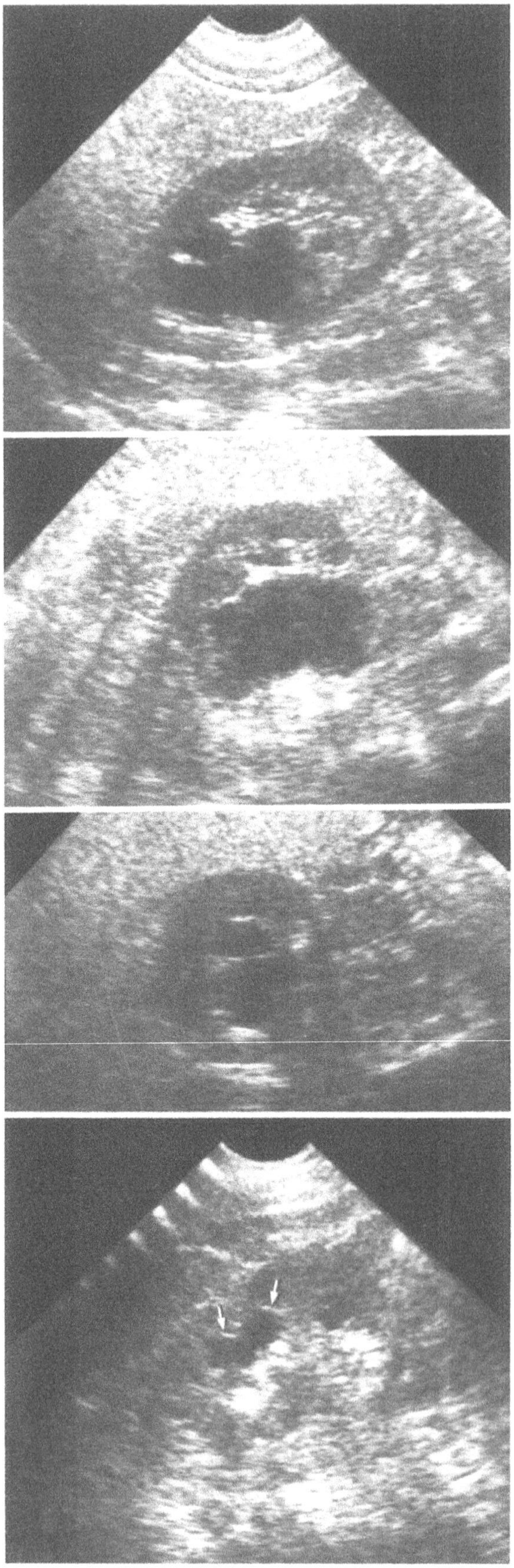

a

b

c

d

Fig. 3.21. a–c Pseudohydronephrotic pattern of multiple juxtapyelic cysts, of which one is particularly large. **a** Sagittal scan; **b** intercostal scan; **c** transverse scan; **d** another process: papillary necrosis. The fluid-filled cavities are not mere dilated minor calices. Location of the fluid, adjacent to the arcuate arteries (*arrows*) demonstrates that the fluid extends further than the calices through the destroyed pyramids, in the direction of cortex

3.5 Ureteral Dilatation

We have already dealt with the junction and initial segment of the ureter. Despite a few successes (Figs. 3.12, 3.13, 3.22, 3.23), the lower abdominal ureter itself is usually not visualized. The anterior approach is compromised by intestinal gas, whereas the iliac bone impedes coronal and posterolateral sections. Sometimes, however, the dilated abdominal ureter can be displayed by parasagittal scans (Fig. 3.24). A dilatation of the juxtavesical ureter can be observed through the acoustic window of the full urinary bladder (Fig. 3.25, see also Fig. 12.3 d, e).

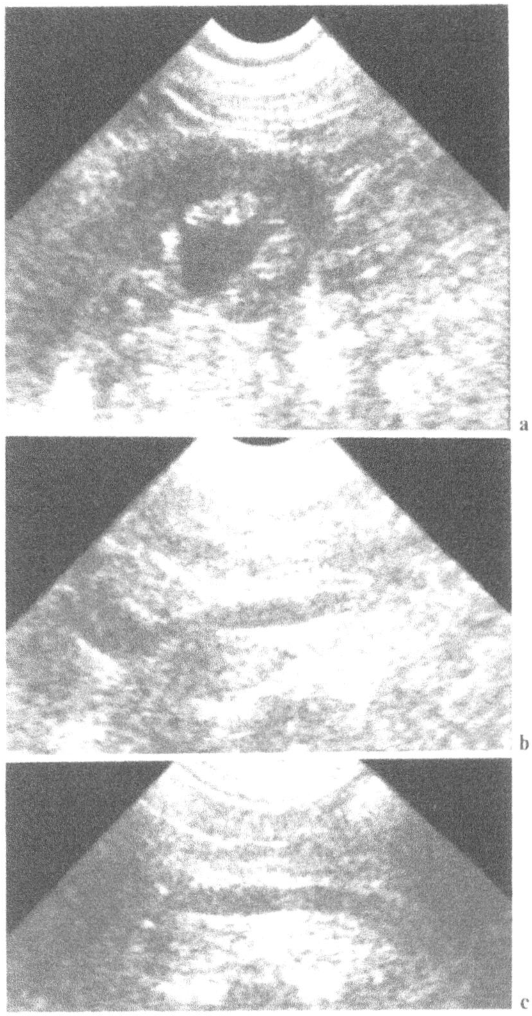

Fig. 3.22 a–c. Left hydronephrosis with dilatation of the ureter. **a** Coronal scan of the kidney; **b** junction and abdominal ureter; **c** abdominal ureter – dilatation accompanies anastomosis with the sigmoid colon

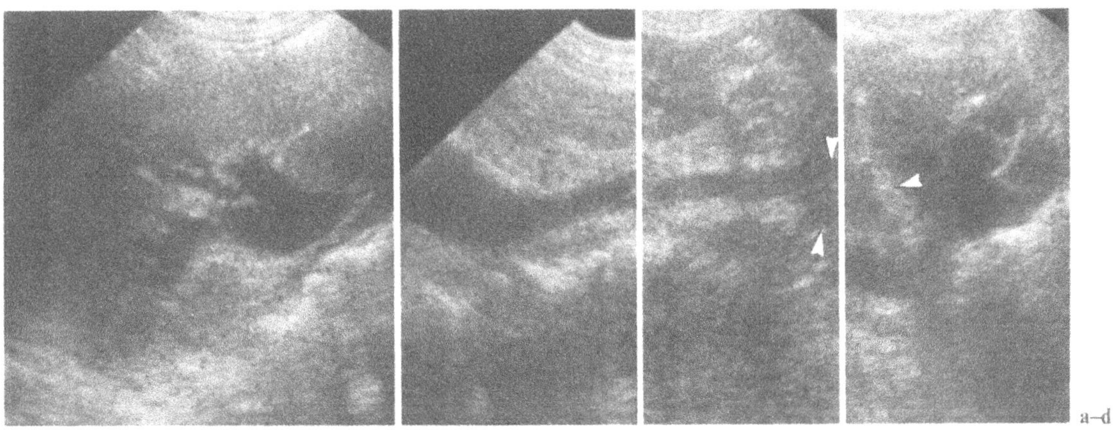

Fig. 3.23 a–d. Totally dilated right urinary tract, discovered at the occasion of acute renal insufficiency with bilateral hydronephrosis. Ureteral scans show stop due to ureteral extension of the bladder carcinoma (*arrowheads*)

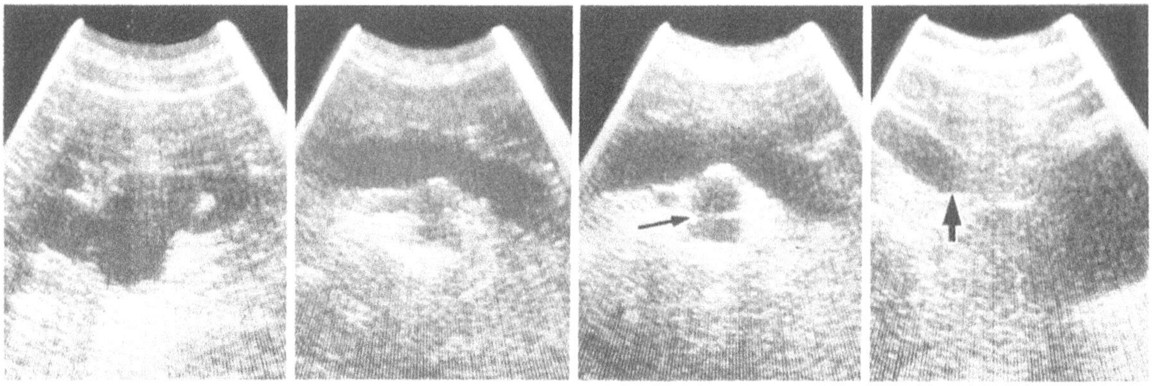

a–d

Fig. 3.24 a–d. Ureterohydronephrosis: IVU showing nonsecreting left kidney in patient complaining of dysuria. **a** Coronal scan shows pelvic dilatation. **b, c** Two left parasagittal sections demonstrate dilatation of the ureter. Note in **c** section of the iliac vessels (*arrow*) posterior to the dilated canal. **d** Parallel section of the bladder shows stop (*arrow*) on the ureter, due to infiltrative tumoral process

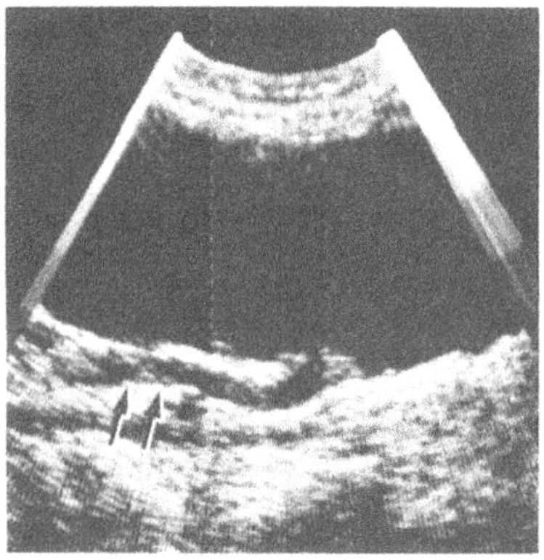

Fig. 3.25. Dilated pelvic ureter (*arrows*) displayed thanks to the acoustic window of the full bladder

3.6 Complementary Pelvic Examination

Whether bilateral or unilateral, hydronephrosis can be due to the presence of a pelvic mass (Figs. 3.26–3.28) or to lower urinary tract abnormalities. The pelvic examination may disclose a pelvic mass, a dilated bladder with postmictional residue, or a prostatic or bladder lesion (see Chap. 12). As stated above, a dilated ureter can be visualized thanks to the fluid window provided by the bladder (Fig. 3.25).

In many cases, a primary ultrasonic diagnosis of hydronephrosis will lead (except in pregnant women) to the performance of a conventional intravenous urogram. If, after intravenous injection of contrast medium, the kidney is found to be nonsecreting, sonography can still help in the realization of antegrade opacification by guided puncture (see Fig. 8.15).

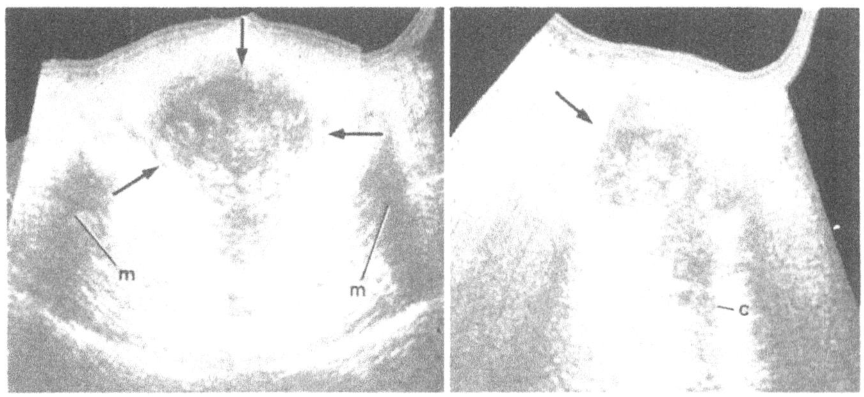

a b

Fig. 3.26 a, b. Large pelvic mass: corporeal uterine carcinoma (*arrow*). **a** Transverse scan; **b** sagittal scan; *c*, cervix; *m*, shadow of iliac bone

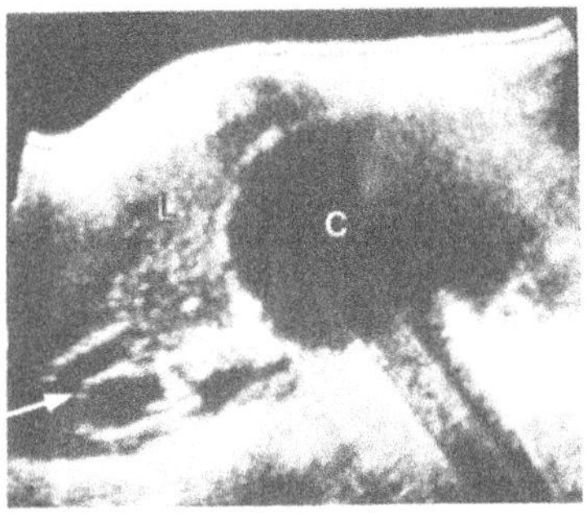

Fig. 3.27. Large pelvic mass: right sagittal scan shows hydronephrotic kidney (*arrow*) and compressing ovarian cyst (*C*). Note acoustic shadow arising from the cyst. *L*, liver

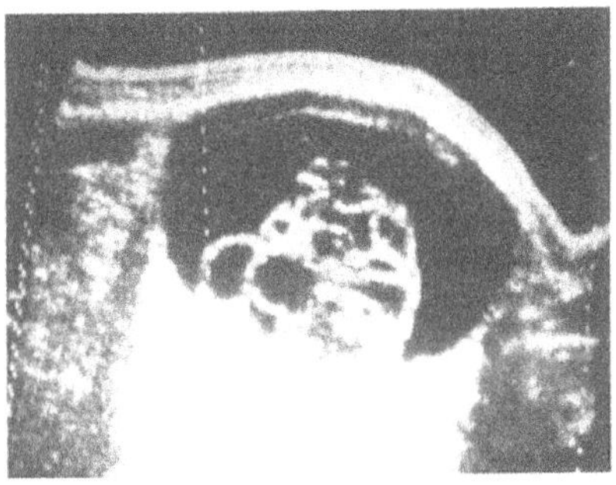

Fig. 3.28. Complementary transverse caudal scan shows intracystic growths

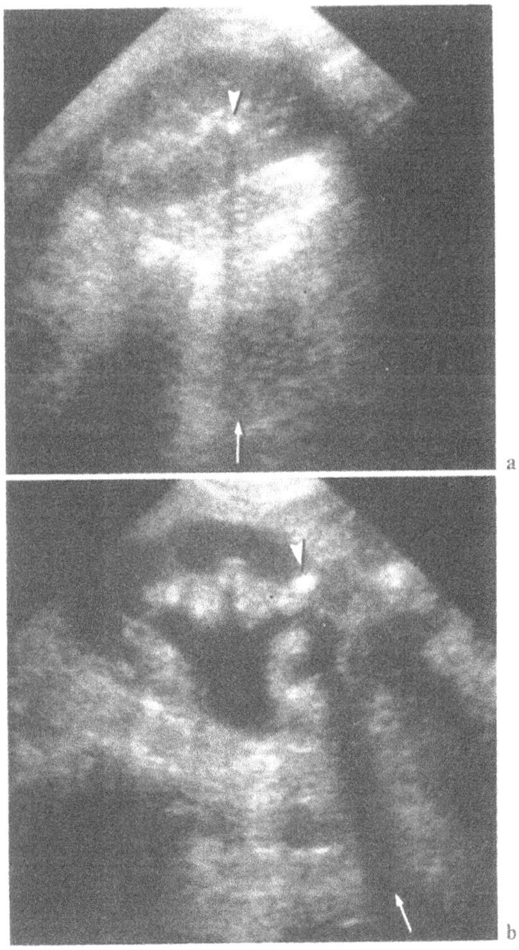

Fig. 3.29 a, b. Bilateral lithiasis. **a** Right kidney: small echogenic focus (*arrowhead*) with posterior shadow (*arrow*). **b** Left kidney. Similar image in minor calix

3.7 Renal Lithiasis

In most cases renal stones, like gallstones, produce their own reflective area, with an acoustic shadow behind it. The images are nevertheless different according to the presence or absence of a pelvicaliceal dilatation.

Without associated dilatation, lithiasis gives rise to an intense echo, pelvicaliceal in topography, with posterior acoustic shadowing (Figs. 3.29–3.32). Since the central zone is strongly echogenic, the proper contrast of the stone can be low (Fig. 3.30). Correct analysis of the shadow is therefore of utmost importance; lithiasic shadows persist despite changes in the scanning direction, whereas refractive shadows arising from intrasinusal elements are fugacious. Lithiasic shadowing is related to extrinsic and intrinsic factors, i.e., coincidence between the ultrasonic beam and the stone, focusing and frequency, the crystalline structure of the stone, and its size. Shadows fail to appear only exceptionally even when dealing with noncalcified calculi. When the collecting system is dilated, urine around stones introduces a particular contrast (Figs. 3.33, 3.34).

Staghorn calculi disrupt the pelvicaliceal ultrasonic architecture. Due to their size, the ultrasonic beam does not coincide everywhere with the calculus. The shadowing is therefore often much less intense than expected (Fig. 3.35). Some staghorn calculi are much less evident than small stones with a thin, intense shadow.

The presence of a peripheral area of reflection, at a distance from the infundibula, with an acoustic shadow, signifies parenchymal calcification (Fig. 3.36).

Intrarenal arterial calcifications, fortunately rare, can cause difficult diagnostic problems (Kane 1983).

The threshold of visibility of renal stones, in our experience, is 3–4 mm. Sweeping real time scans can even show the thin acoustic shadow of smaller stones.

Sonography is finally, in this respect, as sensitive, if not more, as a plain X-ray of the abdomen, the more so since most noncalcified stones cast acoustic shadows.

That optimistic opinion must be balanced by the failure of ultrasound in the ureteral calculi – with the exception of juxtavesical calculi, which can be demonstrated thanks to the acoustic window of the repleted urinary bladder. Such impacted stones bulge within the lumen of the bladder (Figs. 3.37, 3.38). A sudden or recent impaction is not necessarily accompanied by a ureteric dilatation (Fig. 3.37), since it appears only progressively. However, ultrasound associated to a plain film of the abdomen, yields sufficient results in most cases of renal colic (Hill 1985); if the display of the stone is clear, IVU has no utility. Follow-up examinations will monitor the evolution of the pelvic and ureteral dilatation, whereas plain films will demonstrate the stone migration. Some diagnostic problems can arise from weakly reflective stones, which do not cast acoustic shadows. Intrapelvic or caliceal reflection due to blood clots must then be discussed. Positional changes and follow-up examinations are likely to disclose modifications of the dubious areas. Urothelial tumors can also give rise to intrapelvic reflective areas without acoustic shadowing. Here we are confronted for the first time (but not for the last) with the limitations of ultrasound, used alone, when ultrasonic patterns are not specific. CT is instrumental in such cases. Finally, let us also keep in mind the peroperative ultrasonic localization of calculi (Cook 1977).

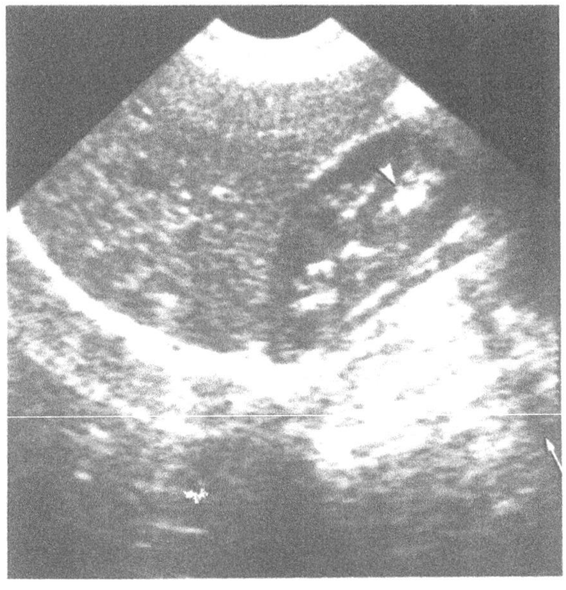

Fig. 3.30. Lithiasis (*arrowhead*) with shadow (*arrow*). (Sagittal scan of the right kidney)

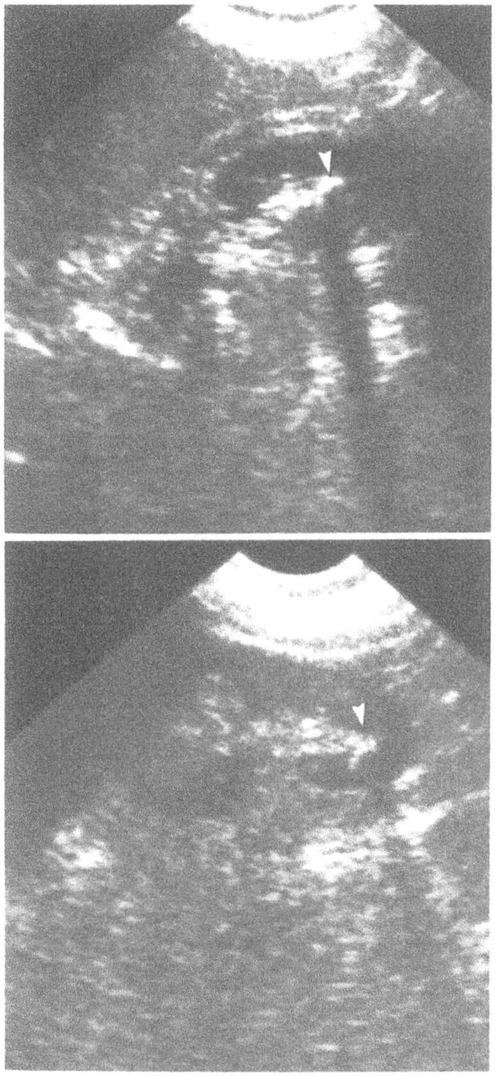

a

b

◂ **Fig. 3.31 a, b.** Lithiasis (*arrowhead*): the shadow is more relevant than the proper image of calculus. **a** Right sagittal scan; **b** coronal scan

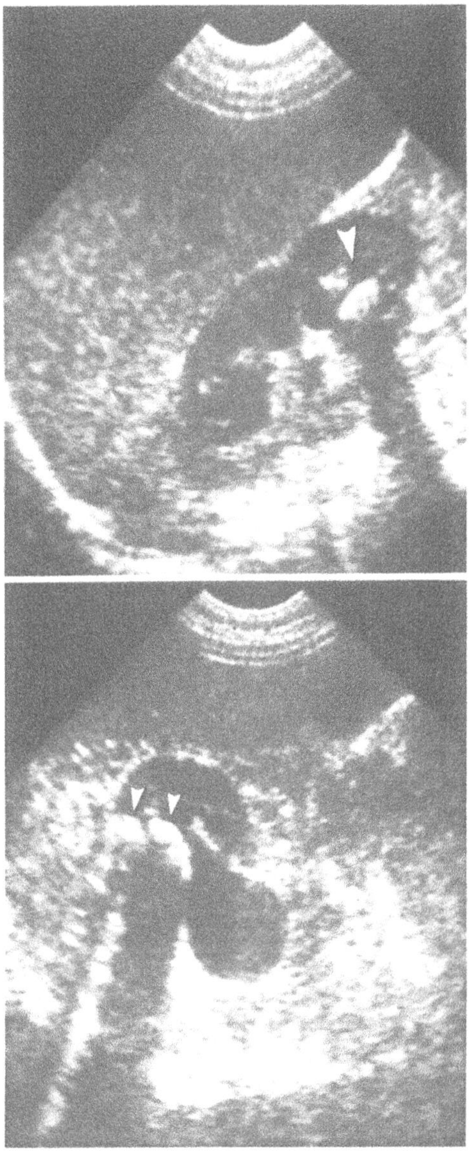

a

b

Fig. 3.33 a, b. Lithiasis (*arrowhead*) within hydronephrosis in the right kidney. **a** Sagittal scan; **b** transverse scan

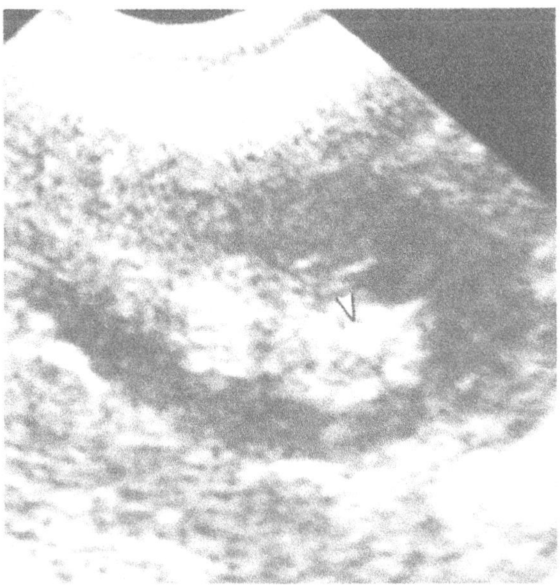

◂ **Fig. 3.32.** Lithiasis (*arrowhead*). Shadow is ill defined

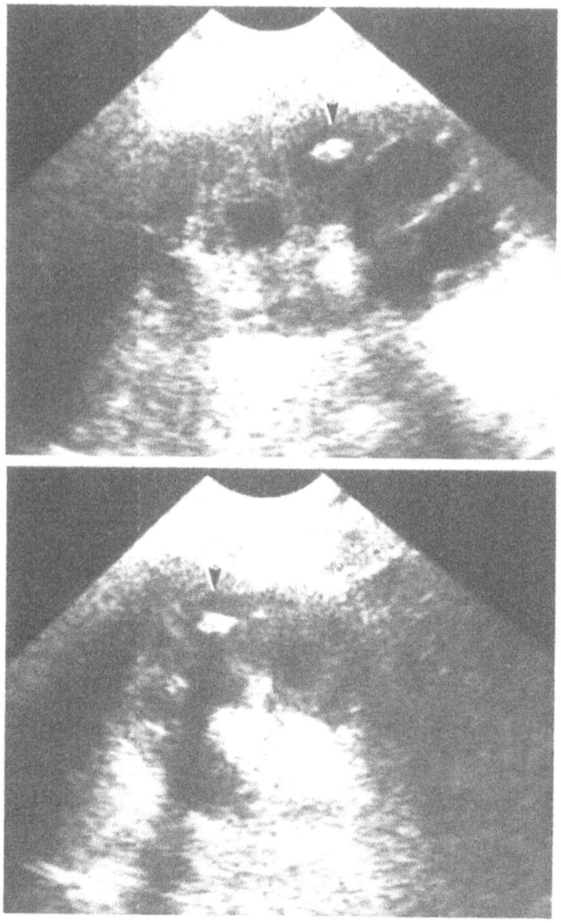

Fig. 3.34 a, b. Lithiasis (*arrowhead*) within left hydronephrosis

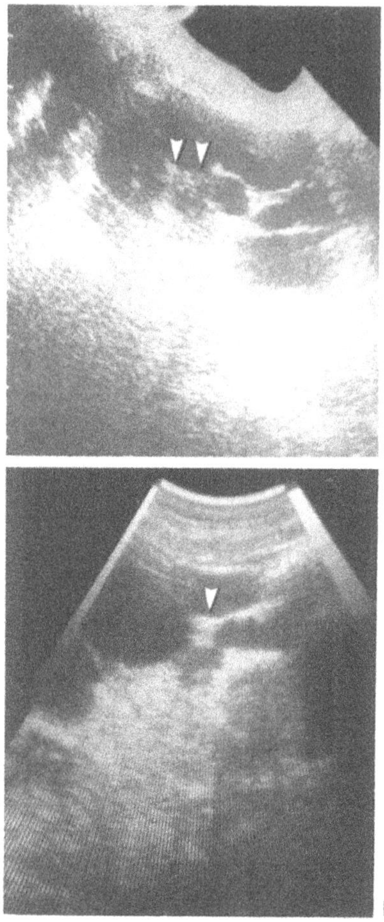

Fig. 3.35 a, b. Left staghorn calculus in hydronephrosis. **a** Posterior sagittal scan; **b** intercostal scan; calculus (*arrowheads*) and shadows are ill defined

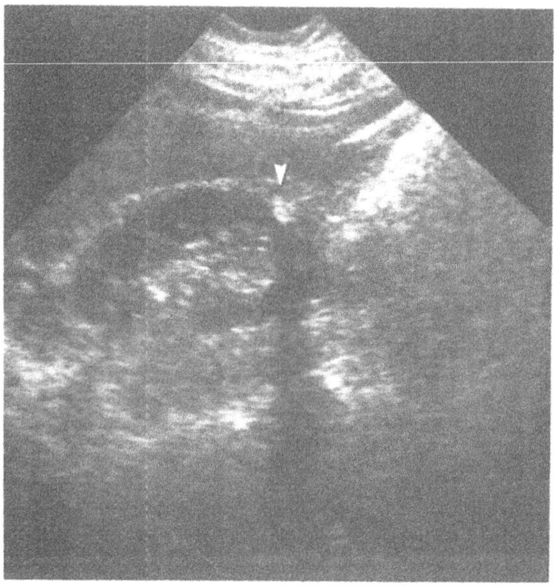

Fig. 3.36. Extracaliceal calcification (*arrowhead*)

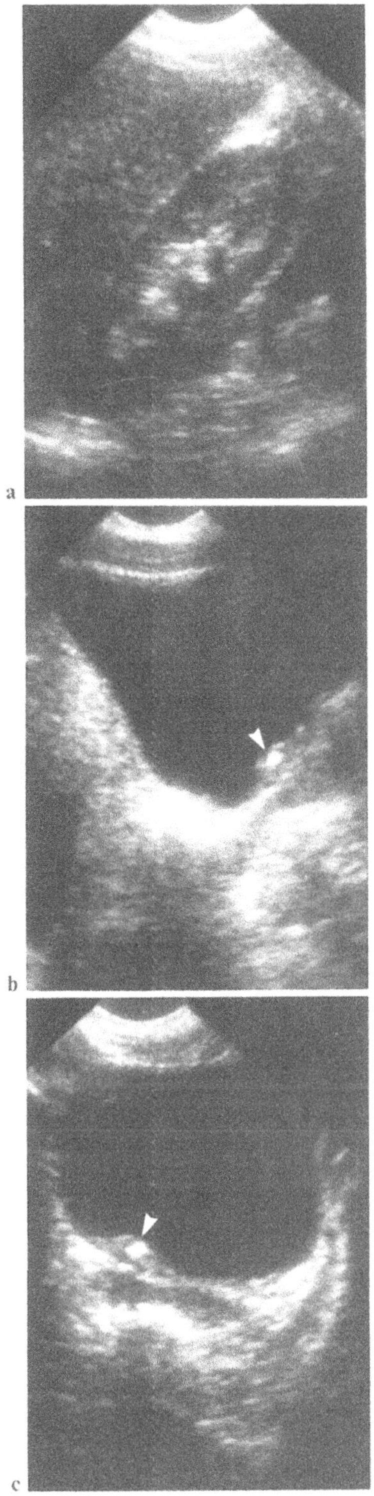

Fig. 3.37 a–c. Juxtavesical lithiasis. **a** Right kidney: there is no dilatation; **b** sagittal scan of the urinary bladder shows stone (*arrowhead*) impacted in terminal ureter; **c** transverse scan of stone

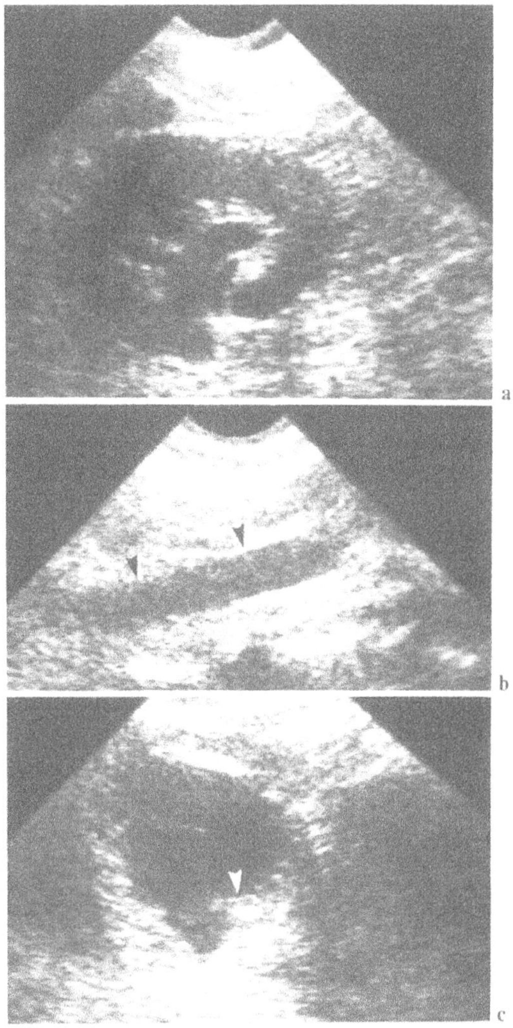

Fig. 3.38 a–c. Juxtavesical lithiasis. **a** Left collecting system is dilated; **b** ureter is also dilated; **c** section of urinary bladder show stone impacted in terminal ureter (*arrowhead*)

4 Renal Cysts

This chapter basically deals with one type of image: the ultrasonic cystic pattern. But that image can be the expression of many different lesions:
- Benign cysts, solitary or multiple
- Parapelvic cysts
- Multicystic and polycystic processes of the infant and adult
- Acquired cystic disease of the hemodialyzed patient
- Parasitic cysts
- Cystic tumors

Moreover, we shall still have to consider, in addition to these different kinds of true renal cysts, several varieties of pseudocystic lesions. We shall discuss them at the end of this chapter, when dealing with the differential diagnosis of cysts.

In Table 4.1, we have grouped the pathogenesis of different cystic processes, as reported by GROSSMANN et al. (1983). MELLINS (1984) has also contributed with a comprehensive developmental approach.

Table 4.1. Pathogenesis of different cystic processes

Type of cystic process	*Pathogenesis*
Multicystic displastic kidney	Developmental hydronephrosis consecutive to pelvic or ureteral atresia
Multilocular renal cyst	Pathogenesis unknown
Infantile polycystic disease	Congenital, recessive; dilatation of tubules
Adult polycystic disease	Congenital, dominant, medullary cysts
Benign cysts, solitary or multiple	Pathogenesis unknown
Parapelvic cysts	Pathogenesis unknown; lymphangiectasia considered
Acquired polycystic disease of the hemodialyzed patient	Tubular ectasia? Basal membrane alteration?

The Renal Cystic Pattern

This pattern associates an echo-free area, remaining echo-free at higher gain and higher frequency; a well-delineated, continuous smooth limit, due to the cyst's thin proper wall; and an enhancement of the posterior interface, with a posterior area of increased reflection, due to free sound transmission through the fluid contents (Fig. 4.1). Despite this typical pattern, the ultrasonic cystic image is nonspecific. It merely indicates the presence of a fluid-filled pouch with poorly attenuating contents.

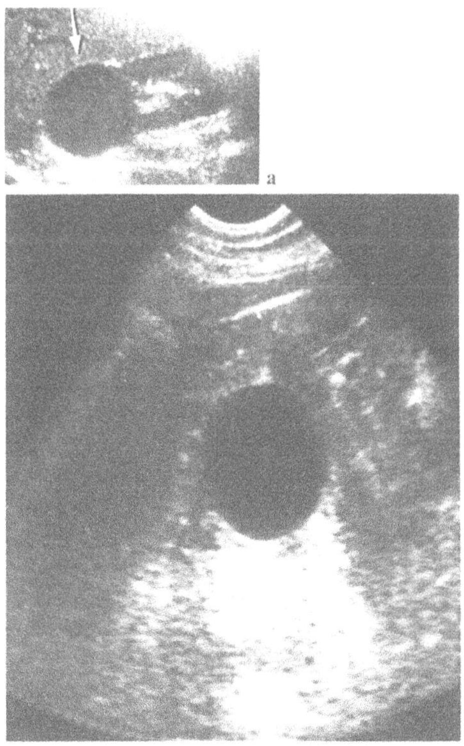

Fig. 4.1. a Typical cystic pattern: contents of right upper pole cyst (*arrow*) are echo-free. Note perirenal fat, thin proper wall, and posterior reinforcement. **b** Central cyst. Note posterior enhancement and refractive shadows

4.1 Benign Cysts

Diagnostic Circumstances

The ultrasonic diagnosis of simple cysts is usually made in one of the following clinical conditions: (a) a mass disclosed on an IVU (a "urographic" mass); (b) (rarely) abdominal pain or palpable mass; and (c) abdominal ultrasonic screening. Ultrasound and CT in daily routine demonstrate the frequency of benign cysts, particularly in older patients. Exceptional, but possible, in children, benign cysts are usually encountered in adults over 30 years of age. They are encountered in 20% of patients over 60 years of age.

Ultrasonic Pattern

This pattern is of course exactly the pattern we just depicted above. Possible morphological variations are related to the cyst's size and location.

Size. As we shall see again later, familial studies of polycystic kidneys show the smallest diameter of visualized cysts to be 3 mm. Conversely, a giant cyst may grow up to a diameter of 15 cm. Any intermediate size may be encountered (Figs. 4.2–4.4).

Location. Any location is possible: cortical, the cyst bulging out of the renal cortex (Figs. 4.2a–e, 4.3b, c), cysts of the renal poles (Fig. 4.1a), intraparenchymal cysts (Fig. 4.3), or central cysts (Figs. 4.1b, 4.2f). Such central cysts are different from parapelvic cysts, which develop within the fat of the renal sinus itself. We shall study them later on.

Anterior and posterior cortical cysts are readily visualized, whereas on conventional urograms they are often overlooked. The relation of a cortical cyst to the proximal parenchyma must be assessed: in a simple benign cyst the neighboring parenchyma makes a clear angle with the cystic wall, exactly as it does on a conventional nephrotomogram (Fig. 4.2b). This pattern is particularly evident in peripheral cysts arising from the renal margin (Fig. 4.2e). Cortical cysts bulge within the perirenal fat, which remains continuous; they do not traverse it beyond the perirenal fascia.

The discovery of a cystic pattern calls for multidirectional scans in order to evaluate the entire surface of the cystic wall and confirm the absence of tumoral growths. On the other hand, complementary high-gain scans may show the presence of intracystic echoes; the significance of this particular intracystic pattern will be discussed later.

After completion of these two complementary technical steps, it is possible to confirm that the cyst is benign. At least for asymptomatic cysts of the adult, no other diagnostic procedure has to be considered, with the exception of a follow-up examination a few months later. Such a conservative attitude is supported by the reliability of ultrasound and by the high frequency of asymptomatic simple cysts in patients over 50 years of age, a frequency disclosed both by ultrasonic examinations and by CT. Nevertheless, we shall later discuss in greater detail the management of ultrasonic cystic images.

Multiple Benign Cysts

This multicystic process is different from the polycystic disease, which we shall study later on. Multiple benign cysts are not congenital; they are much less evolutive and do not bring about renal insufficiency. All the cystic patterns described above can associate (Fig. 4.5).

Atypical Cysts – Tumoral Cysts

The appearance of a cyst may be atypical, when compared with the standard pattern depicted above, because it has a different shape or a different pattern of contours or contents. The *shape* may be less circular, less regular (Fig. 4.6a).

The *cystic wall* may lose its smooth, thin pattern (Fig. 4.6b). This can be due merely to a progressive collapse. Parietal elevations could be consistent with an intracystic tumor. In fact, most elevations correspond to incomplete septations (Figs. 4.3a, 4.8, 4.9).

The *fluid contents* may be moderately reflective, sometimes even at low frequency, sometimes only on high-frequency cuts. The abnormal reflection may consist either in scattered echoes, or in grouped echoes constituting a dependent layer (Fig. 4.7). These patterns are encountered in the presence of intracystic hemorrhage or infection (Jackman and Stevens 1974; Chon et al. 1976).

The cystic contents may even show a solid pattern, due to blood clots (Weill 1974; Fridey 1975); the diagnosis of cyst then risks not being considered. Such confusions are exceptional thanks to the density resolution of present equipment. The cystic wall can now be readily displayed. CT imaging and densitometry are helpful in such cases.

In a few cysts the wall may calcify, giving rise to a shell sign, that is, a strong linear reflection with acoustic shadowing behind it. Special diagnostic

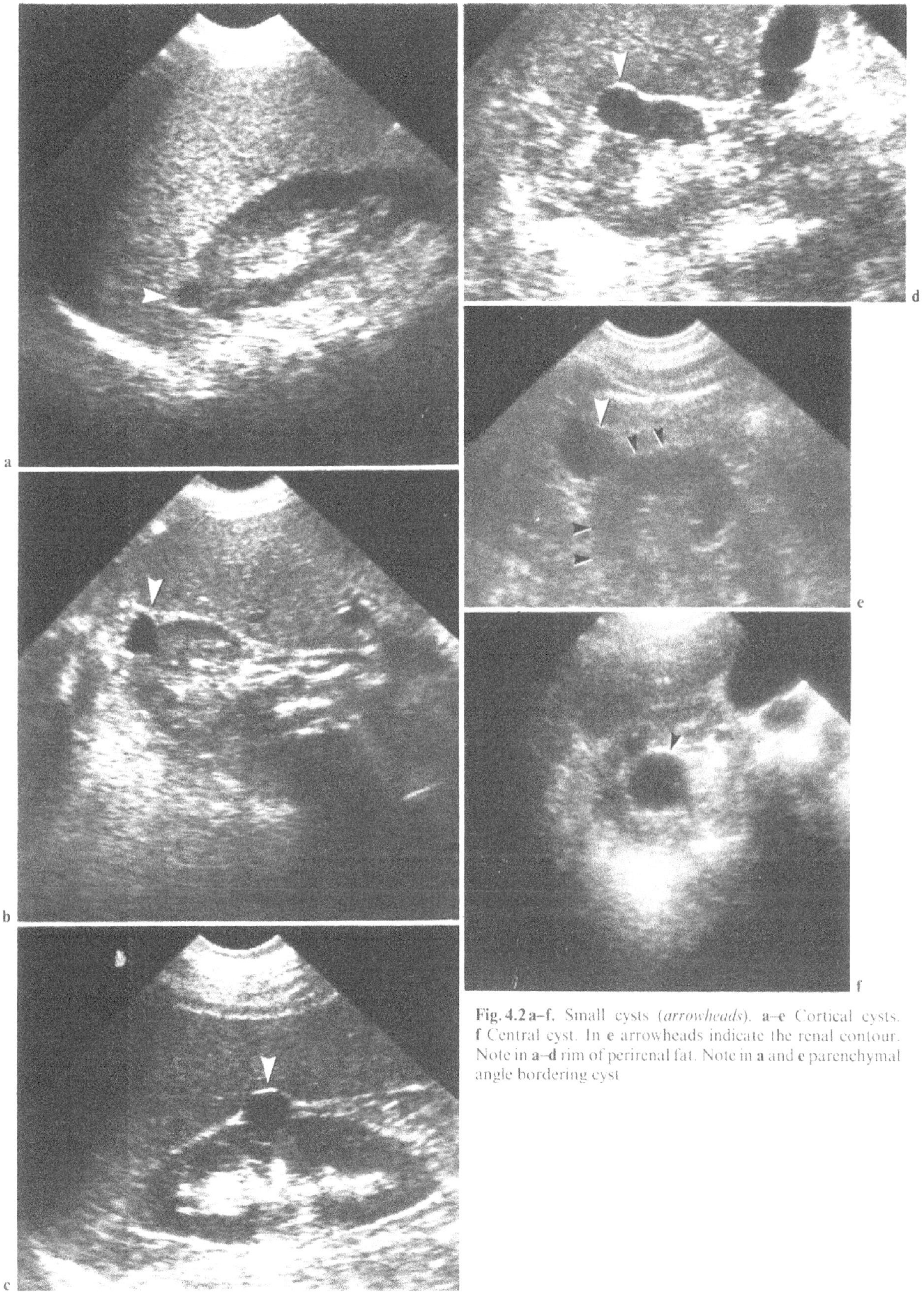

Fig. 4.2 a–f. Small cysts (*arrowheads*). **a–e** Cortical cysts. **f** Central cyst. In **e** arrowheads indicate the renal contour. Note in **a–d** rim of perirenal fat. Note in **a** and **e** parenchymal angle bordering cyst

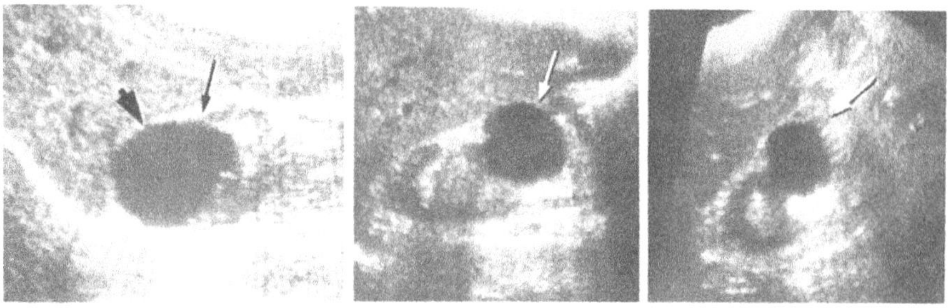

a–c

Fig. 4.3 a–c. Different cystic sizes and locations. **a** Six-centimeter cyst in right upper pole, bulging slightly out of the renal contour (*arrow*). A thin strip of perirenal fat still delineates cystic upper limit. Note parenchymal angle (*thin arrow*). **b** Six-centimeter cysts in right lower pole, bulging out of the renal contour (*arrow*). Fatty limit is hardly seen. **c** Same cyst in transverse section. Development of the cyst is internal. Perirenal and pericystic fat is better outlined

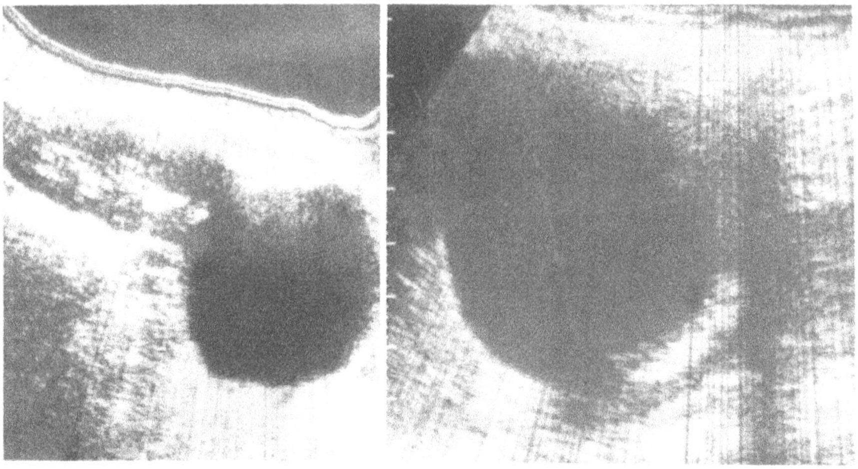

a b

Fig. 4.4 a, b. Larger cysts. **a** Left lower pole cyst (posterior scanning in prone position), 8 cm in diameter. Cyst, of cortical origin, is almost pediculated. **b** Giant right anterior cortical cyst, 12 cm in diameter, pushing the kidney downward (anterior scanning). No proper limit other than the cystic wall is displayed between the cyst and renal cortex. A reflective cleavage plane, corresponding to perirenal fat, would indicate an extrarenal cyst

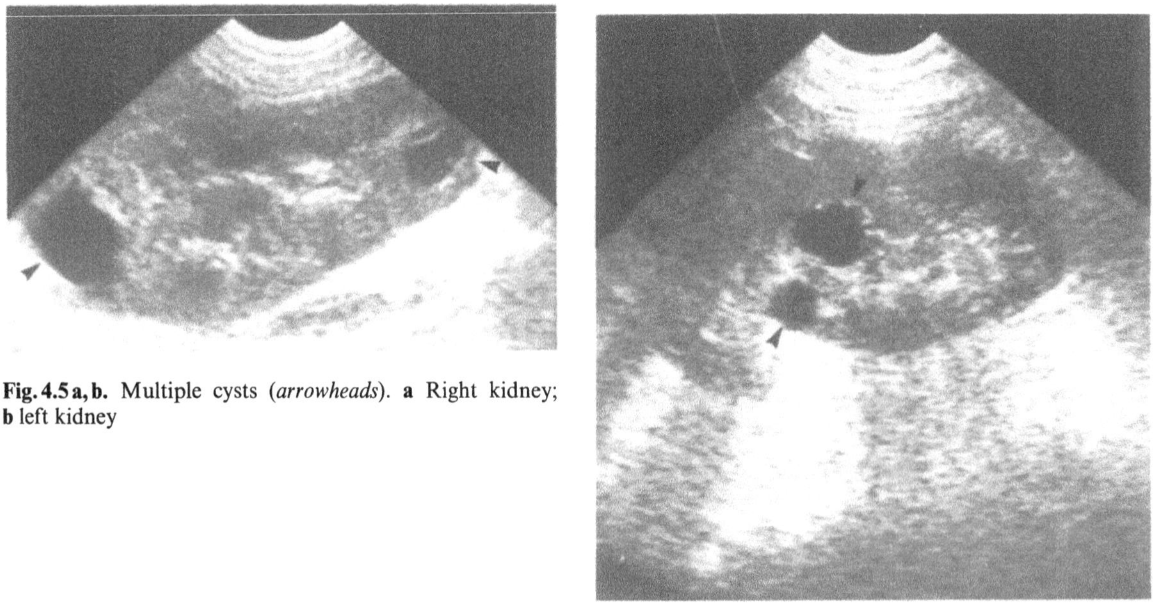

a b

Fig. 4.5 a, b. Multiple cysts (*arrowheads*). **a** Right kidney; **b** left kidney problems arise from calcified cysts, which we shall discuss later.

Some cysts are *multilocular* (Fig. 4.8). Their diagnosis is easy if their components have benign features. Image interpretation is more difficult if septations are interrupted (Fig. 4.9) or incomplete. A small intracystic elevation can also be present (Fig. 4.10) which, if irregular, can require a puncture (Fig. 4.11), since misdiagnosing a small intracystic malignant tumor is always of concern (see Fig. 5.25). Larger intracystic tumors are of course readily recognized (Fig. 4.15).

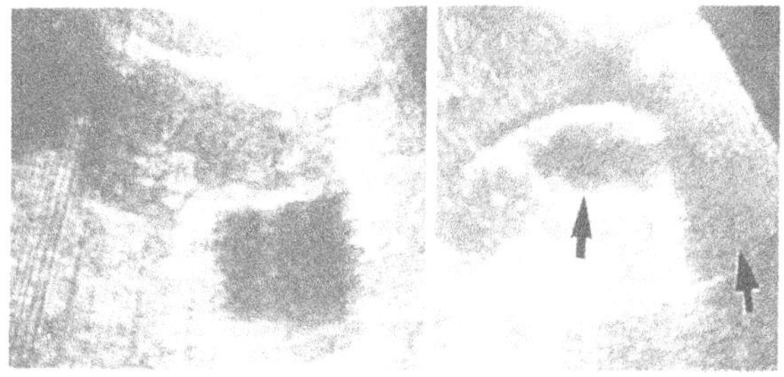
a, b

Fig. 4.6 a, b. Atypical cysts. **a** Shape of lower pole cyst is irregular. **b** Flattened cyst with irregular walls (*arrow*). This is collapsing cyst. There is also a moon crescent sign, a sonolucent strip between liver and kidney indicating fluid in Morison's pouch. Acoustic shadow (*arrow*) is due to colonic gas

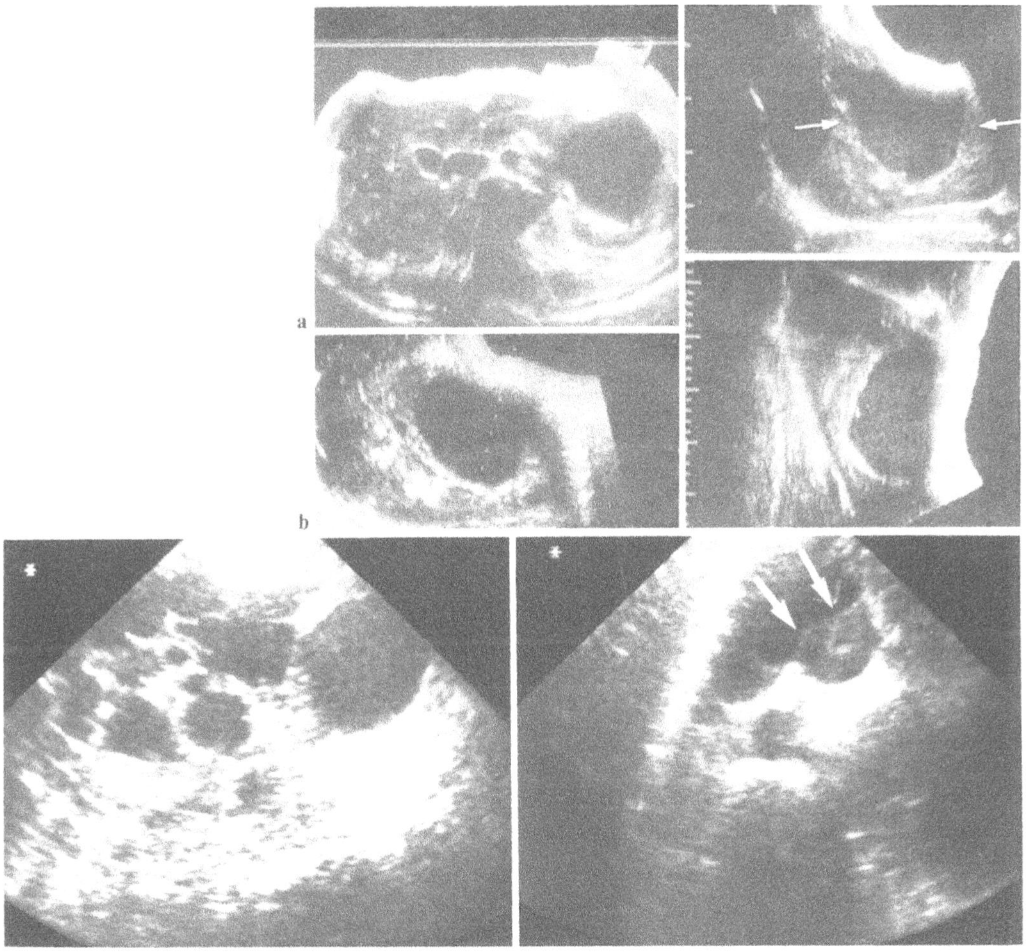
a b c d e f

Fig. 4.7 a–f. Atypical cyst. **a, b** Transverse **a** and left sagittal **b** sections display giant anterior cyst in left kidney. **c** New sagittal scan with 5 MH tranducer instead of 2.5 shows dependent echoes with horizontal line of separation (*arrows*). **d** Patient is placed in erect position. Horizontal level of separation is displayed again; this indicates presence of thick fluid. Puncture confirms puriform contents. **e, f** Another case. Patient with adult polycystic disease complains of acute pain in right flank. **e** Multiple renal cysts; **f** parallel scan shows echogenic pattern within cyst (*arrows*) in sensitive area, due to hemorrhage

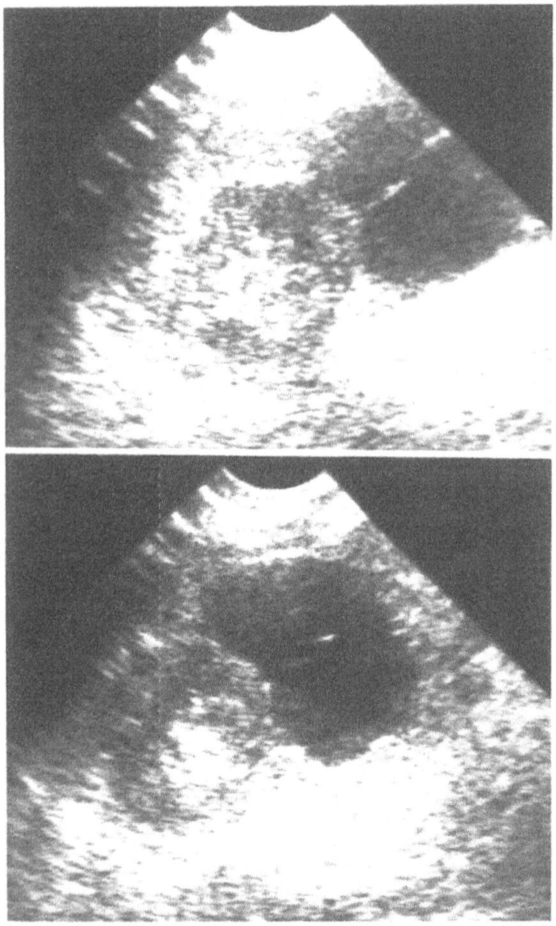

Fig. 4.8 a, b. Septated cortical cyst of the left kidney

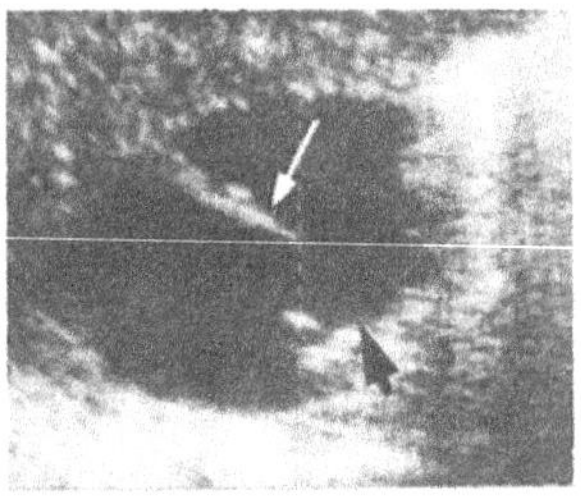

Fig. 4.9. Septated cyst (*arrows* septation). Posterior septum mimics growth

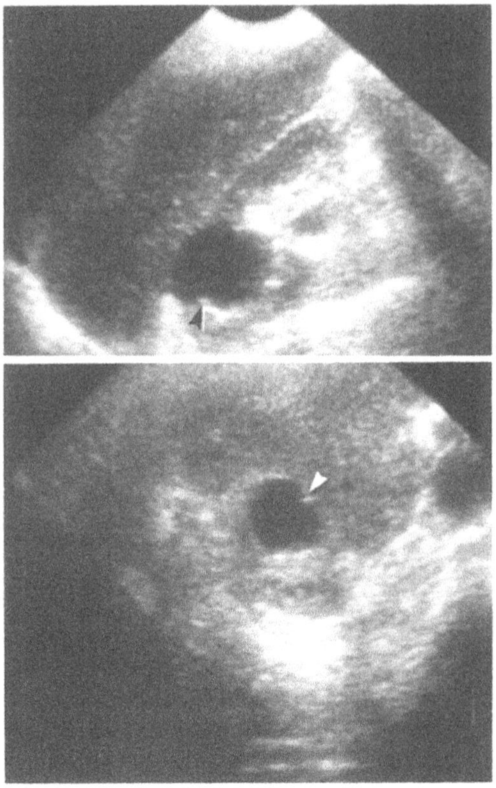

Fig. 4.10 a, b. Cyst with incomplete septation: parietal elevation (*arrowhead*). **a** Sagittal scan; **b** transverse scan

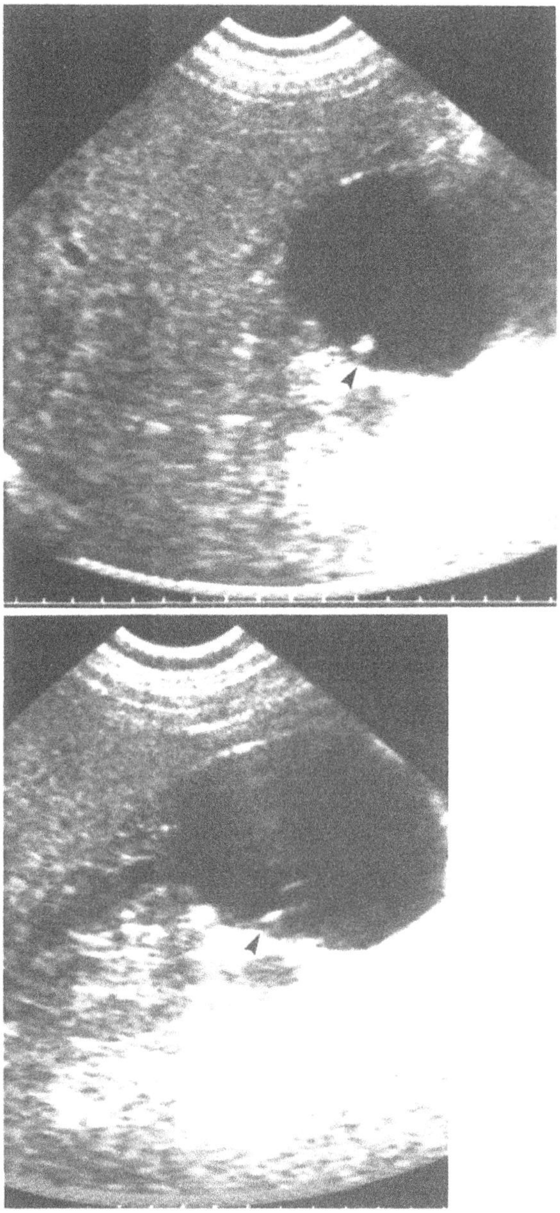

Fig. 4.11 a, b. Atypical cyst. a, b Two parallel scans show parietal elevation (*arrowhead*) which could correspond to a tumoral process. No abnormal cell was found at puncture

Parapelvic Cysts

Parapelvic cysts correspond perhaps to lymphangiectesia, but in fact their precise pathogenesis remains uncertain. They develop within the sinus and when small remain surrounded by echogenic fat (Fig. 4.12). They are often multiple (Figs. 4.13, 4.14). If adjacent they can mimic a hydronephrosis; however no confluence between the cystic elements is observed (see Fig. 3.3 and 3.4, p. 40).

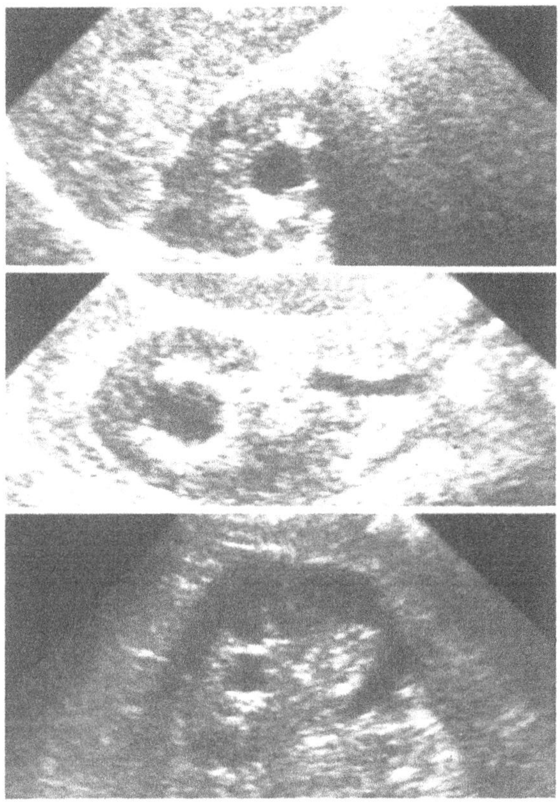

Fig. 4.12 a–c. Parapelvic cyst. **a** Sagittal section; **b** transverse section; **c** coronal section finally shows two cysts

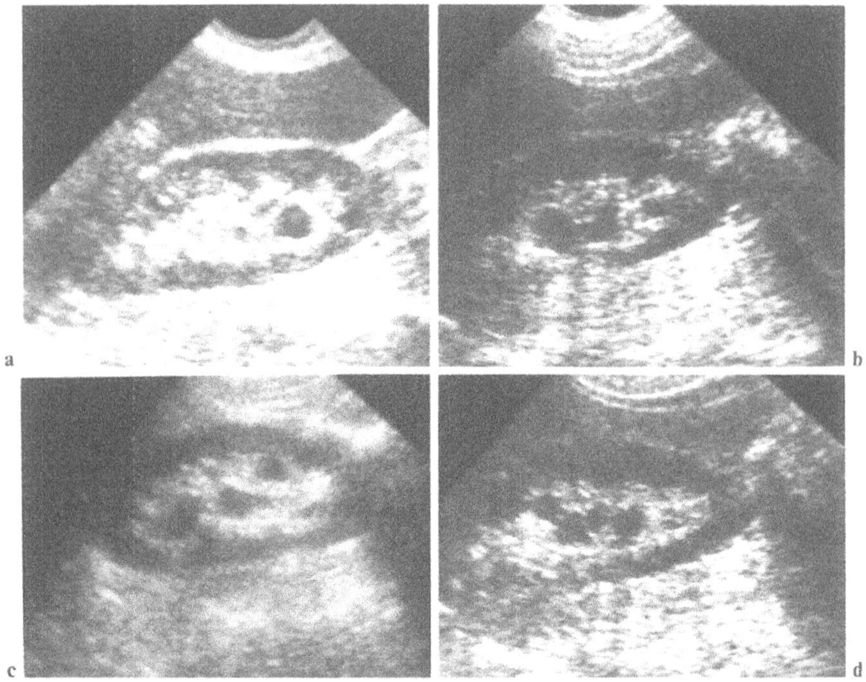

Fig. 4.13 a–d. Several examples of multiple parapelvic cysts. **a, b** First case; **a** sagittal section; **b** coronal section; **c, d** another case – coronal sections show multilocular pattern in the central zone

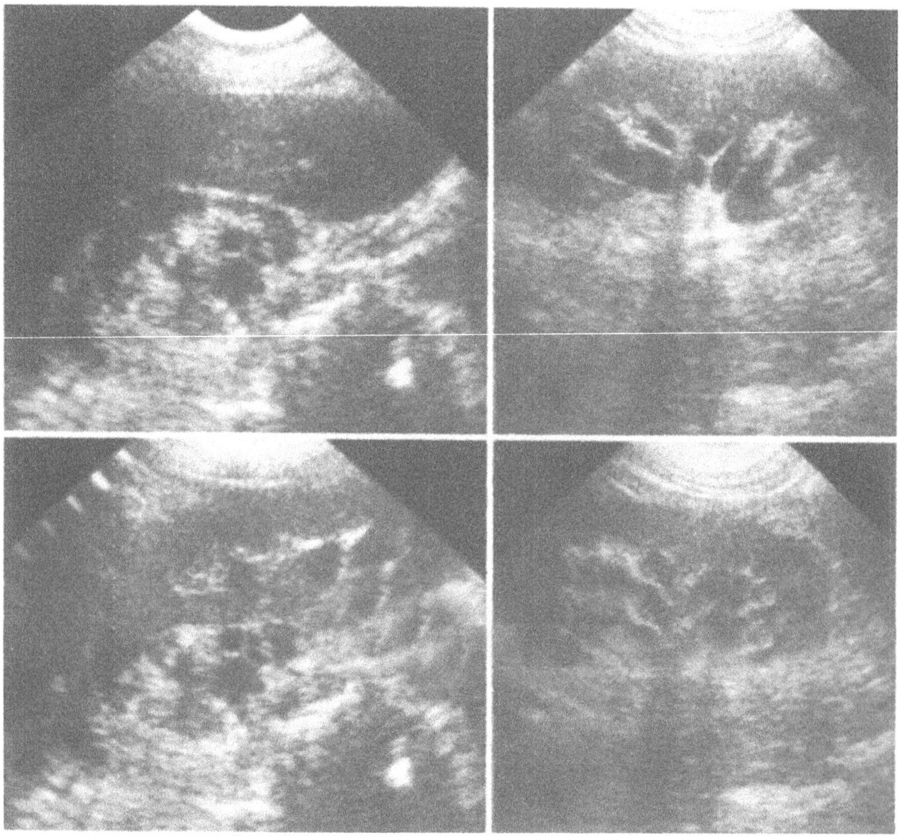

Fig. 4.14 a–d. Multiple parapelvic cysts. **a, b** First case; **a** sagittal section; **b** coronal section; **c, d** another case: left coronal sections show a sinusal multilocular pattern

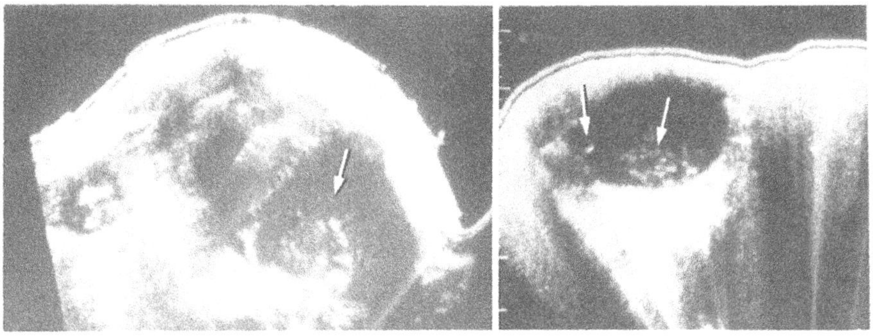

Fig. 4.15 a, b. Malignant cysts (intracystic carcinomas). a Transverse section shows enlarged right kidney with external fluid collection. Large tumoral growth (*arrow*) bulges into cystic mass. b Another case: oblique posterior section shows several intracystic growth (*arrows*). Positional changes are necessary to confirm such reflective areas to be tumoral, and not merely dependent echoes in thick, heterogeneous fluid

Differential Diagnosis

Diagnosis of Small Cysts

Small cysts may be misinterpreted as dilated infundibula. In such cases a follow-up examination after water intake, showing an increasing dilatation, may give relevant results (ROSENFIELD 1980). However, IVU remains mandatory in most cases whenever a definite differentiation is required.

Diagnosis of Medium-Sized Cysts

Exceptionally, a *localized infundibular dilatation* may possess a cystic-like pattern. Usually a multidirectional real time examination will also show a dilated calix and permit differentiation. A similar problem arises when *hydronephrotic dilatation* occurs in one of the nephrons of a *duplicated kidney*. If the relief of the dilated infundibula and calices is not apparent, the hydronephrotic pattern will mimic a cyst (see Fig. 3.11). An IVU will show an incomplete collecting system. Last but not least, a cyst can be *associated with hydronephrosis* (Fig. 4.16). Unless the cyst is bulging out of the cortex, this diagnosis is very difficult with ultrasound alone.

In areas where the parasite is endemic, *echinococcal cysts* must be considered. There is no possibility of ultrasonic differentiation between a young echinococcal cyst and a simple cyst. We shall discuss this problem later. *Collected abscesses*, which we shall discuss in Chap. 7, may have echo-free contents mimicking a cyst. However, atternation is usually higher within abscesses than in simple cysts. The abscess wall is thicker than that of simple cysts, while the clinical data are usually

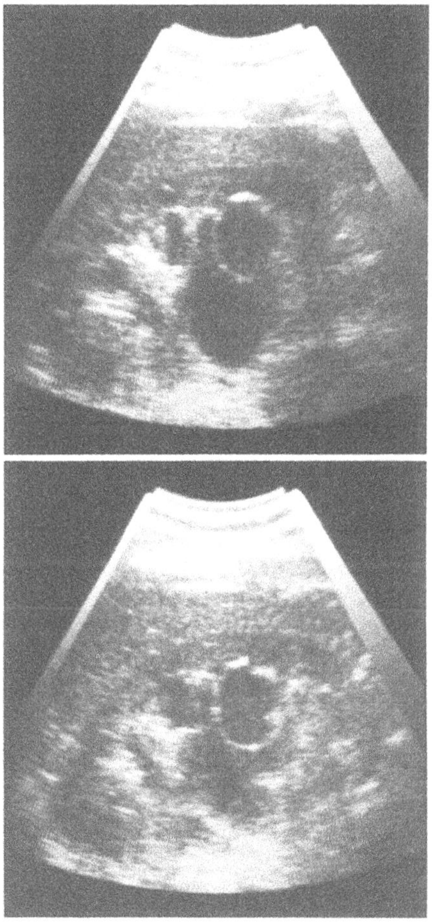

Fig. 4.16 a, b. Association of cyst with hydronephrosis

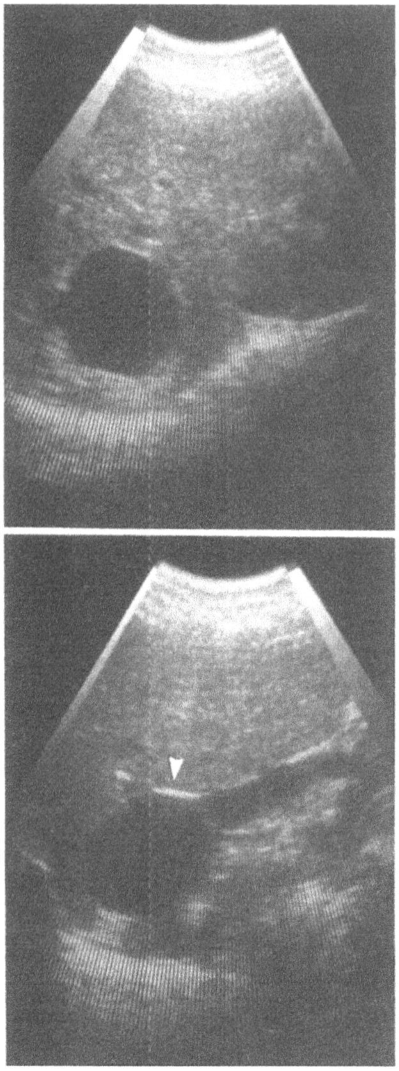

a

b

Fig. 4.17 a, b. Cyst of the upper pole of the right kidney. **a** Right recurrent subcostal section: the cyst could be hepatic. **b** Sagittal section confirms the renal location of the cyst (*arrowhead*)

quite relevant. When clinical features are less relevant, a puncture will confirm the diagnosis. A similar problem can arise from a *tuberculous abscess*. In such cases IVU usually displays different foci of abnormalities. The sonolucent pattern of a *sinus lipomatosis* cannot be misinterpreted, if high frequency is used, as a parapelvic cyst.

A few years ago we misinterpreted an anterior cortical cyst as a *dilated gallbladder*. Such a gross error can be ruled out by a comprehensive study of the different organs of the right upper quadrant.

Another critical point is the differentiation between cysts in the renal upper pole or anterior cortex, and *intrahepatic posterior cystic* lesions. A layer of reflective perirenal fat can constitute a well-delineated limit at the level of the renal upper pole. But the anterior fat layer is sometimes too thin to outline a separation (Fig. 4.17). Cysts of the adrenal are more difficult to identify.

On the left side, *splenic cysts* must be discussed in cases of upper pole lesions; cysts of the *mesentery root* may mimic an anterior cortical renal cyst. If the topographic diagnosis is important, CT will help. A rare pitfall is the presence of an *aneurysm* (Fig. 4.18). Real time may show the arterial confluence with the aneurysmal sac, as well as lesional pulsations. Duplex Doppler yields in such cases involuable information. Evidence of a calcified wall on a plain X-ray of the abdomen (a mode of information which is not forbidden to ultrasound users) may prove conclusive, although simple cysts may exceptionally possess a calcified wall. In fact calcified walls are also encountered in echinococcal cysts and in a few renal cell carcinomas.

Finally, contrasted, enhanced CT or digitized angiography will give specific images, avoiding puncture, a procedure not usually recommended in aneurysms. When calcified, echinococcal cysts have usually lost their liquid pattern, since they are mature. But the acoustic shadowing of the calcified

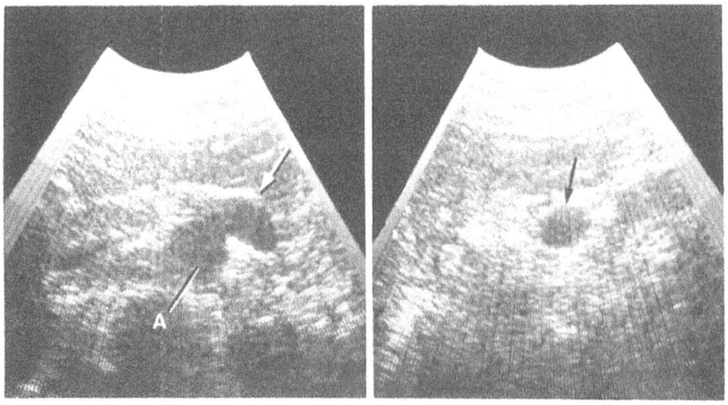

a

b

Fig. 4.18 a, b. Aneurysm of the left renal artery. **a** Transverse section shows, on the left side of the aorta (*A*), an enlarged renal artery (*arrow*). Pulsations enabled it to be differentiated from the left renal vein. **b** Sagittal section of aneurysm. Such a pattern can mimic a cyst if it is closer to the renal sinus wall can mask the solid pattern of the old daughter vesicles. Some tumors, such as cystadenomas, have a cystic pattern. The presence of some thick septations, and of solid elements, is relevant, and should lead to CT and puncture.

Diagnosis of Large Cysts

Large and giant cysts, like any large abdominal mass, are liable to cause topographic diagnostic problems, since their true origin may remain unclear. The kidney is deformed and flattened exactly as it would be by an adrenal, hepatic, or splenic cyst of similar size (Fig. 4.4 b). The triangle-shaped parenchymal margin adjacent to the cyst is not always evident. As mentioned for smaller cysts, a strip of perirenal fat may persist and delineate the cyst, but otherwise conventional procedures (CT rather than IVU or hepatosplenic nuclear imaging) will be considered. The huge dilatation of some hydronephroses should not be confusing thanks to the analysis of intercaliceal septations (see Chap. 3).

Diagnosis of Atypical Cysts

The most difficult diagnostic problems arise from atypical cysts corresponding, as stated above, to infected lesions, or hemorrhage, or *pseudocystic lesions*. Collected abscesses (see Chap. 7) may mimic a cyst – but the clinical conditions are quite different. A very difficult problem arises with pseudocystic, necrotized tumors. The cystic walls are less smooth, and thicker. There are usually debris floating in the fluid contents, or at least scattered echoes (Fig. 4.19, see also Figs. 5.23 and 5.24). Anyway, in the presence of an atypical cyst, an ultrasonically guided puncture is mandatory in order to collect material. If the cystic fluid is hemorrhagic, CT and/or selective angiography must be considered.

Some atypical pancreatic pseudocysts may enter the renal capsule and mimic a cyst. Here again, puncture is the key to diagnosis.

The possibility of "sentinel" cysts must be kept in mind (Fig. 4.19 b); discovery of a true simple cyst does not dispense with the need for complete renal scanning, to search for a tumor.

a b c d

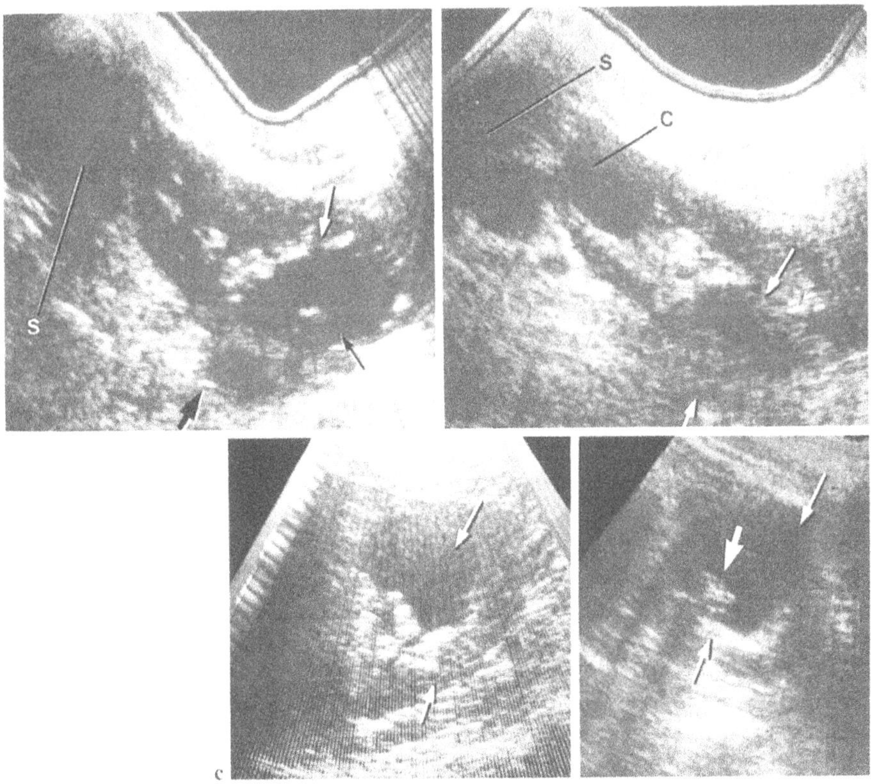

Fig. 4.19 a–d. Cyst-like necrotized tumors. **a, b** First case. **a** Sagittal scan in the prone position shows fluid collection (*small arrow*) in the lower pole. Limits are irregular; contents are heterogeneous with floating debris. The lesion bulges anteriorly (*broad arrow*) (*S*, spleen). **b** Parallel more internal scan also shows a sentinel cyst (*C*). **c, d** Another case. **c** Anterior cystic lesion (*small arrow*). The shape of the cyst is irregular. So is the posterior lesional limit (sagittal scan in supine position). **d** Scanning in the prone position shows better the intracystic tumoral growth (*braod arrow*)

The points discussed above are brought together in Table 4.2. Our own results are reported in Table 4.3. They show a reliability similar to that published by other authors.

Table 4.2. Differential diagnosis of cystic patterns

Pseudocystic patterns	Dilated infundibulum
	Partial hydronephrosis in a duplicated kidney
	Collected abscess
	Tuberculous abscess
	Renal artery aneurysm
	Intracapsular extension of pancreatic fluid collection
Pitfalls	Gallbladder hydrops
	Neighboring hepatic, splenic, or adrenal cysts
	Neighboring cyst in mesenteric root
Atypical cysts	Collapsed old benign cysts
	Septated benign cysts
	Hemorrhagic benign cysts
	Cyst with intracystic carcinoma
	Infected benign cysts
	Necrotized and cystic tumors
	Echinococcal cysts
Calcified "cysts"	Calcified aneurysm
	Calcified renal cell carcinoma and other tumors
	Calcified echinococcal cyst
	Calcified benign cyst
	Calcified old multicystic dysplastic kidney old abscesses

Table 4.3. Reliability of diagnosis of cysts (personal results)

Successful diagnosis of simple cyst	167
False-positive (necrotized carcinoma)	1
False-negative (solid pattern due to hemorrhage)	3
Correct diagnosis of atypical cyst (tumor, infection)	7
Atypical cysts which proved benign after puncture	12
	190

Clinical and Radiological Management

The different points discussed above lead to the following management policies:

- The cyst is clearly renal, evidently benign, solitary, asymptomatic: no other examination procedure has to be considered, except a follow-up examination a few months later. Any increase in size or any change in echotexture should lead to a puncture, taking into account the slight risk of small intracystic carcinoma arising from the cystic wall.
- The cyst is accompanied by abdominal pain; the size and location of the cyst are such that they may give rise to pelvic compression: CT will be carried out, followed if necessary by puncture. An active policy is also commendable in young patients.
- The cyst is atypical: puncture is performed. In the case of hemorrhagic content, a CT scan will be carried out, complemented if necessary by angiography.
- The size of the cyst is such that its renal origin is not certain: CT scanning, and in some case angiography, will be considered.
- We shall consider later the particular case of cysts diagnosed in countries with endemic echinococcosis.

Finally, complementary procedures will be necessary in about 1% of cases only.

Puncture

The area of entry, posterior or lateral, will be chosen so that the minimal volume of parenchyma is pierced. It should be as far as possible from the hilus. If the puncture route is not strictly posterior it is wise to check that no intestinal loop is interposed, particularly before inserting a catheter.

After precise localization, puncture is easy if the cyst is over 3 cm in diameter (Figs. 4.20, 4.21). The smallest cyst we have punctured had a diameter of 2 cm. A follow-up examination after the procedure enables one to check the emptiness of the cyst, taking into account the possibility of injecting ethanol in order to prevent recurrence (Fig. 4.20a) (note that, paradoxically, even ethanol must be sterilized).

In fact, cysts are punctured essentially to collect material for cytological study. Complete evacuation is almost impossible when a fine needle is used, which is the best way to prevent puncture complications.

As we said above, careful ultrasonic analysis of cysts permits the confirmation of a benign cyst in most cases, thus reducing dramatically the number of punctures.

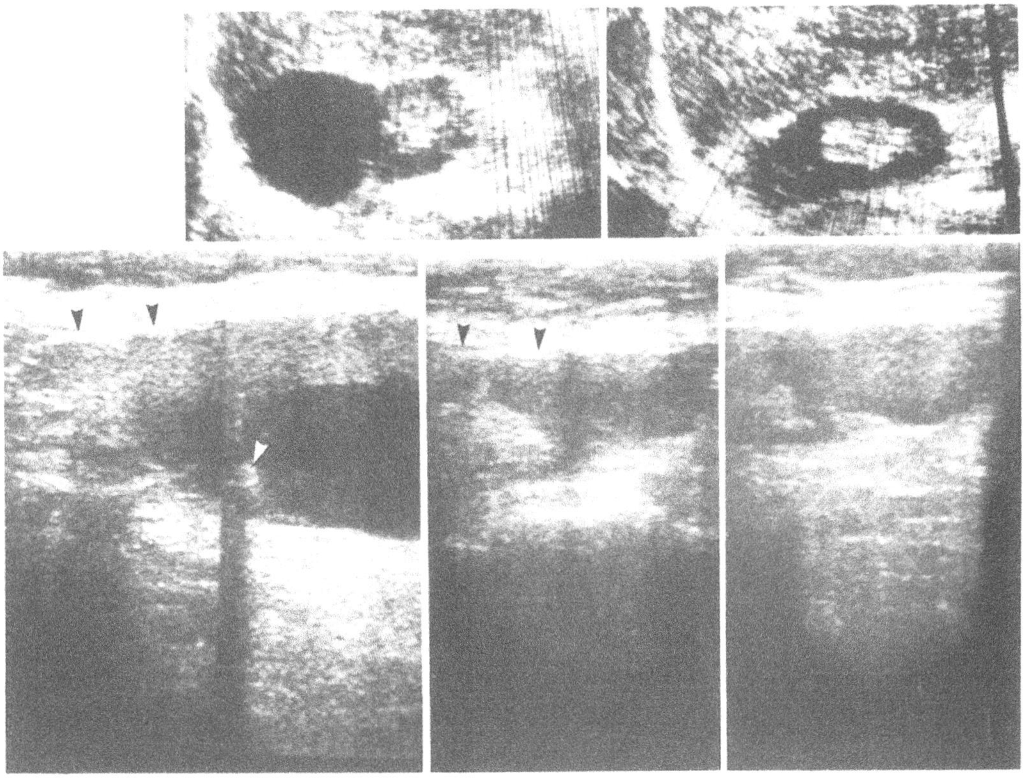

Fig. 4.20 a–e. Puncture. **a, b** First case. **a** Upper pole cyst. **b** Follow-up examination after puncture. **c–e** Another case. **c** Sagittal scan of huge cyst of the lower pole of the kidney, which is indicated by *black arrowheads. White arrowhead* points to tip echo of the needle. **d** Kidney (*black arrowheads*) and cyst at the end of the procedure. **e** Cyst after injection of 15 ml sterile alcohol

4.2 Polycystic Processes

Polycystic Processes of the Neonate and Child

We shall deal briefly only with the rarest of such processes.

Multicystic Dysplasic Kidney

Multicystic dysplasic kidney is the most common of renal masses in the neonate (GROSSMANN 1983). It is unilateral and has the pattern of a multilocular cystic mass (Fig. 4.21 a, b). It corresponds (Table 4.1) to a hydronephrosis arising in utero from ureteral or pelvic atresia. The cystic elements correspond to dilated calices. They can display confluences in the pelvic area. If not operated on, or misdiagnosed, multicystic dysplasia can decrease in volume during the first years of life. It appears later on as a unilateral cystic process, sometimes within calcified walls.

Multilocular Cysts

This is a benign tumoral entity, which has sometimes been confused with Wilms' tumor. It has been termed "cystic nephroma," "cystic hemartoma," "cystic lymphangioma," "Perlmann tumor," and even "Wilms' tumor." Pathology can show areas of nephroblastoma. Multilocular cysts are perhaps a benign variety of Wilms' tumor. Encountered in the child and adult, its pattern is usually more cystic in children, with rather thick and echogenic septations and solid areas (Fig. 4.21 c, d).

Infantile and Juvenile Polycystic Disease

In this rare anomaly, there may be small cysts. The size of the kidney is increased. But the main features arise from diffuse tubular ectasia: multiple reflections on the enlarged tubules give rise to an increased reflectivity of the medulla. The parenchyma becomes diffusely reflective, with a loss of

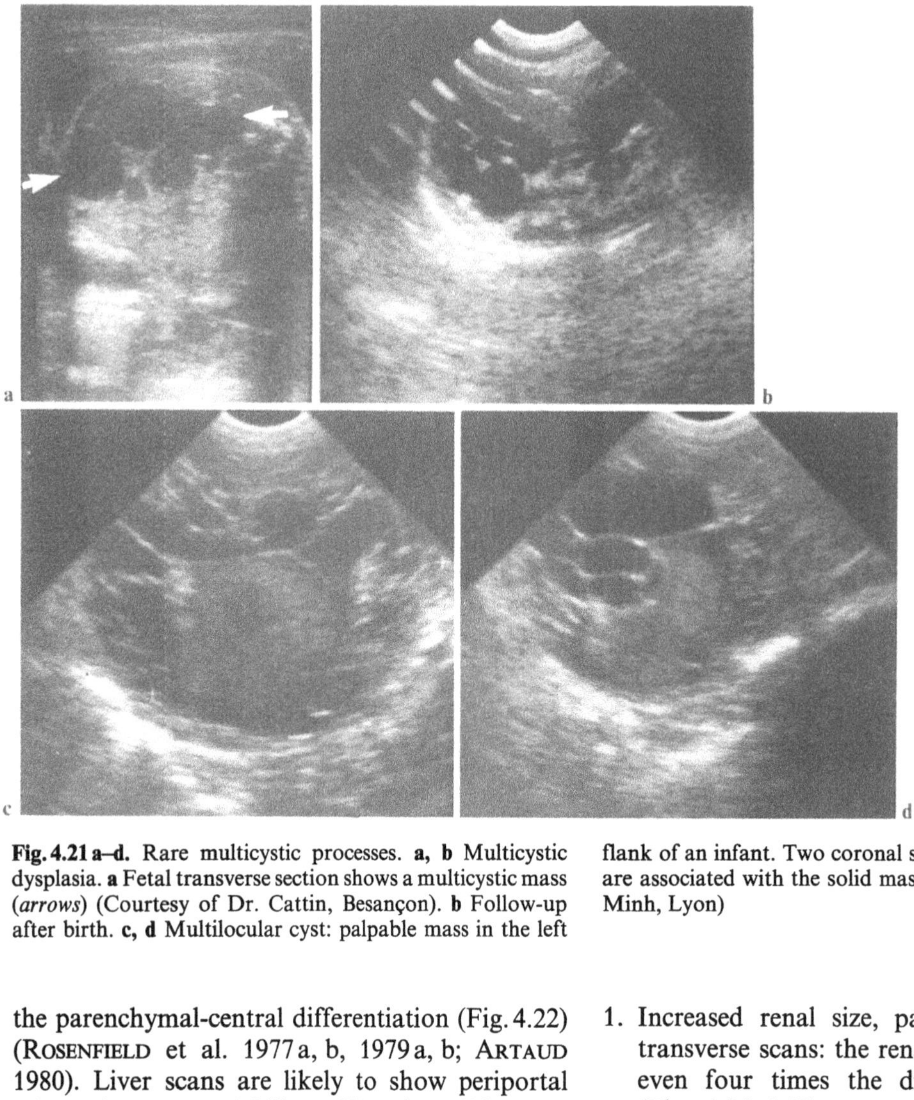

Fig. 4.21 a–d. Rare multicystic processes. **a, b** Multicystic dysplasia. **a** Fetal transverse section shows a multicystic mass (*arrows*) (Courtesy of Dr. Cattin, Besançon). **b** Follow-up after birth. **c, d** Multilocular cyst: palpable mass in the left flank of an infant. Two coronal sections. Multilocular cysts are associated with the solid mass. (Courtesy of Prof. Tran Minh, Lyon)

the parenchymal-central differentiation (Fig. 4.22) (ROSENFIELD et al. 1977a, b, 1979a, b; ARTAUD 1980). Liver scans are likely to show periportal echogenic areas and biliary dilatations (Fig. 4.23) (ROSENFIELD et al. 1977a, b, 1979a, b; ARTAUD et al. 1980) due to the associated congenital fibrosis. The prognosis is very poor, a few days usually. Survival for several months or years is exceptional.

Adult-Type Polycystic Disease of the Infant

Adult-type polycystic disease of the infant shows the same features (Fig. 4.24) as the polycystic disease of the adult, which we shall consider next.

Polycystic Disease of the Adult (PCD)

Typical Patterns

The multiple cysts of polycystic disease (PCD) give rise to:

1. Increased renal size, particularly evident on transverse scans: the renal diameter is three or even four times the diameter of the spine (Figs. 4.24, 4.25).
2. Multiple cortical bulgings (Fig. 4.26).
3. A multilocular pattern, with fluid-filled areas of variable size (Figs. 4.26, 4.27).

This pattern of abnormally large, multilocular kidneys, which may occupy the entire half of the abdomen (Fig. 4.24), is typical.

Asymptomatic Polycystic Disease

Large and giant kidneys represent the later evolution of the multiple cysts' growth. Systematic study of the members of a family in which a case of PCD has been discovered permits diagnosis of less-advanced cases – and, incidentally, is a good test of the image quality of your machine. Along with obvious cysts, several centimeters in diameter, multidirectional real time scans frequently show very small cysts whose diameter is only a few millimeters (Figs. 4.28, 4.29). We ceased screening families of

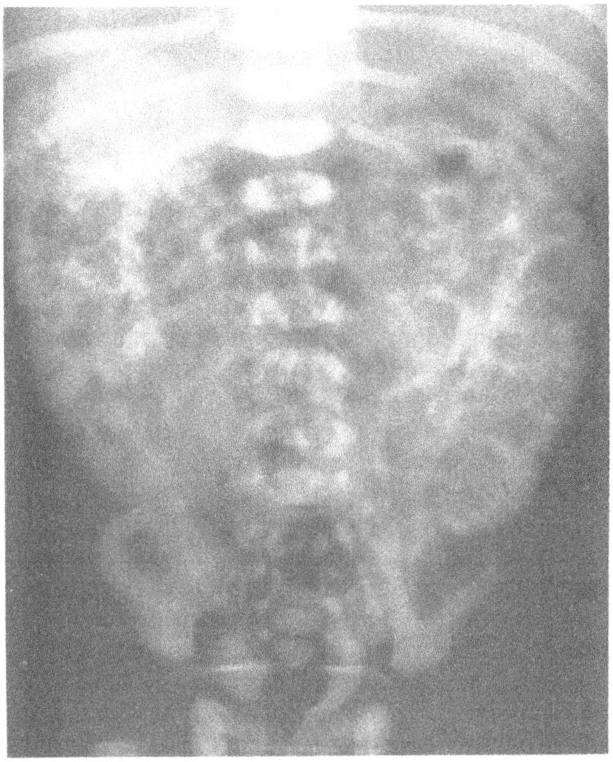

a

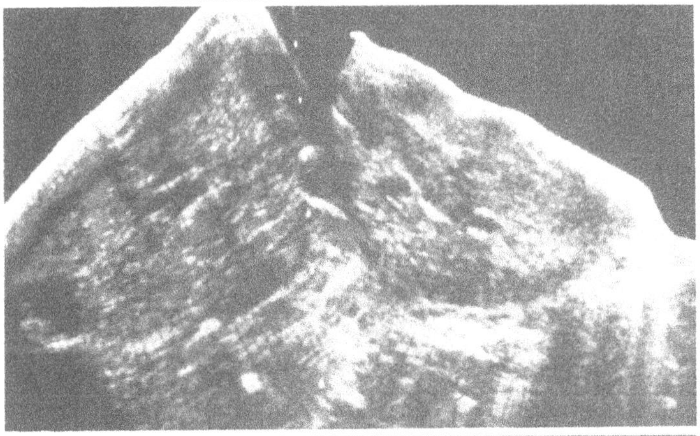

b

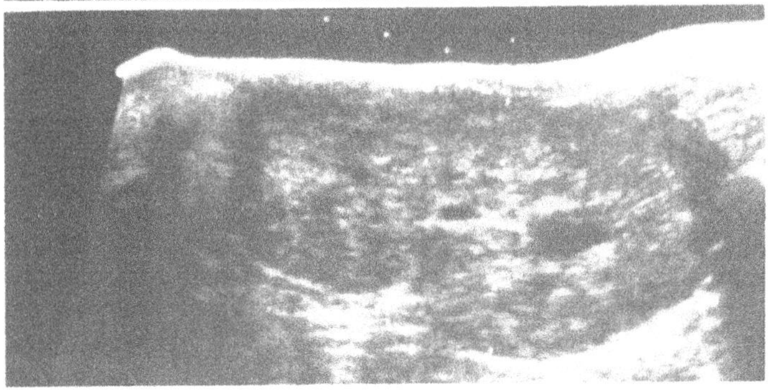

c

Fig. 4.22 a–c. Infantile polycystic disease. **a** IVU shows enlarged kidneys with tubular ectasia. **b** Transverse scan in the prone position shows massively enlarged kidneys. Parenchymal-central differentiation has almost disappeared. **c** Sagittal scan of the right kidney in the prone position shows the same echotexture. (Courtesy of Prof. Diard, Bordeaux)

PCD patients, since the disclosure of the disease generates anxiety in young subjects.

Atypical Polycystic Disease

The interfaces of multiple adjacent microcysts give rise to numerous echoes, and on occasion to a misleading echotexture of solid type (Weill et al. 1974). We have encountered that echotexture only once, before the gray-scale era, and we made a false diagnosis of solitary cyst. A partial pattern of that kind is illustrated in Fig. 4.29. Like that of simple cysts, the pattern of some of the cysts of a PCD may alter, especially after a hemorrhage or infection (Fig. 4.30).

The ultrasonic diagnosis of adult polycystic disease is so reliable that other procedures are not usually necessary. Ultrasound enables one to avoid IVU, which could aggravate a renal insufficiency. However, other pathological processes can be associated. Precise analysis of the remaining renal tissue, laminated and deformed, is hazardous in the case of multiple large cysts. CT is valuable, particularly after onset of pain, in order to localize a hemorrhagic cyst, demonstrate a calculus, or show an exceptional renal cell carcinoma.

Associated Extrarenal Cysts

In about 20% of cases there are associated hepatic cysts, either solitary or multiple (Figs. 4.30–4.33). Posterior hepatic cysts are difficult to differentiate from anterior right renal cysts. We have already discussed this problem in connection with simple cysts. Other locations, pancreatic for instance, are exceptional.

Differential Diagnosis

We shall consider comprehensively the differential diagnosis of multiple cysts at the end of this chapter (see Table 4.4).

Acquired Polycystic Disease of the Chronically Dialyzed Patient (APD)

Sonographic follow-up of chronically dialyzed patients showed the frequency of acquired cysts in dialyzed patients (Fetisoff 1981; Monnet-Guichard 1982; Andersen 1983). Such cysts become more numerous as dialysis is pursued.

Table 4.4. Diagnosis of multiple renal collections

Extrarenal collections	Multiple hepatic cysts
	Multiple splenic cysts
	Septated ascites
	Multilocular ovarian cyst
	Cystic lymphangioma
	Malignant mesenchymoma
Intrarenal collections	Multiple benign cysts
	Cystic tumors
	Unilateral multicystic disease
	Polycystic disease
	Multiple echinococcal cysts
	Hydronephrosis
	Benign cysts associated with other abnormalities:
	Cyst + hydrocalices
	Cyst + hydronephrosis
	Cyst + pseudocystic tumor
	Multiple abscesses
	Multiple tuberculous abscesses
	Tuberculous abscesses associated with dilated calices
Pitfalls	Tumor with multiple necrotized cavities
	Lymphomatous nodules

In some series, cysts are found in over 70% of patients. APD has essentially two patterns:

1. Cysts in small altered kidney (Fig. 4.34a)
2. A polycystic pattern, with external bulges, in swollen kidneys, resembling congenital polycystic disease (Fig. 4.34b).

Chronically dialyzed patients require a regular ultrasonic follow-up: hemorrhage can occur in some cysts; but the main complication is renal cell carcinoma, which seems to develop only in patients who have acquired cysts.

Echinococcal Cysts

In countries where echinococcosis is endemic, discovery of a renal cyst requires immunological tests. Only young echinococcal cysts can mimic simple cysts, whose pattern is exactly the same. Echinococcosis can even mimic hepatorenal PCD: we have encountered multiple renal and liver echinococcal cysts in three cases. The multilocular pattern of large echinococcal cysts due to giant daughter vesicles is, however, rather typical (Fig. 4.35). Mature echinococcal cysts contain daughter vesicles which give rise to a solid echotexture (Weill et al. 1973b). In the case of calcified walls a shell sign is seen. The gamut of cysts with calcified walls is depicted in Table 4.2, p. 70.

Differential Diagnosis of Multiple Cysts

Extrarenal Processes

Discussion of multiple hepatic cysts adjacent to the kidney is of little interest in cases of PCD, since multiple renal cysts are also present anyway. The discussion is more important in the case of multiple echinococcal cysts. CT is the best complementary procedure in such cases. A hepatic cyst can compress a kidney in exactly the same way as an upper pole cyst would, and vice versa; IVU and scintigraphy are absolutely unspecific in this regard. Multilocular patterns are encountered in septated ascites, in intraperitoneal tumors (abdominal ovarian cyst, cystic lymphangioma), and also in retroperitoneal tumors (malignant mesenchymoma). Multiple ultrasonic scans will show the kidney as an individual image, even if it is flattened. In the case of inconclusive images, CT will lead to a correct diagnosis.

Intrarenal Processes

Hydronephrosis is diagnosed by the images of communication between adjacent fluid-filled septations. Very confusing patterns arise from associated lesions: hydrocalices and cyst, hydronephrosis and cyst, benign cysts, and pseudocystic tumors. Any doubtful pattern must lead to a puncture. The pattern of some tumors (cystadenomas, hemartomas) can be multicystic; here again, CT and/or puncture are required.

Difficulties can also arise from multiple abscesses (bacterial or tuberculous – see Chap. 7). Puncture will ensure a correct diagnosis if IVU is not specific or if clinical symptoms are irrelevant. Polycystic disease can also be mimicked by quite a different process – at least if the examination is not thorough: Multiple sonolucent nodules are encountered, in enlarged kidneys, in some cases of renal localization of lymphoma (see Fig. 8.11) (KAUDE 1978, Chap. 8). Even if such nodules are pseudocystic at first glance, a high-sensitivity study, which is mandatory for all liquid masses, will show a lack of posterior reinforcement, and a few scattered echoes. Differentiation of true multicystic tumors, as cystadenomas, is achieved by CT and puncture. The differential diagnosis of multiple cysts is summarized in Table 4.4.

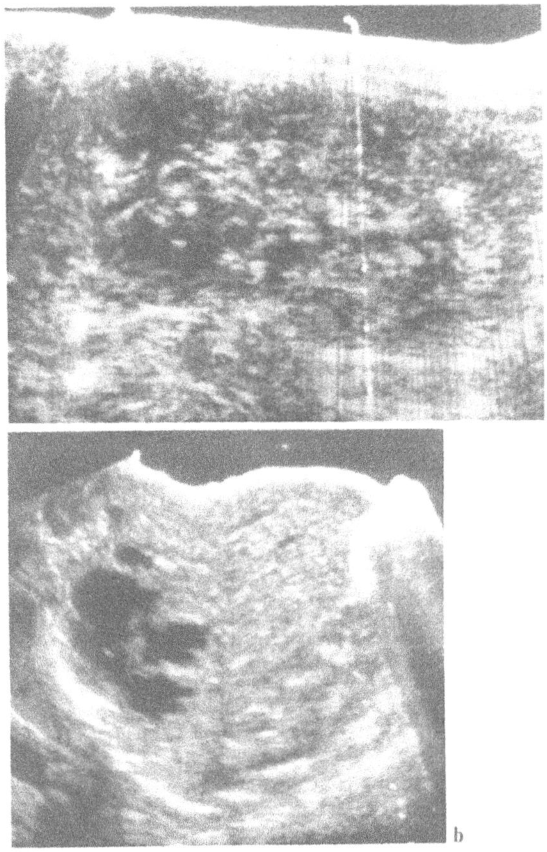

a

b

Fig. 4.23 a, b. Infantile polycystic disease. **a** Sagittal cut of left kidney in prone position shows abnormal echoes in parenchyma. Parenchymal-central differentiation is altered. **b** Sagittal section of liver displays fluid-filled elements corresponding to enlarged bile ducts accompanying congenital fibrosis (courtesy of Prof. Diard, Bordeaux)

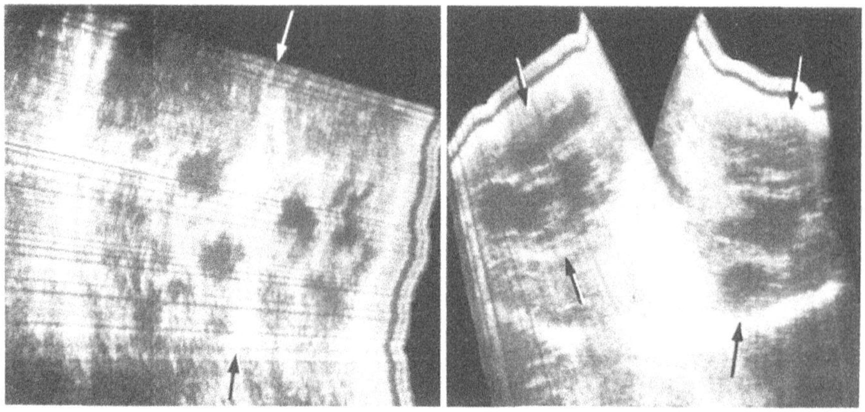

a b

Fig. 4.24 a, b. Polycystic disease, adult type, in infant 11 months old. **a** Coronal scan. Section is presented with cranial side above, as in conventional X-ray tomography. The polycystic kidneys are so enlarged that the internal contours (*arrow*) are in contact (*arrow*); their volume occupies the entire abdomen. **b** Transverse scan (*arrows* kidneys)

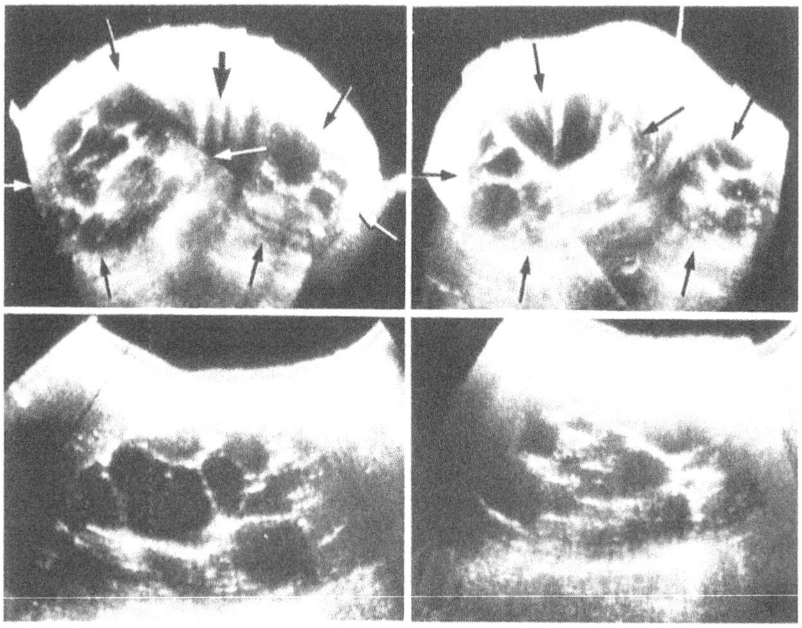

a b c d

Fig. 4.25 a–d. Polycystic disease. **a** Transverse scan in the prone position. Both kidneys (*arrows*) are enlarged (compare diameter with spine) (*broad arrow*). Both renal sections show multiple adjacent typical cysts. **b** Parallel, more caudal scan. **c** Sagittal scan of the right kidney (prone position). **d** Sagittal scan of the left kidney (prone position)

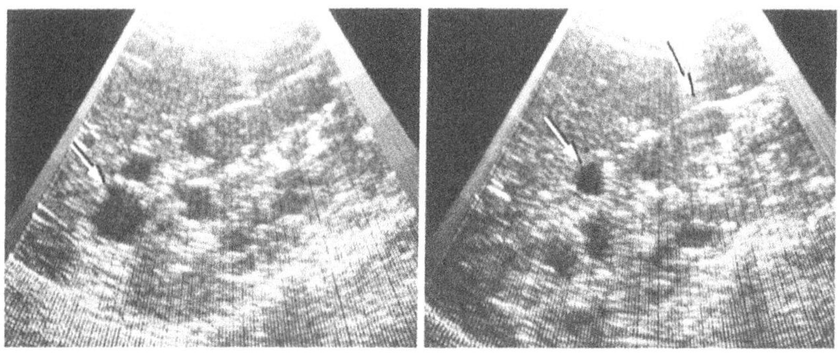

a b

Fig. 4.26 a, b. Polycystic disease. Parallel sagittal real time scans. Cysts are smaller than in Fig. 4.25. Note cortical bulges (*arrows*)

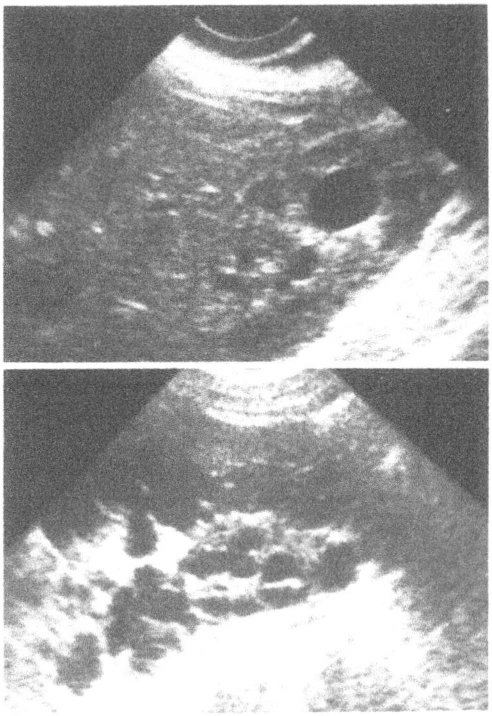

Fig. 4.27 a, b. Polycystic disease with cysts of varying size. **a** Right kidney; **b** left kidney

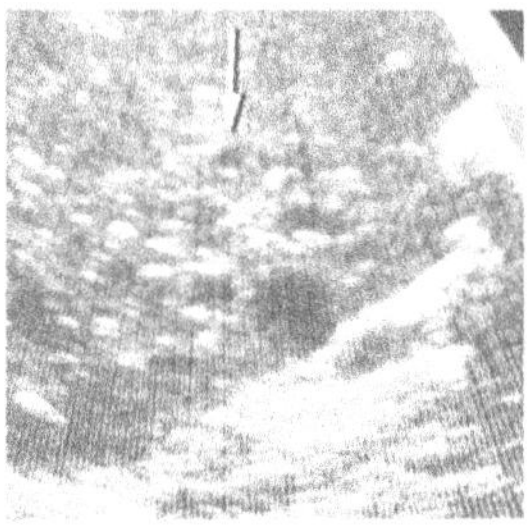

Fig. 4.28. Polycystic disease. Small cysts disclosed by systematic familial examination after diagnosis of typical pattern in sister. Note 3-mm cyst (*arrow*)

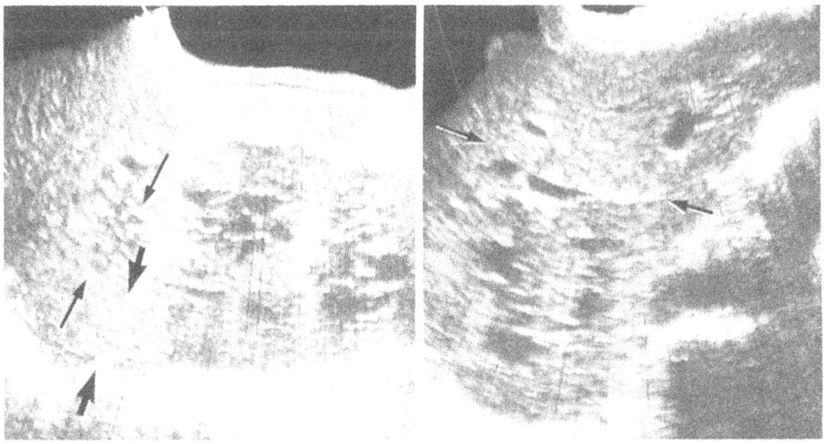

Fig. 4.29 a, b. Polycystic disease. Small cysts. **a** Sagittal section: along with frank cysts, there are small elements (*small arrow*) in several areas. Cysts are so small that multiple cystic walls bring about solid pattern (*broad arrow*). In such areas renal tissue is not easily differentiated from liver. **b** Transverse section: note the unsharp cleavage plane (*arrow*) with liver

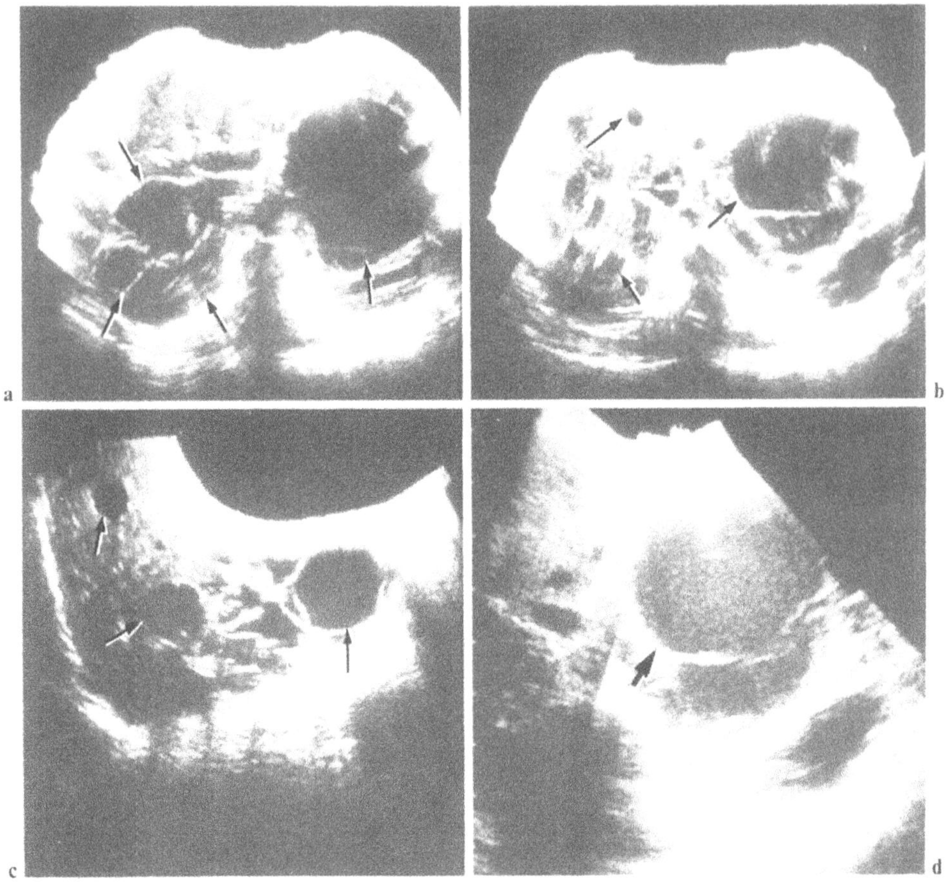

Fig. 4.30 a–d. Polycystic disease. **a–c** Transverse and sagittal scans show multiple hepatic and renal cysts (*arrows*). **d** Left oblique section with postprocessing demonstrates intracystic echoes due to infection (*arrow*)

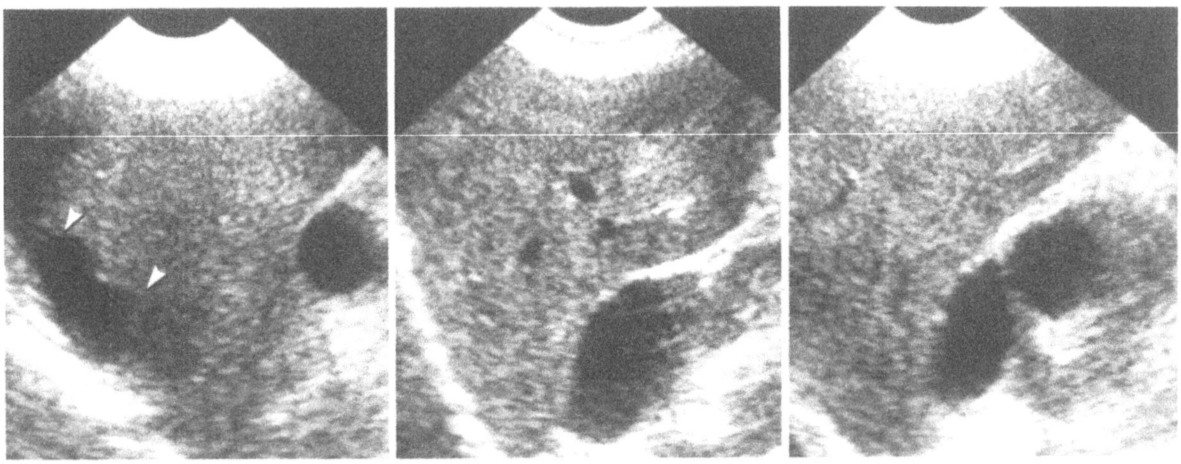

Fig. 4.31 a–c. Polycystic disease of liver and kidneys. **a–c** Three right parasagittal scans. **a** Hepatic (*arrowheads*) and renal cysts. **b, c** Renal cysts

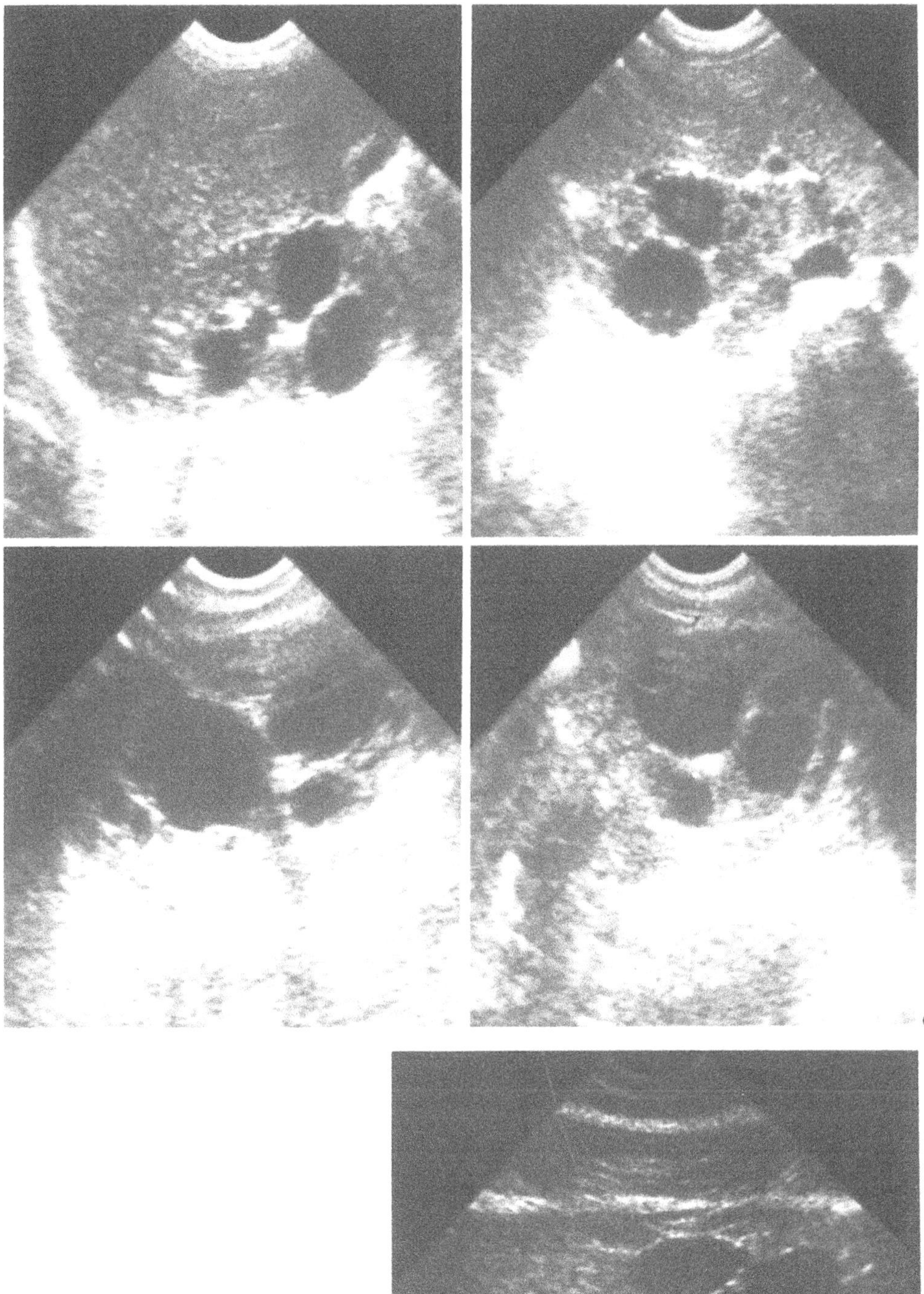

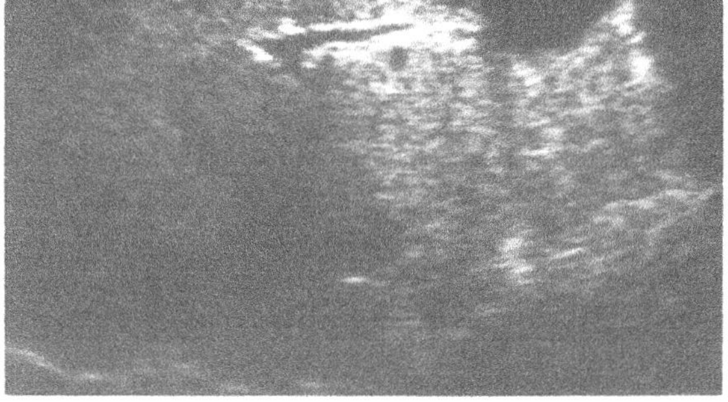

Fig. 4.32 a–e. Polycystic disease of liver and kidneys. **a, b** Sagittal and transverse scans of right kidney. **c, d** Coronal and transverse scans of left kidney. **e** Transverse scan of cysts in left lobe of liver

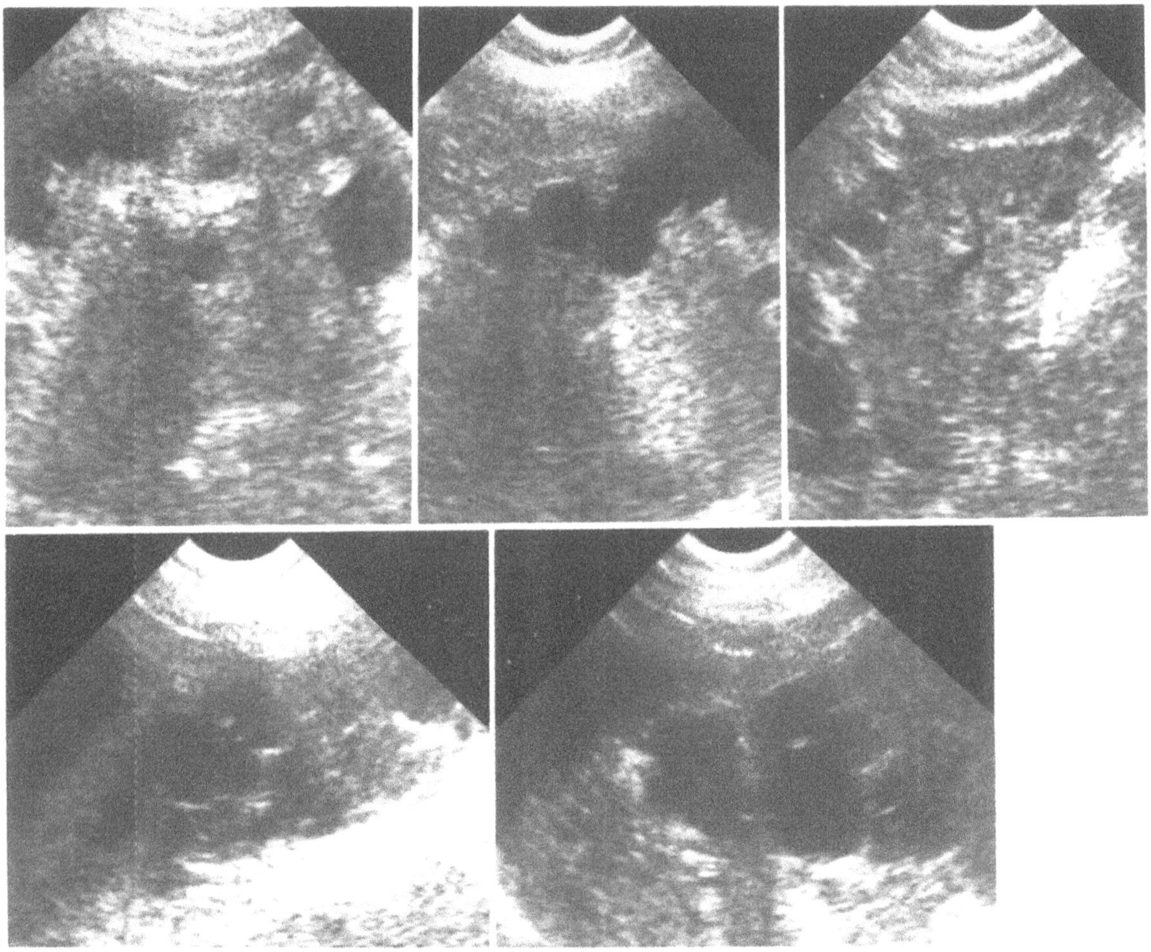

a–c

d, e

Fig. 4.33 a–e. Polycystic disease of liver and kidneys. **a, c** Liver sections; **d, e** renal sections; **a** subcostal recurrent scan; **b** transverse scan; **c** medial sagittal scan; **d** right kidney; **e** left kidney

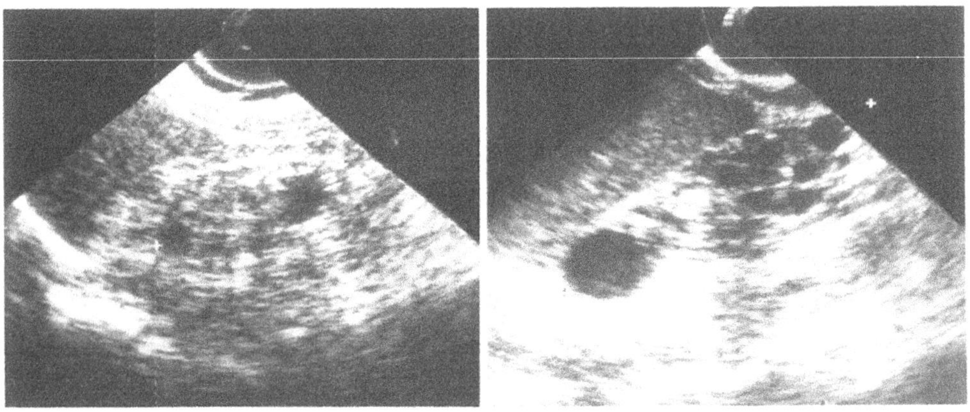

a

b

Fig. 4.34 a, b. Acquired polycystic disease of the chronically dialyzed patient. **a** Cysts in small kidney with loss of differentiation. **b** Polycystic pattern mimicking congenital polycystic disease. (Courtesy of Dr. Monnet-Guichard, Annecy, France)

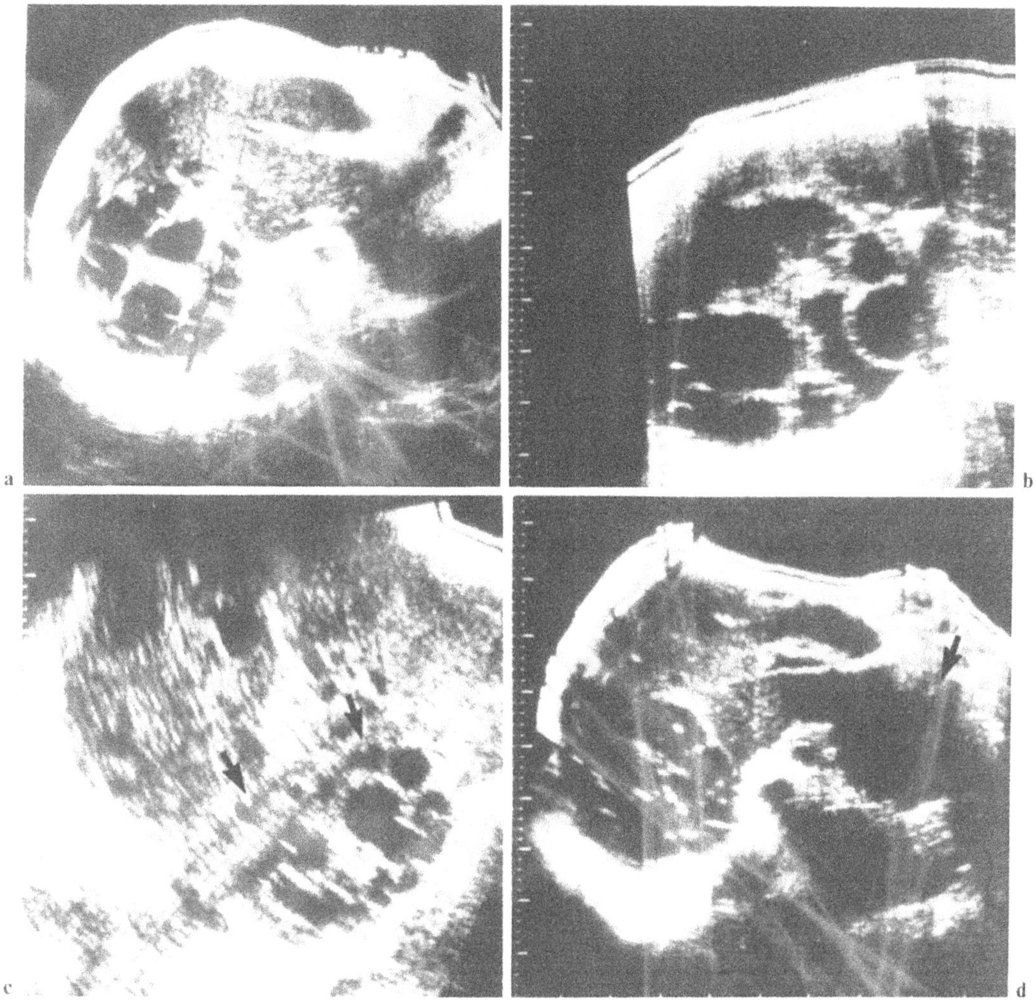

Fig. 4.35 a–d. Multiple cysts in the right kidney and liver. **a** Transverse scan. **b** Close-up view. **c** Normal characters. **d** More caudal transverse section also discloses cyst in the pancreatic tail (*arrow*). Your diagnosis? (Answer at bottom of page*)

* Such grape-like multiple adjacent cysts are typical of giant daughter vesicles in echinococcal cysts.

5 Renal Tumors

5.1 Malignant Tumors

Renal Cell Carcinoma

Renal tumors give rise to changes in the organ's size (in the case of the largest tumoral masses), the organ's shape (except in the case of small parapelvic tumors), and the balance between the parenchyma and the central pyelovascular area. The contours and echotexture of the tumor are the next points of analysis, as well as, finally, the proximal relations of the tumoral process.

Changes in Size

When the tumor is wider than the kidney, and moreover when its craniocaudal development is greater then the organ's axial length, its appearance is that of a mass of variable shape (Fig. 5.1). Most tumors, however, only give rise to a partial, local tumefaction (Figs. 5.2, 5.3).

Changes in Shape

The various morphological changes are illustrated in Fig. 5.4. Whether central or peripheral, once the tumor has developed beyond the parenchyma, it gives rise to a superficial bulge, breaking the kidney's even contours. Small tumors produce a localized relief (Fig. 5.5). Larger tumors cause more striking changes. A localized swelling of the distal or medial part of the kidney is then associated with distortion of the contours (Fig. 5.6). In some cases the tumoral bulge is sharp enough to form a definite angle with the neighboring cortex (Fig. 5.5 a).

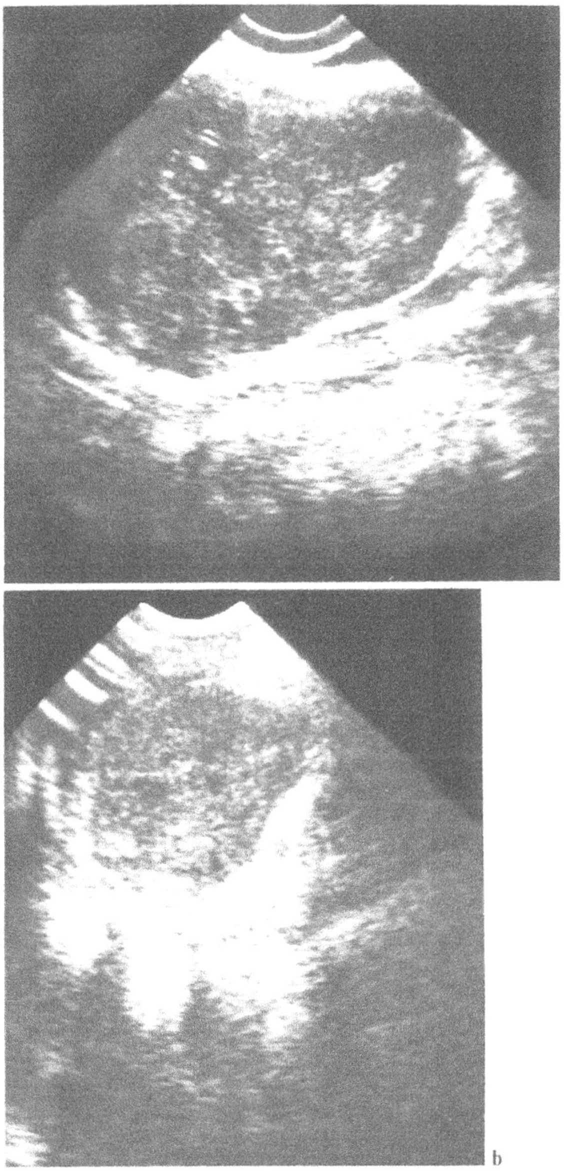

a

b

Fig. 5.1 a, b. Huge renal cell carcinoma swelling whole right kidney. Perirenal fat is ill defined around upper pole of mass. **a** Sagittal scan; **b** transverse scan

Relative Proportions of Parenchyma and Central Area

We described in Chap. 1 the even thickness of the parenchyma, the smooth, if scalloped, limits of the

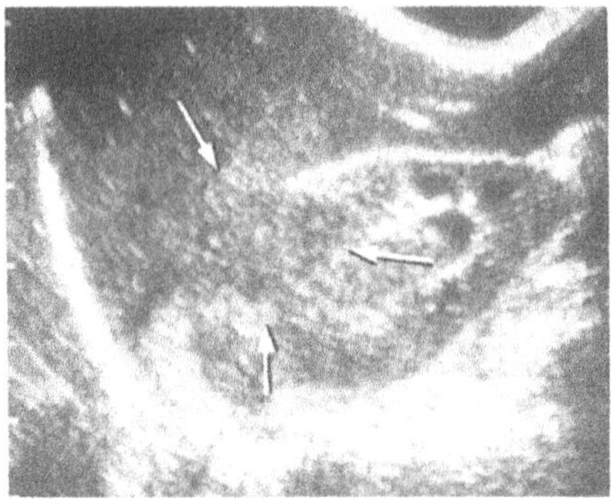

Fig. 5.2. Small renal cell carcinoma. Tumoral nodule (*arrows*), 3 cm diameter, bulges slightly out of anterior cortex of right kidney. Fatty limit has disappeared

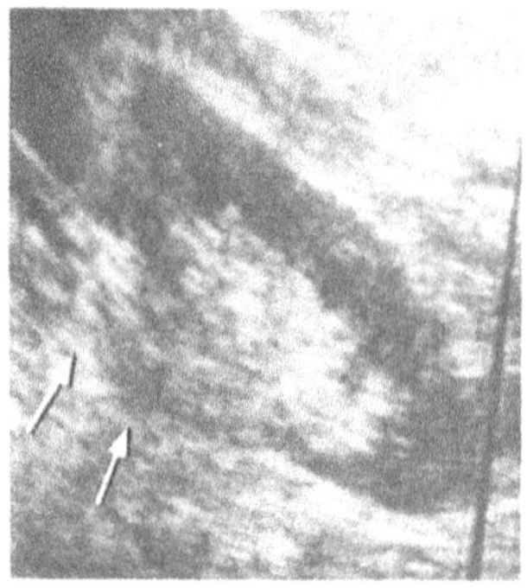

Fig. 5.3. Small renal cell carcinoma: anterior cortex of left kidney bulges forward (*arrows*). The tumoral area is abnormally echogenic

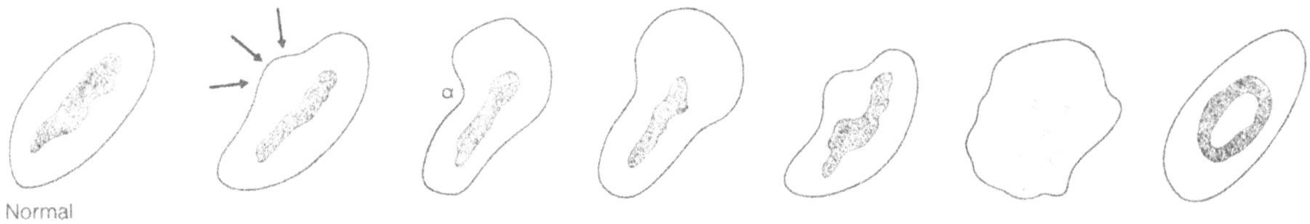

Fig. 5.4. Shape of the kidney in different tumoral locations

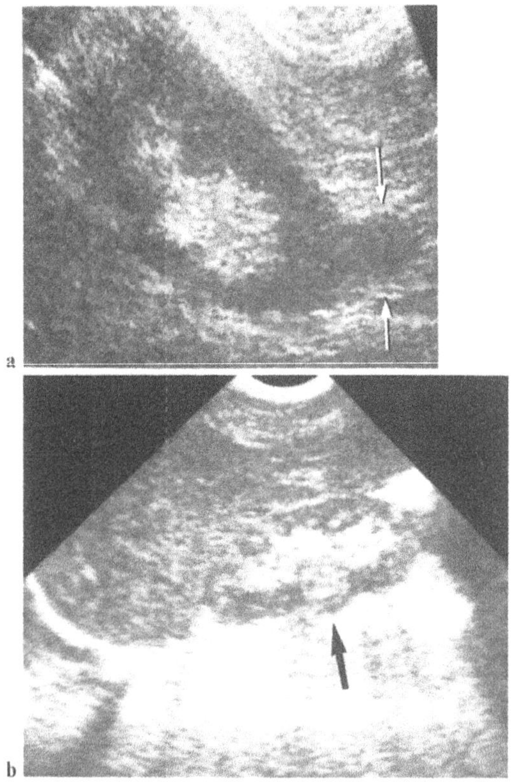

Fig. 5.5 a, b. Marginal tumors. **a** Lower pole renal cell carcinoma gives rise to prominent bulging (*arrows*). This kind of external development is hardly seen on IVU images, unless frankly hypervascularized. **b** Posterior nodule (*arrow*). Nodule is separated from depressed perirenal fat by thin layer or normal cortex. Central zone is frankly depressed

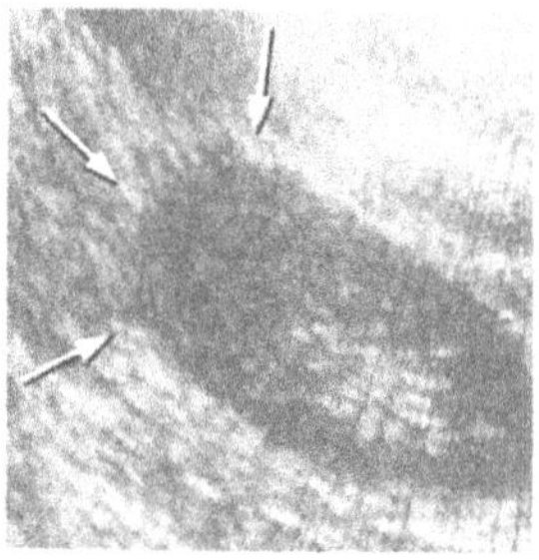

Fig. 5.6. Left renal cell carcinoma: global swelling (*arrows*) of upper lobe

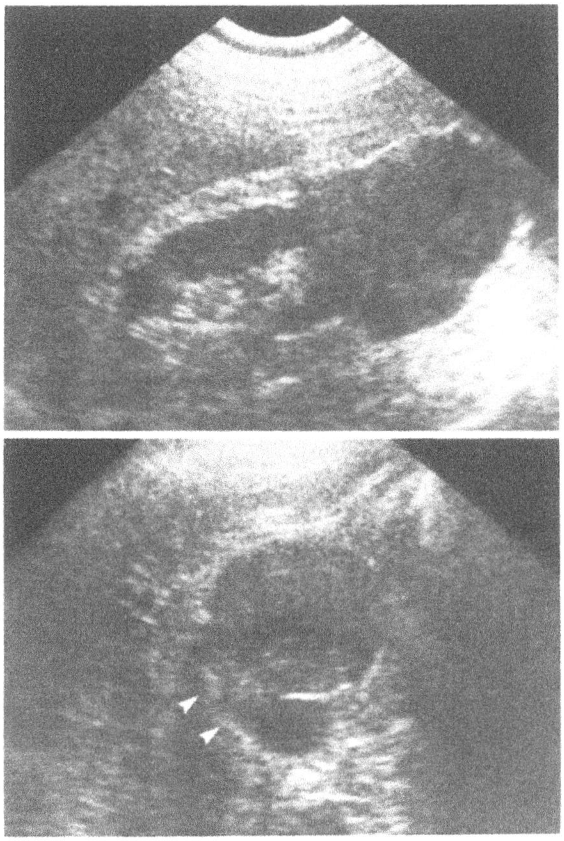

a

b

◂ **Fig. 5.7 a, b.** Large carcinoma of right lower pole. **a** Sagittal scan; **b** transverse scan. In **a**, fatty rim is well delineated; in **b**, extension through perirenal fat is visualized (*arrowheads*)

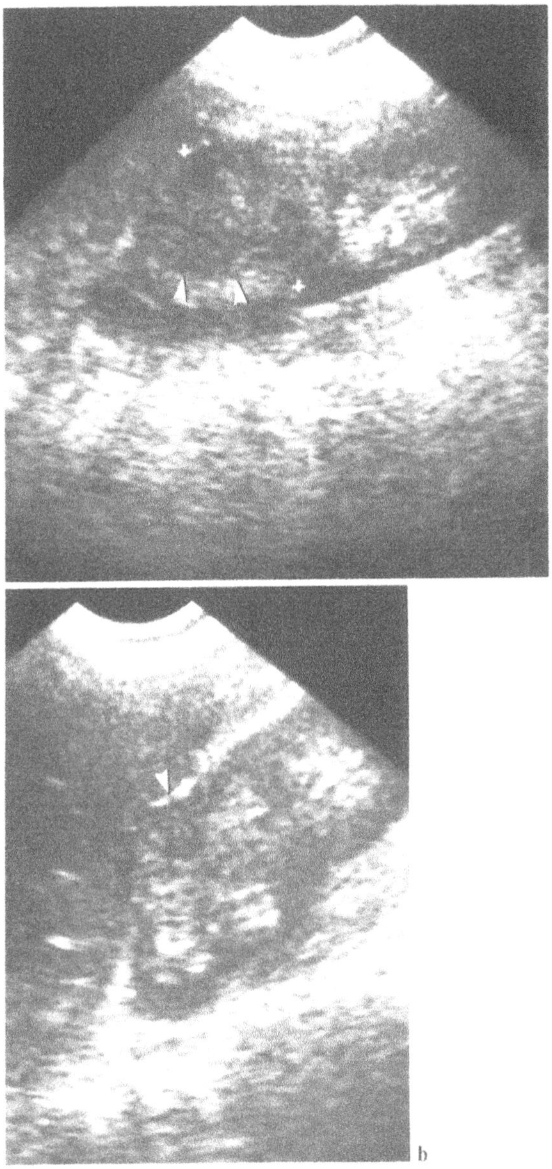

a

b

Fig. 5.9 a, b. Cortical tumors. **a** Small mass, poorly echogenic, bulges out of anterior contour and produces impression on central zone (*arrowheads*); perirenal fat is thinned. **b** Small cortical carcinoma (*arrowhead*) with impression on thinned perirenal fat

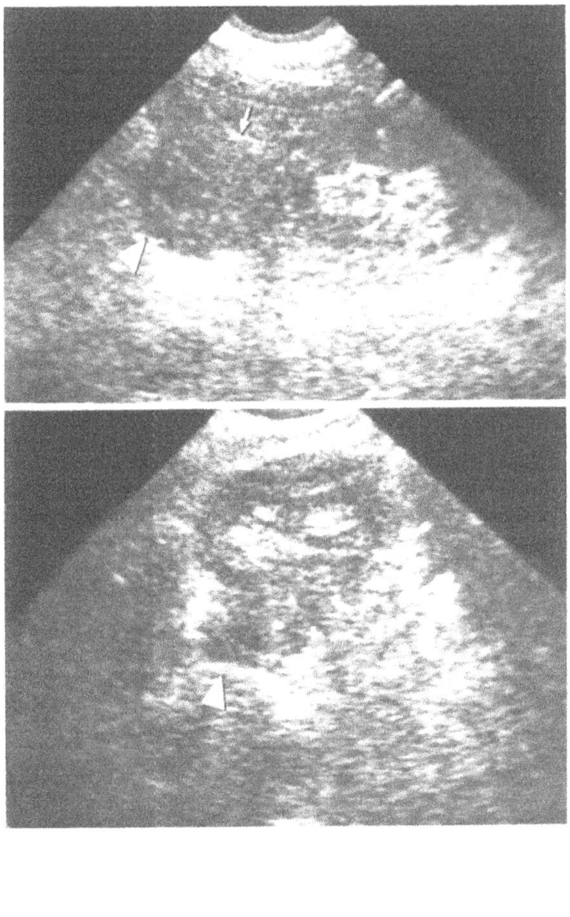

a

b

◂ **Fig. 5.8 a, b.** Renal cell carcinoma of left upper pole. **a** Coronal scan shows mass (*arrowhead*) bulging out of internal cortex. Central zone is depressed (*arrow*). **b** Transverse scan

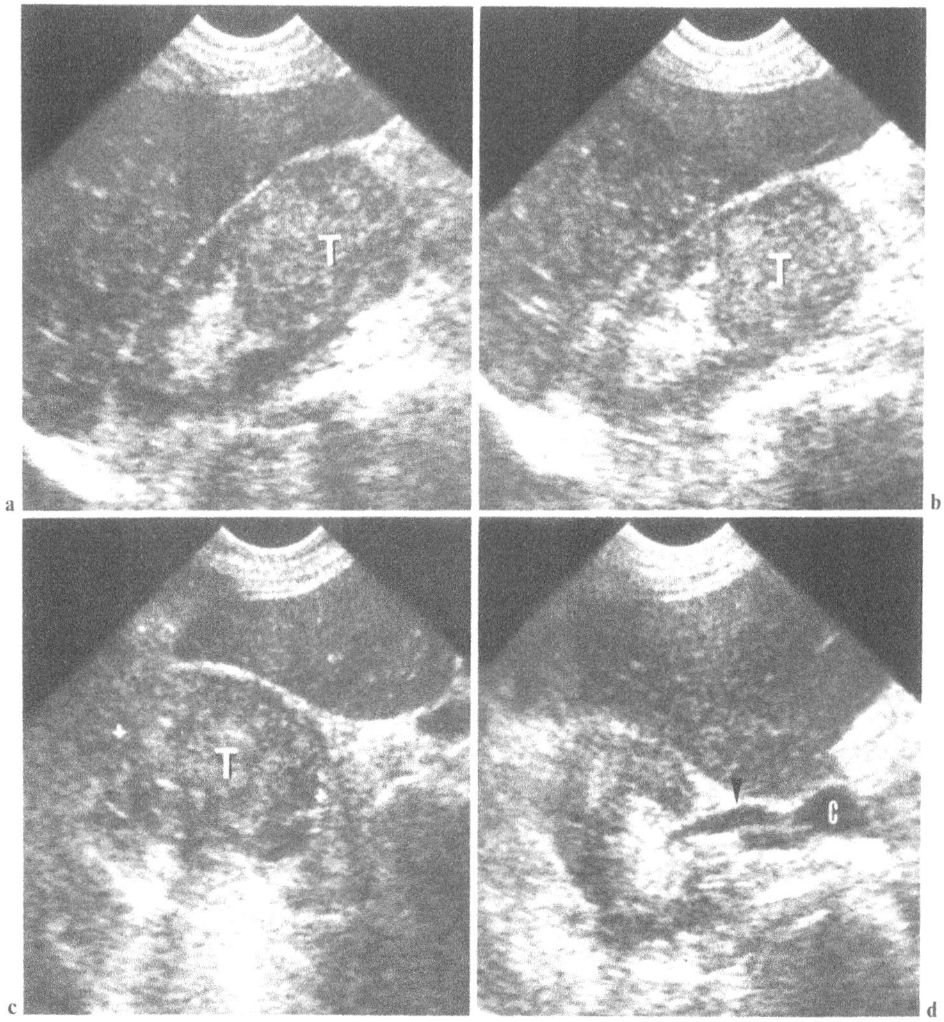

Fig. 5.10 a–d. Tumor of upper pole (*T*). **a, b** Two sagittal scans; **c** transverse scan of mass; **d** parallel scan, more caudal through renal vein (*arrowhead*) and cava (*c*). Note in **a** and **b**, impression of mass on central zone. Note also integrity of perirenal fat

pyelovascular central area and its intense, homogeneous reflectivity. Like the parenchyma, the central area has equal thickness along most of its longest axis (Fig. 1.2). That regular appearance is subject to specific changes in the case of marginal and of central tumors.

Marginal Tumors. The parenchymal thickness is increased at the level of the tumor, changing the ratio *parenchyma/central area*. This can be observed in the medial part of the kidney or at the level of the upper or lower pole (Figs. 5.7, 5.8 a, b). This abnormality is related to the classical observation of cortical index changes on conventional urograms. A related abnormality is the *impression of the tumoral nodule* on the limit of the pyelovascular central area (Figs. 5.5 b, 5.9, 5.10 a, b). This type of abnormality can be quite similar to the pattern of a columnar hypertrophy (Fig. 5.10 c, d; see also Fig. 1.8 d), not taking into account changes in echotexture.

Central Tumors. These develop inside the central area and press outward, broadening and distorting it (Figs. 5.11, 5.12). If the tumor is completely outlined by the limits of the central echogenic area, it possesses a regular pattern quite similar to that of a sinusal lipomatosis.

Tumor Contours

If the tumor bulges out of the renal cortex, its contours are usually well delineated. In fact, at least for a while, this sharp delineation is due to the permanence of echogenic perirenal fat (Figs. 5.5, 5.7 and 5.10). Sometimes the tumor bulges, coming into

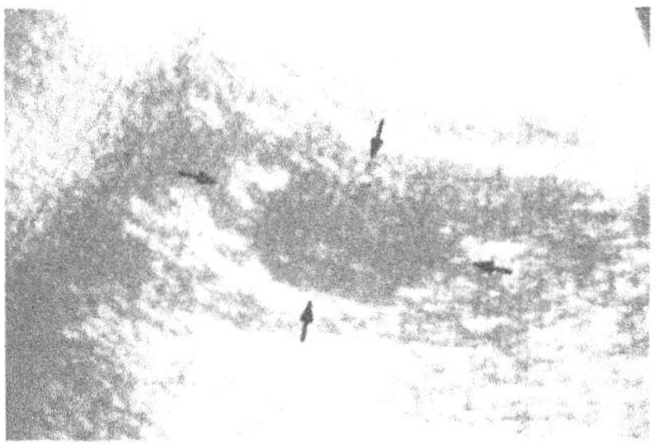

Fig. 5.11. Central, parapelvic renal cell carcinoma (*arrows*) developing inside central echogenic area

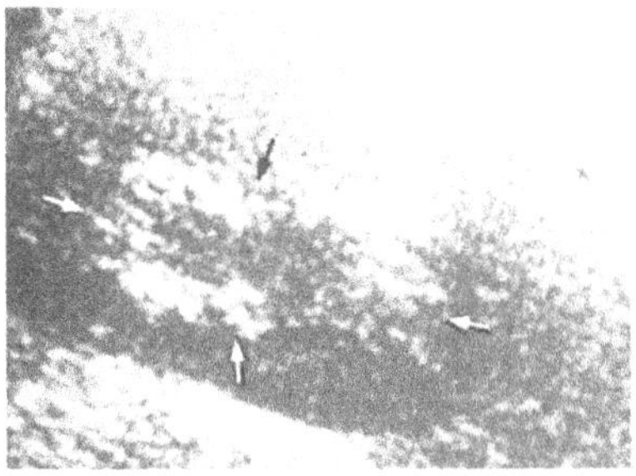

Fig. 5.12. Central tumor (*arrows*): urothelial tumor arising from renal pelvis

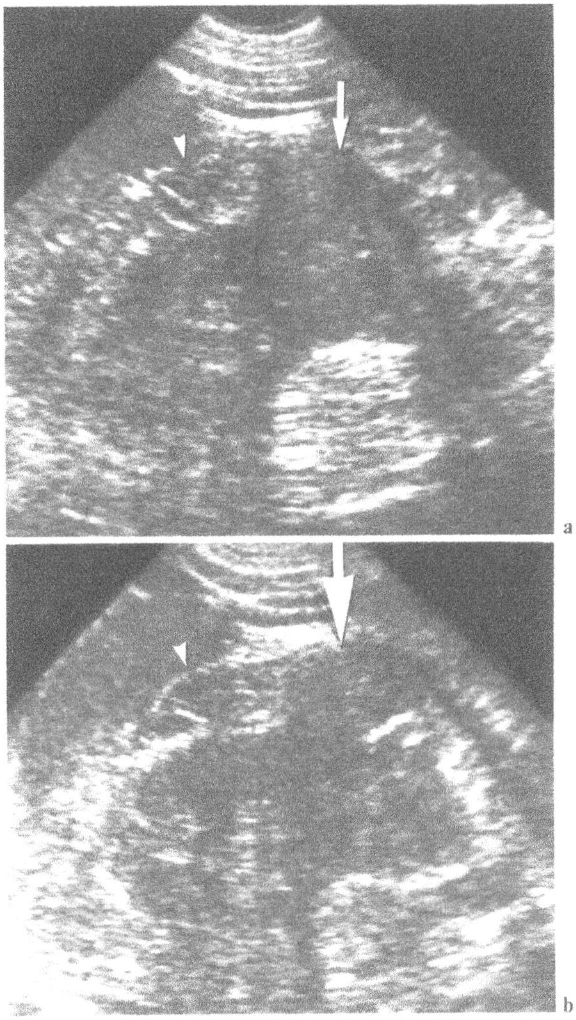

Fig. 5.13 a, b. Left lower pole carcinoma: two coronal scans. The tumor invades the perirenal fat (*arrow*) and comes into contact with the fascia (*arrowhead*)

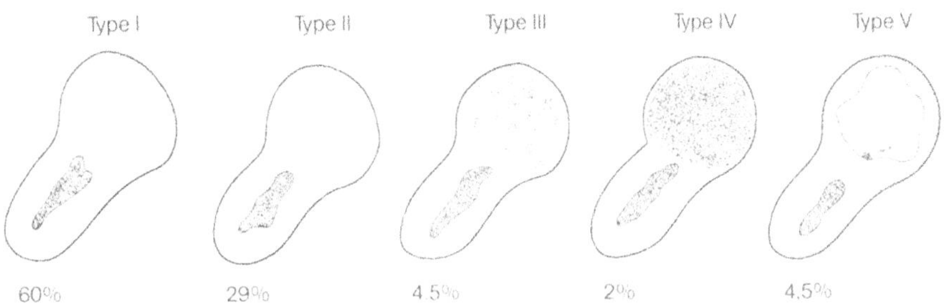

Fig. 5.14. Schematic representation of varying tumoral echotextures

contact with the perirenal fascia (Fig. 5.13). Once the tumor has expanded beyond the renal area the contours are much more difficult to assess (Fig. 5.1); we shall discuss this again later.

The delineation of the limits of intraparenchymal tumoral nodules also depends on the tumor's echotexture: strongly echogenic, homogeneous nodules possess a sharper boundary than heterogeneous nodules or sonolucent nodules (Fig. 5.10), whose only clear limit may be constituted by the central pyelovascular area (Figs. 5.9, 5.10), or by the perirenal fat.

Echopatterns of Tumors

We differentiate five types of tumoral echotexture (Fig. 5.14):

Type I: sonolucent, of the semisolid type (Figs. 5.6 and 5.15).

Type II: corresponding to the presence, in an echotexture of type I, of a few echogenic nodules (Figs. 5.7, 5.8 and 5.13).

Type III: heterogeneous, associating multiple echogenic areas and sonolucent (or sonotransparent) areas (Figs. 5.1 and 5.9). Calcified foci can induce acoustic shadows.

Type IV: containing areas of frank and diffuse echogenicity (Figs. 5.5b, 5.10, 5.18, 5.19).

Type V: necrotized tumors – to be dealt with later (see also Fig. 4.19).

A personal study (1980) of 45 cases, constituting a technically homogeneous series examined with the latest generation machines (but representing only a small part of our series of over 250 cases) showed the following distribution among the different types:

Type I	60%
Type II	29%
Type III	4.5%
Type IV	2%
Type V	4.5%

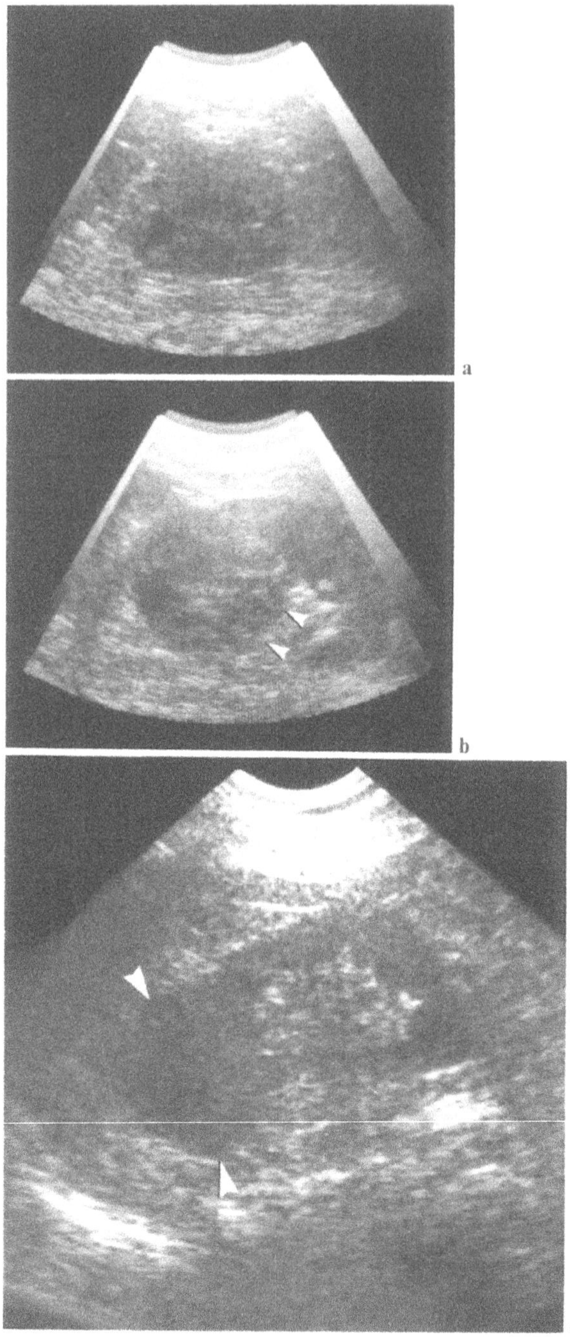

Fig. 5.15 a–c. Two carcinomas of the left upper pole. **a, b** First case: two intercostal scans. The mass is mostly sonotransparent, with few echogenic areas. It produces an impression on the central zone (*arrowheads*). **c** Another case: sonotransparent echotexture (*arrowheads*)

Necrotized Tumors

The advent of a necrotizing process in large tumors (over 6 cm in diameter, in our experience) brings about a liquid echopattern. Such a pseudocystic echopattern constitutes classically a major concern for the sonologist dealing with renal cystic images, owing to the risk of misinterpreting a malignant process as a benign lesion. In fact, the pattern of these rare necrotized lesions is quite different from that of simple cysts (Hill and Sanders 1978). Instead of being thin, with the same thickness every-

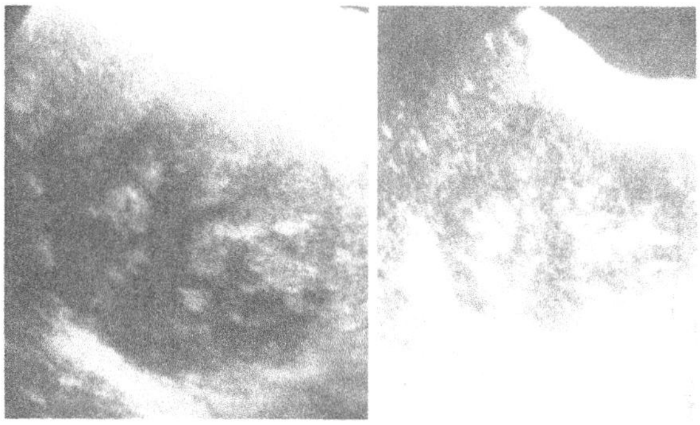

Fig. 5.16 a, b. Tumoral echotexture of type II: presence of a few echogenic nodules

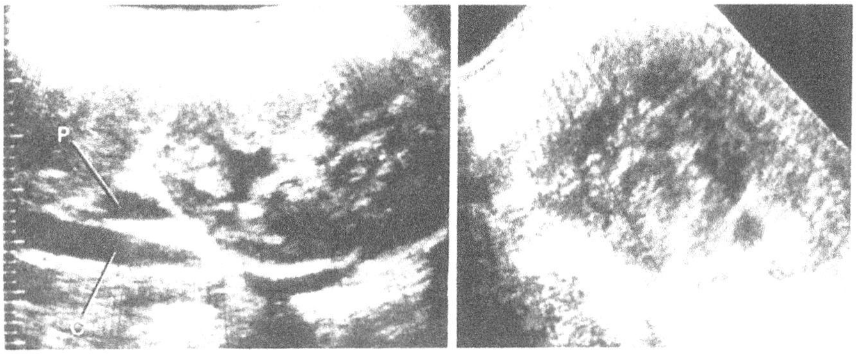

Fig. 5.17 a, b. Tumoral echotexture of type III: heterogeneous pattern with strongly reflective areas and sonolucent zones. Note, in **a,** compression of vena cava (*C*) and mesenteric-portal confluence (*P*)

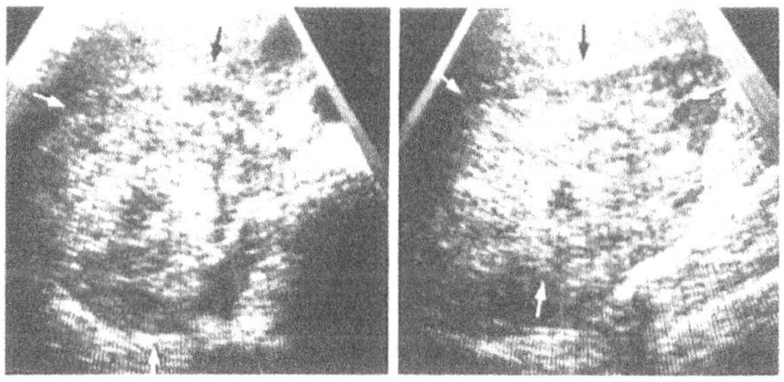

Fig. 5.18 a, b. Tumoral echotexture of type IV: presence of fields of diffuse reflectivity (*arrows,* tumor)

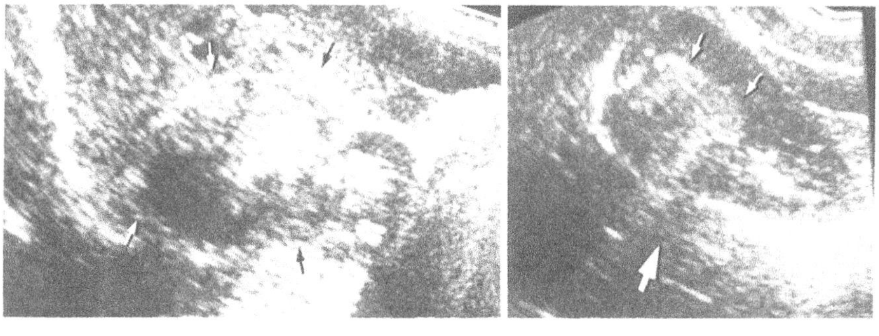

Fig. 5.19 a, b. Tumoral echotexture of type IV (*arrows,* tumor). Note, in **b,** acoustic shadow (*broad arrow*) due to tumoral calcification

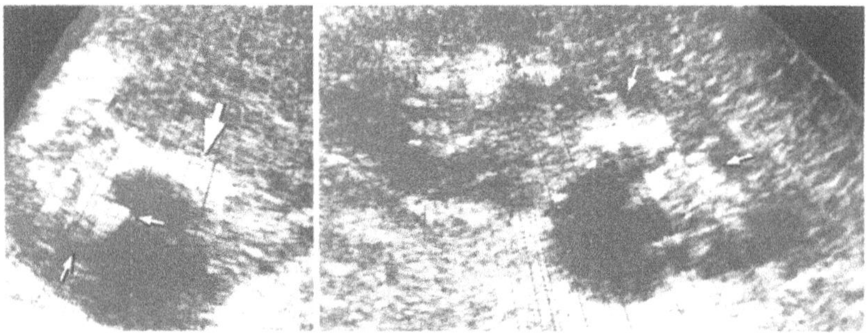

a b

Fig. 5.20 a, b. Echotexture of type V: necrotized tumor. **a** Oblique scan display area of sonolucency (*broad arrow*). Growth (*arrows*) bulges out of upper limit. **b** Sagittal scan in prone position also show thick and irregular wall (*arrows*). (Courtesy of M. Lafortune, Montréal)

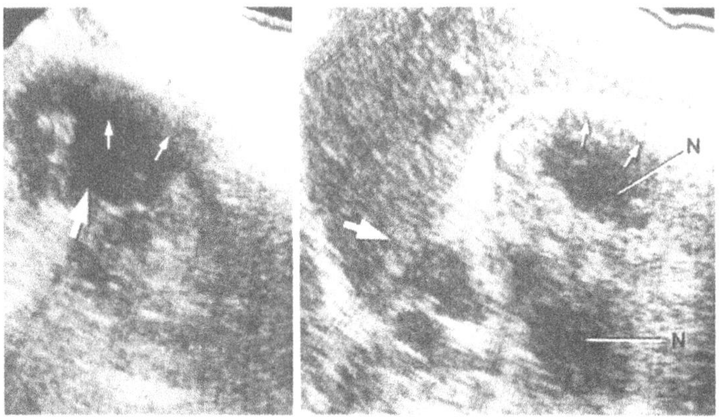

a b

Fig. 5.21 a, b. Echotexture of type V: necrotized tumors. **a** Area of sonolucency (*broad arrowhead*) occupies upper pole. Posterior wall delineation is irregular. Anterior wall is thick and blurred (*arrowheads*). **b** Another case. Two necrotized areas occupy upper half of the right kidney (*N*). Anterior wall of anterior necrotized zone is 1 cm thick (*arrows*). Sonolucent nodules indicate involvement of perirenal fat (*broad arrow*)

where, the "cystic wall" is several millimeters thick, while its thickness varies from place to place. The inner limit of the wall is irregular, or, at least, has lost its smoothness (Fig. 5.20), with rare exceptions. Lastly its contents are not really sonotransparent (Fig. 5.21), especially when a higher frequency is used. There may even be necrotic debris, either floating or dependent.

Only once have we observed a renal cell carcinoma of true cystic appearance. Its wall was a thin and smooth as that of a benign cyst, except in a small area. The contents were echogenic, since it was hemorrhagic (Fig. 5.22), as proven by puncture.

In large necrotized renal cell carcinomas, several cavities of necrosis may be encountered.

Necrotized tumors are one of the different kinds of atypical cysts we studied in Chap. 4; such cysts require puncture. Hemorrhagic content is sufficient evidence to suspect a tumoral process, even before a cytological study. CT scanning will then follow the puncture; it would be carried out anyway in order to evaluate the tumoral extension.

Other liquid patterns may accompany tumoral processes: hemorrhage arising from a renal mass, whether benign or malignant, can induce subcapsular hematomas – which are sometimes the first symptom of the disease (Barret et al. 1980).

Cystic Tumors

True cystic patterns are encountered exceptionally in renal cell carcinomas (Fig. 5.23). Cystic patterns are more common in cystadenocarcinomas. In that type of tumor some septations are thick, whereas solid tissue is displayed in some areas. Contrast-enhanced CT enables that particular pattern to be precisely analyzed.

Intracystic Carcinomas

In intracystic carcinomas, the cystic image is quite similar to that of a simple cyst, but multidirectional scans can show the presence of growths. The threshold of visibility for tumoral growths is about 4 mm (Figs. 5.24, 5.25). The puncture fluid may be free of blood but cytological studies are usually positive.

Pediculate Tumors

Exceptionally, a renal cell carcinoma may dramatically bulge out of the renal cortex, to which it eventually remains attached only by a pedicle (Fig. 5.26). In such cases, even multidirectional

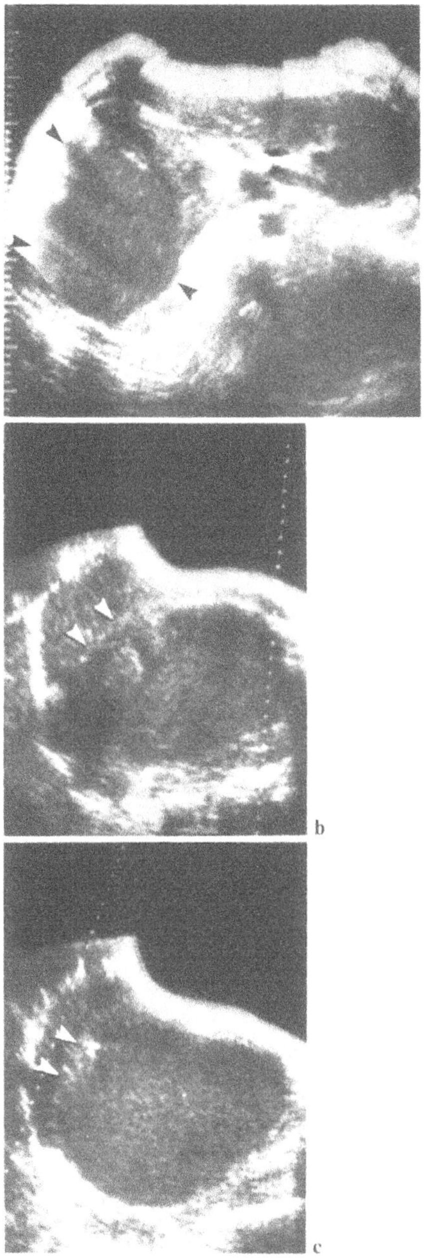

Fig. 5.22 a–c. Cystic carcinoma. **a** Transverse scan shows a large renal mass (*arrowheads*). **b, c** Sagittal scans: echotexture of mass is slightly echogenic, homogeneous, without attentuation, and corresponds to blood, as confirmed by puncture. The wall is thin, except at the upper pole of the mass (*arrowheads*)

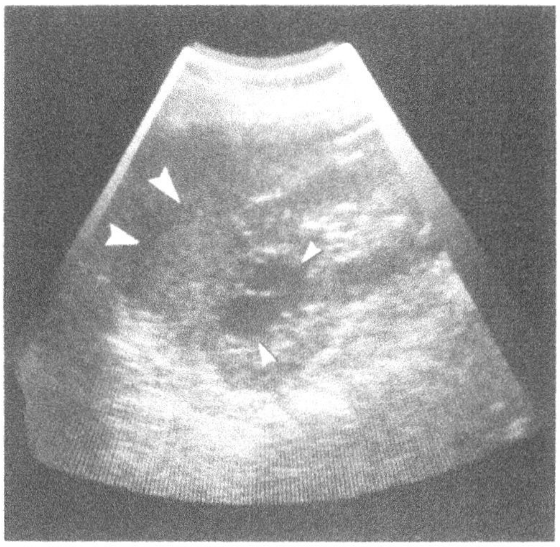

Fig. 5.23. Renal cell carcinoma (*arrowhead*) with cystic component (*small arrowhead*)

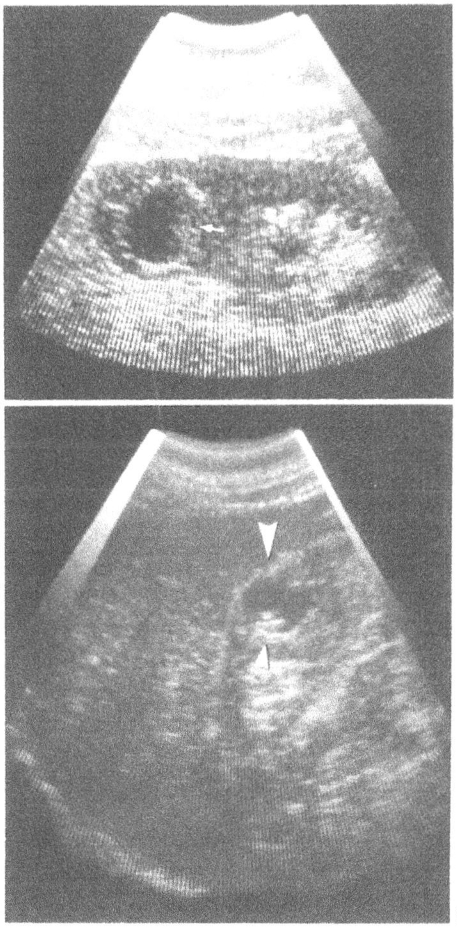

Fig. 5.24 a, b. Intracystic malignant tumors. **a** Elevation (*arrow*) in a cystic element with a thick wall (Courtesy of Dr. Petigny, Audincourt). **b** Elevation (*small arrowhead*) in small cyst. Note rather thick wall with small elevation on other side of cyst (*large arrowhead*)

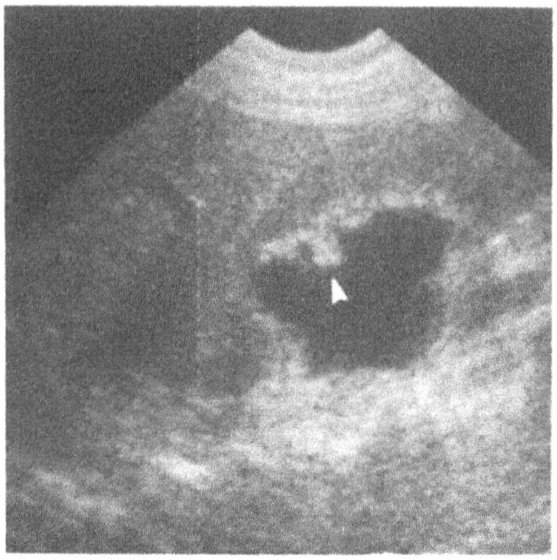

Fig. 5.25. Tumoral growth (*arrowhead*) in cystic renal cell carcinoma (atypical cyst)

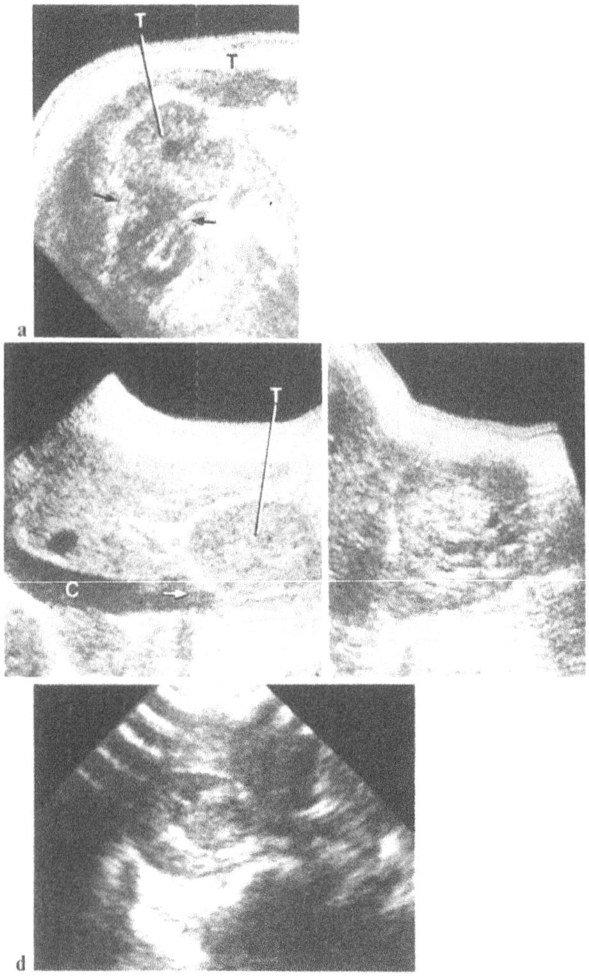

Fig. 5.26. a–c Pediculated renal cell carcinoma. **a** Transverse scan shows tumor (*T*) of type IV, connected to kidney by a narrow anterior pedicle (*arrows*). **b** Sagittal scan shows tumor (*T*) compressing (*arrow*) vena cava (*C*). **c** More external, parallel scan shows a more classical tumoral pattern. **d** Oncocytoma: heterogenous but well delineated intrarenal nodule (transverse scan of right kidney)

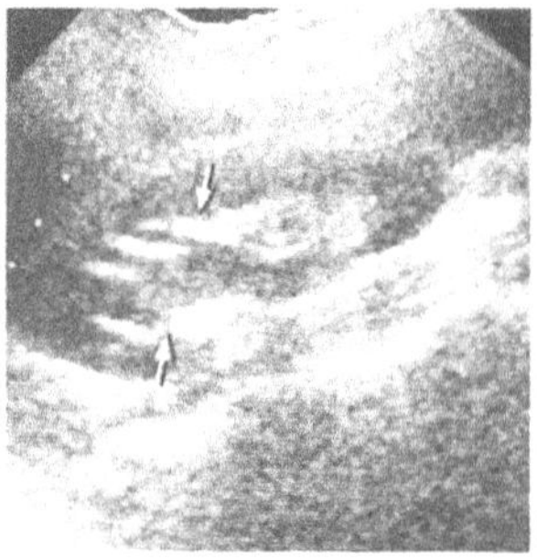

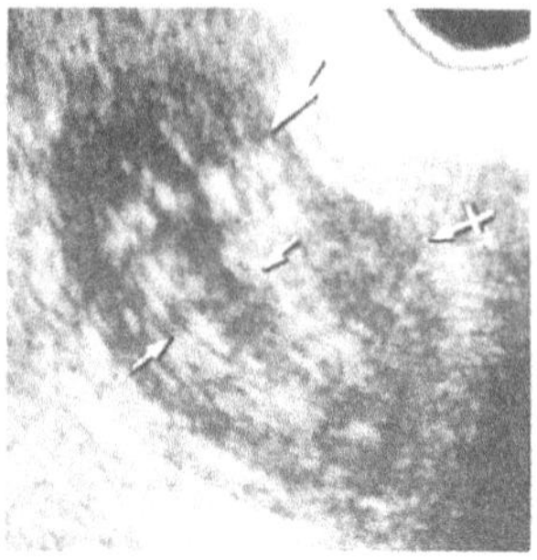

Fig. 5.27. Urothelial tumor. Area of moderate echogenicity (*arrows*) indicates tumoral spread inside the upper part of the echogenic central area. (Courtesy of M. Lafortune, Montréal)

Fig. 5.28. Pelvic urothelial tumor (*small arrows*). In fact, the echogenic nodule (*broad arrow*) and the cortical bulge (*crossed arrow*) indicate a wide spread beyond the pelvic limits

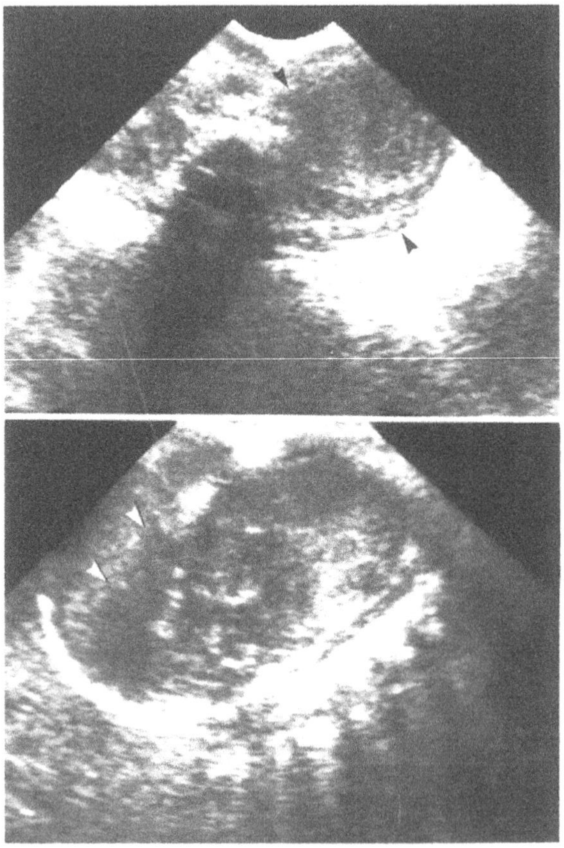

Fig. 5.29 a, b. Left nephroblastoma in a 5-year-old girl. **a** Transverse scan of a mass (*arrowhead*). **b** Sagittal scan. Note ill-defined contour of mass (*arrowhead*) close to liver

scans are likely to show the spleen (or liver), the kidney, and the mass as distinct entities. The final ultrasonic diagnosis is then liable to be falsely that of an independent retroperitoneal mass, arising from muscle, connective tissue, or nervous elements. CT scans will lead to similar conclusions, unless the pedicle itself is cut across. Even angiography can remain inconclusive in such cases. Of course the arterial opacification will show the tumoral network originating from branches of the renal artery; but, since ultrasound and CT showed an independent mass, the angiographic images will be interpreted in favor of a sarcoma arising from the perirenal connective tissue. We have encountered two renal cell carcinomas of this kind. Our diagnosis was that of an extrarenal sarcoma.

Bilateral Tumors

About 5% of renal cell carcinomas are bilateral: even if, in most cases, the occurrence of the tumor is not simultaneous, discovery of a renal tumor does not mean a careful contralateral examination can be dispensed with.

Tumors with subcapsular hematoma: as stated above, rarely, the initial manifestation of a renal tumor is a spontaneous subcapsular hematoma.

Oncocytomas

Often listed among benign renal tumors, oncocytomas are now considered as belonging to the group of renal cell carcinomas, but without generalized malignant potential. They represent about 5% of such tumors; they are usually well delineated, even capsulated (Gorney et al. 1984) (Fig. 5.26 d). They display often a central, scar-like pattern, echogenic on ultrasound scans, hyperdense on CT scans, of specific value (Quinn et al. 1984).

Urothelial Carcinomas

Pelvic

At an early stage, pelvic urothelial tumors appear as intrapelvic growths (Maklad et al. 1977), provided there is sufficient pelvic dilatation to give ultrasonic contrast between the urine and tumoral polyps. We personally have never encountered such images. The tumor will later occupy the entire pelvic cavity, creating a zone of heterogeneity amid the central pyelovascular reflectivity (Fig. 5.27) (Anger et al. 1979). As we said above, sinus lipomatosis can mimic a pelvic tumor.

Intrapelvic growths are particularly well visualized on contrast-enhanced CT sections. After IVP, CT should be performed as the first procedure whenever an intrapelvic urothelial tumor is suspected.

Basically infiltrating, urothelial tumors extend along the calices toward the medulla. They then give rise to areas of reflectivity, contrasting with the dilated infundibula. Reflective areas were predominant in the four cases of diffuse tumors we encountered (Fig. 5.28).

Caliceal

Urothelial caliceal tumors possess the same echopattern as renal cell carcinomas.

Wilms' Tumors and Mesoblastic Nephromas

These tumors, encountered mostly in children, are usually already large when discovered. Their echotexture has been reported as mostly sonolucent, with areas of cystic necrosis (Goldberg et al. 1975 a, b; Gates and Miller 1977). In our experience the echotexture in Wilms' tumors is variable and can correspond to any of the types described under renal cell carcinoma (Figs. 5.29, 5.30). Necrotized cavities, unique or multiple, are possible, as are also bilateral Wilms' tumors.

On the right side, the limits between a large Wilms' tumor and the liver can be poorly delineated. If the tumoral pattern is multifocal (Type III), a false diagnosis of hepatic metastatic nodules is possible (Figs. 5.30, 5.31). Wilms' tumors can arise in horseshoe kidneys (Gay et al. 1983). The pathology of renal tumors is complex: some tumors related to Wilm's tumors are not malignant or have attenuated malignancy.

Mesoblastic nephromas are benign tumors which can reach a large size, with features very similar to those of a Wilms' tumor. Large renal tumors diagnosed before the age of 1 year are usually mesoblastic nephromas (Hartman et al. 1981).

We already mentioned when considering cystic processes (Chap. 4) the relationship existing between Wilms' tumors and multilocular cysts (also termed multilocular cystic nephroma, cystic adenoma benign nephroblastoma, Perlman's tumor). Those cystic tumors are well capsulated (see Figs. 4.21 c, d). Their pattern is less specific when the cysts are smaller and less numerous. The tumor

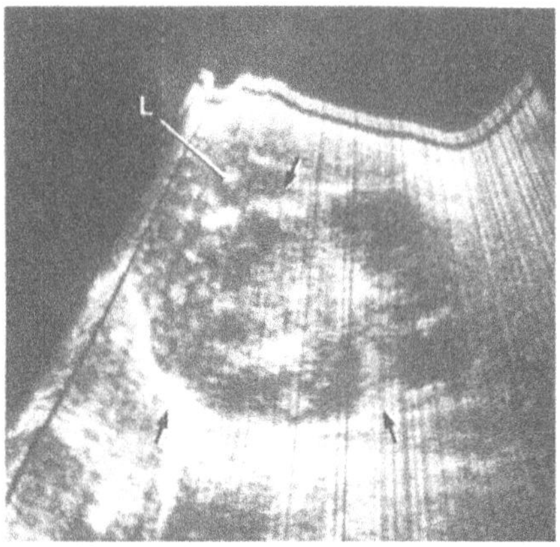

Fig. 5.30. Wilms' tumor in a 5-year-old child. Section of the huge mass (*arrows*) is larger than the liver section (*L*). Echotexture is of type III, with sonolucent areas suggesting necrosis. The cleavage place between the liver and the mass remains delineated

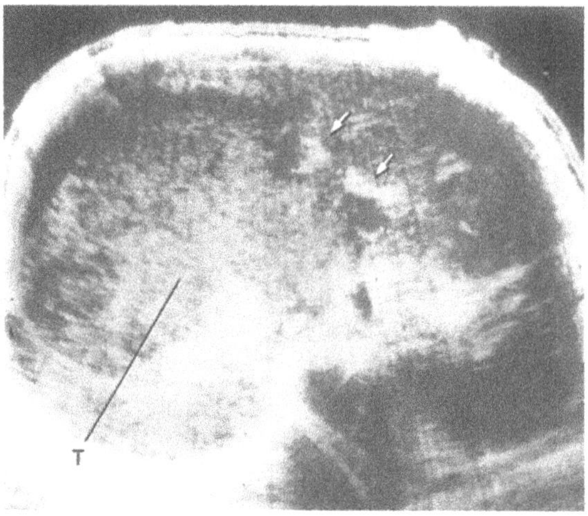

Fig. 5.31. Wilms' tumor in a 14-year-old child. Transverse scan: echotexture of the mass is of type IV. No delineation exists between the renal tumor (*T*) and the liver. Hepatic or renal situation of nodules (*arrows*) is difficult to evaluate. Note enlargement of left lobe of liver

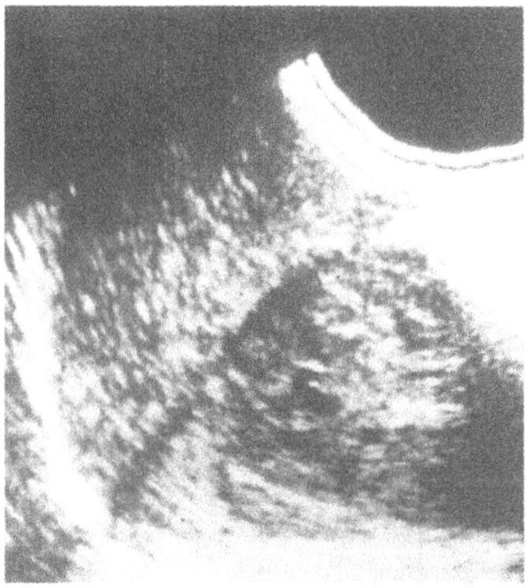

is usually benign but local recurrences and metastases have been reported (BAMER et al. 1983; MADENWELL et al. 1983). Benign and malignant foci can coexist within the same tumoral mass. Thus the complexity of the histology has brought us back to the field of benign tumors while studying malignant tumors. But we still have to examine a few other processes.

Renal Sarcomas

Our experience of renal sarcomas is too limited to permit a description of their ultrasonic pattern. To our knowledge there is no such description in the literature.

Renal Metastases

Renal metastases give rise to changes in the size, shape, and contours of the kidney quite similar to those due to primary tumors. Diffuse infiltration with nephromegaly, as in lymphomas, is also encountered. The echotexture of metastases (Figs. 5.33, 5.34) is variable. As in the field of liver metastases, we would not attempt to propose a histological correlation. The occurrence of bilateral renal cell carcinomas is sometimes discussed since the second tumor could correspond to a metastasis. But there exist true cases of bilateral tumors, with different histological patterns.

Nonfunctioning Kidney

Tumors are responsible for about 5% of nonfunctioning kidneys, by diffuse parenchymal infiltration, by vascular involvement, or by an obstruction of the collecting system. This is the case with renal cell carcinomas as well as with urothelial tumors. The ultrasonic patterns depicted above will enable an etiological diagnosis to be made.

Renal Lymphomas

Multinodular lymphomatous localizations will be studied in Chap. 8. Most lymphomatous infiltrations give rise to localized sonolucent swellings (Fig. 5.35) similar to those arising from other tumoral processes. Diffuse infiltration, with nephromegaly, is also possible.

◂ **Fig. 5.32.** Follow-up after radiotherapy: tumoral volume has decreased. Sharp delineation exists again (sagittal scan). Note shadowing due to sound-bending

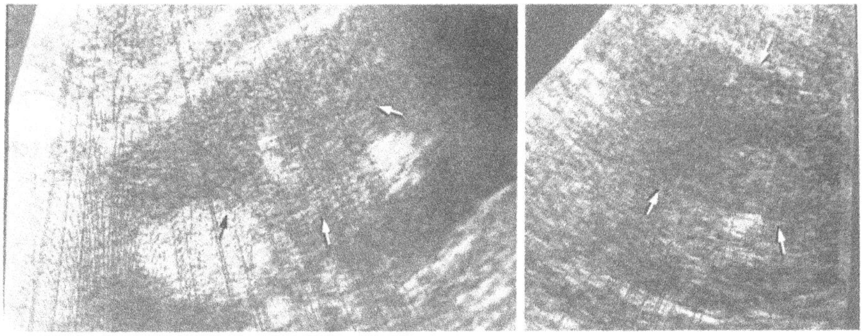

a b

Fig. 5.33 a, b. Renal metastasis (breast carcinoma). **a** Sagittal scan: isoreflective nodule (*arrows*) broadens posterior parenchyma and dislocates echogenic central area. **b** Transverse scan. (Courtesy of M. Lafortune, Montréal)

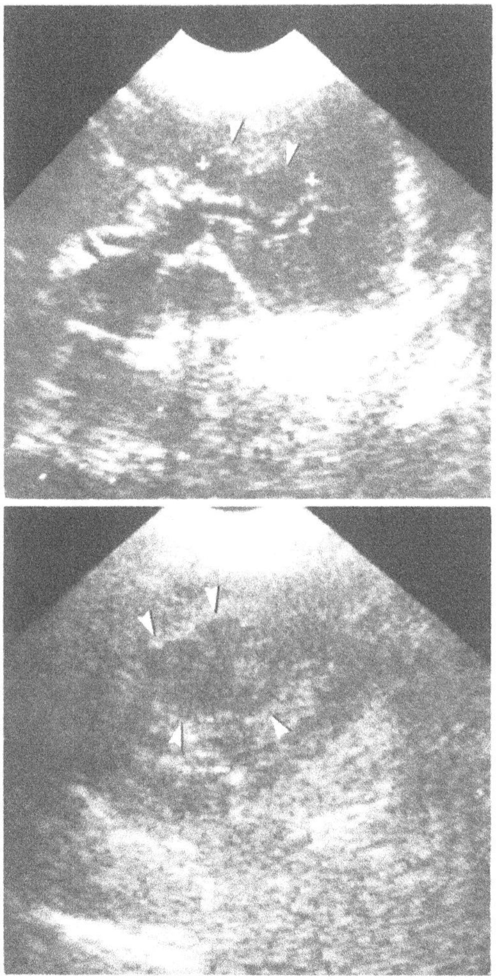

a b

Fig. 5.34 a, b. Metastases of an osteosarcoma. **a** Double nodule (*arrowheads*) in the left lobe of the liver; **b** mass (*arrowheads*) in the left kidney

Diagnosis

Histology

It can be concluded from what has been said that no echotexture study, however thorough, can permit a histological diagnosis. The latter is to be found at the tip of the puncture needle. The puncture of malignant tumors is advocated by the Danish school (Rasmussen, Holm). Their opinion triggers stress and horror in French surgeons, and also, no doubt, in many of their colleagues in other countries. Puncture should nevertheless become a normal step of the diagnosis, at least when ultrasound (and CT) has shown such an extension that no surgical therapy can be endeavored. A cytological or histological diagnosis achieved by means of guided puncture will then allow one to proceed to embolization, radiotherapy, and chemotherapy, without a fruitless surgical operation. Puncture is also invaluable in the case of masses for which the diagnosis of inflammatory process is considered (focal bacterial nephritis, xanthogranulomatous pyelonephritis; see Chap. 7). In focal bacterial nephritis, for instance, no surgery is required.

Relations with Neighboring Tissues

In the next chapter we shall study evaluation of the extension of malignant tumors. But we wish to underscore two points at this stage: The first is the ill-defined character of the limits of some large tumors: the differentiation between hepatic, adrenal, and renal tumors is then difficult (Figs. 5.8, 5.31, 5.32). CT is usually conclusive; selective angiography is only rarely required. The second is the importance of a kinetic study of the kidney during the respiratory cycle. The amplitude of the respiratory displacements of the kidney is easy to display in real time. A loss of mobility suggests spread of the tumor beyond the renal area.

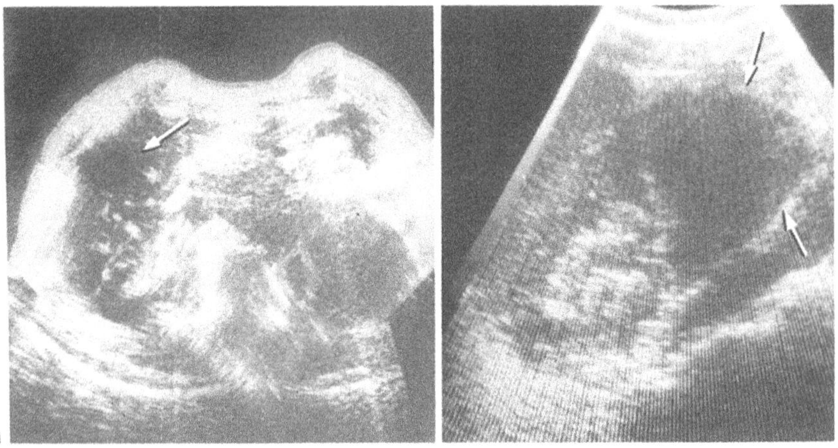

a b

Fig. 5.35 a, b. Renal deposit of lymphoblastosarcoma. **a** Transverse scan shows sonolucent hepatic nodule (*arrow*). The left kidney (*arrowhead*) is enlarged. **b** Intercostal section of left kidney. Lower pole is swollen and sonolucent. Lower part of the central area has disappeared

5.2 Benign Tumors

We shall not involve ourselves in the discussion, still open, about the histological particularities of benign tumors (Table 5.1). Thanks to studies by DUFFY et al. (1977) and LEE et al. (1978) the echopattern of benign tumors has been well clarified. More recently, *angiomyolipomas* have been studied by BOSNIAK (1981), HARTMAN (1981), and KRATZ (1981).

Changes in renal shape and size are not specific in benign tumors. What is more specific is their shape, usually rounded, and their echotexture. Probably because of their rich vascularization, and mainly, because of their fatty contents, they are strongly echogenic. Ultrasonic scans usually show circular areas (Figs. 5.36, 5.37), rather well delineated, or larger fields of reflection (Fig. 5.38). We saw above that this kind of echopattern (type IV) is encountered in only 4% of renal cell carcinomas:

Table 5.1. Classification of benign renal tumors according to GOUYGEN et al. 1976

Epithelial tumors: adenomas	
Non-epithelial tumors	• *with one kind of tissue only*
	lymphoangioma
	hemangioma
	fibroma
	biomyoma
	hemangiopericytoma
	• *with several kind of tissue*
	embryonic
	teratoma
	tumoral dysplasia
	angiomyolipoma
	multiocular cyst
	cystadenoma
	hamartoma

in the presence of a strongly echogenic mass, a benign tumor must be considered, and, in first place, an angiomyolipoma. For once, histological confirmation is available without a microscope, thanks to density evaluation on CT scans (HANSEN et al. 1978): the presence of fat is very specific for these tumors. This diagnosis is important since it can lead to a partial, instead of a total, nephrectomy – or even to no surgery at all.

Angiomyolipomas can be multiple (Fig. 5.37). We once encountered an ultrasonic pseudoimage of angiomyolipoma which, according to CT, merely corresponded to the extension of perirenal fat within a cortical depression (Fig. 5.39). The appearance of angiomyolipomas of the adrenal is similar to that of such tumors arising from the renal upper poles: the fatty cleavage plane which often enables one to recognize the suprarenal location of a mass is ill defined. Exceptionally angiomyolipomas can have a sonotransparent echotexture (Fig. 5.40), without any specificity.

Adenomas usually appear as rounded masses, with an echogenic pattern (Fig. 5.41), but CT does not display fatty contents. CT will also make it possible to consider, if not to confirm, a diagnosis of renal *hemangioma*. Rarely, a cystic or multicystic pattern is also encountered. Such patterns lack specificity regarding the benign tumor's precise nature: benign cystic cystadenoma, cystic hamartoma, multilocular cyst – a variety of tumoral processes which we studied already above. Careful multidirectional studies can display associated solid areas or intracystic growths. CT will contribute to the morphological analysis. But only puncture and cytological studies are able to lead to a precise diagnosis. However, the final diagnostic management is rather simple: the most important step is to separate angiomyolipomas, which never degenerate, from other so-called benign tumors, which can have a malignant potential. Removal of adenomas, for instance, is mandatory, whereas angiomyolipoma are not necessarily operated on. On the other hand, the precise histological diagnosis between malignant and less malignant processes (with the exception of angiomyolipoma) requires a detailed pathologic analysis – often surgery. Thus, all non-fatty tumors will be removed.

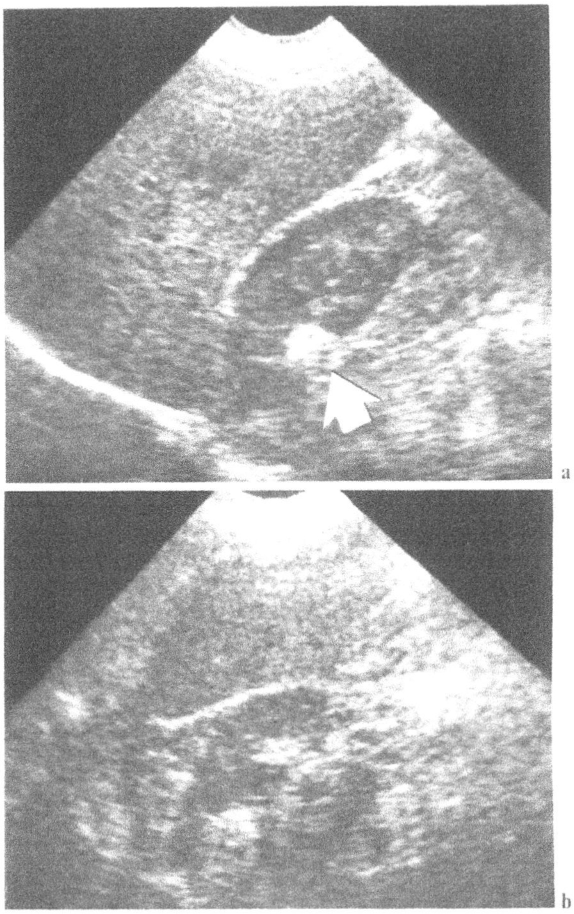

Fig. 5.36 a, b. Angiomyolipoma (*arrow*). **a** Sagittal scan shows an echogenic nodule, **b** transverse scan

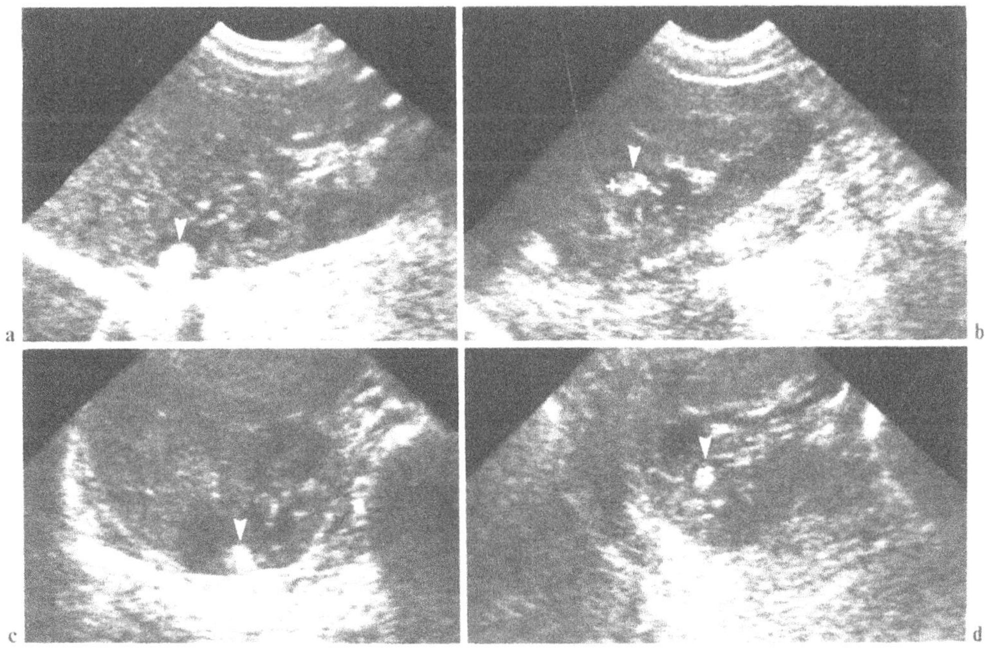

Fig. 5.37 a–d. Multiple small angiomyolipomas in right kidney. The left kidney was removed because of a large angiomyolipoma. **a** Sagittal scan: nodule in upper pole (*arrowhead*); **b** coronal scan: another nodule (*arrowhead*); **c, d** transverse scans

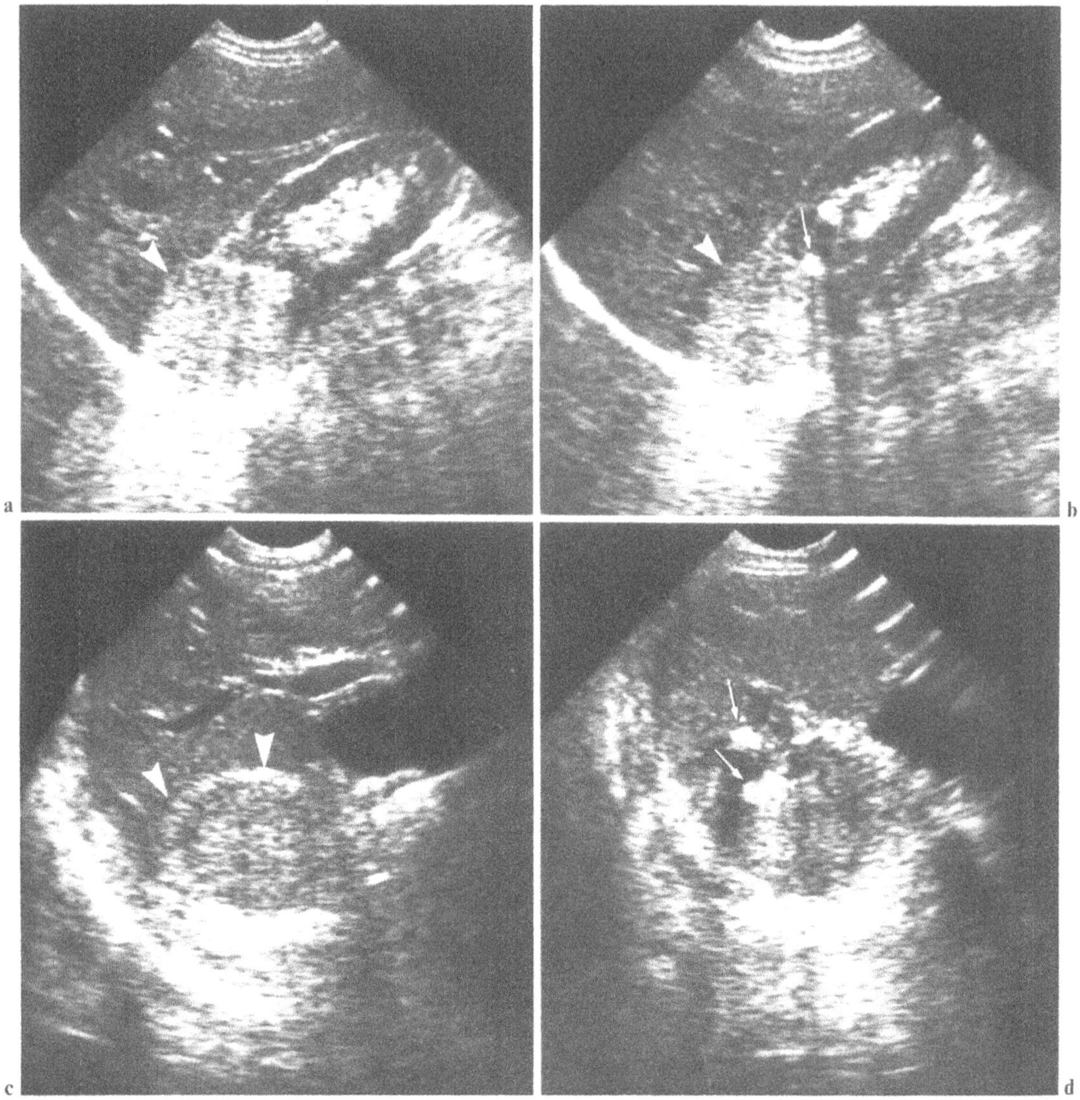

Fig. 5.38 a–d. Angiomyolipoma (*arrowheads*). **a, b** Two sagittal scans; **c, d** two transverse scans. Note associated lithiasis in **b** and **d** (*arrows*)

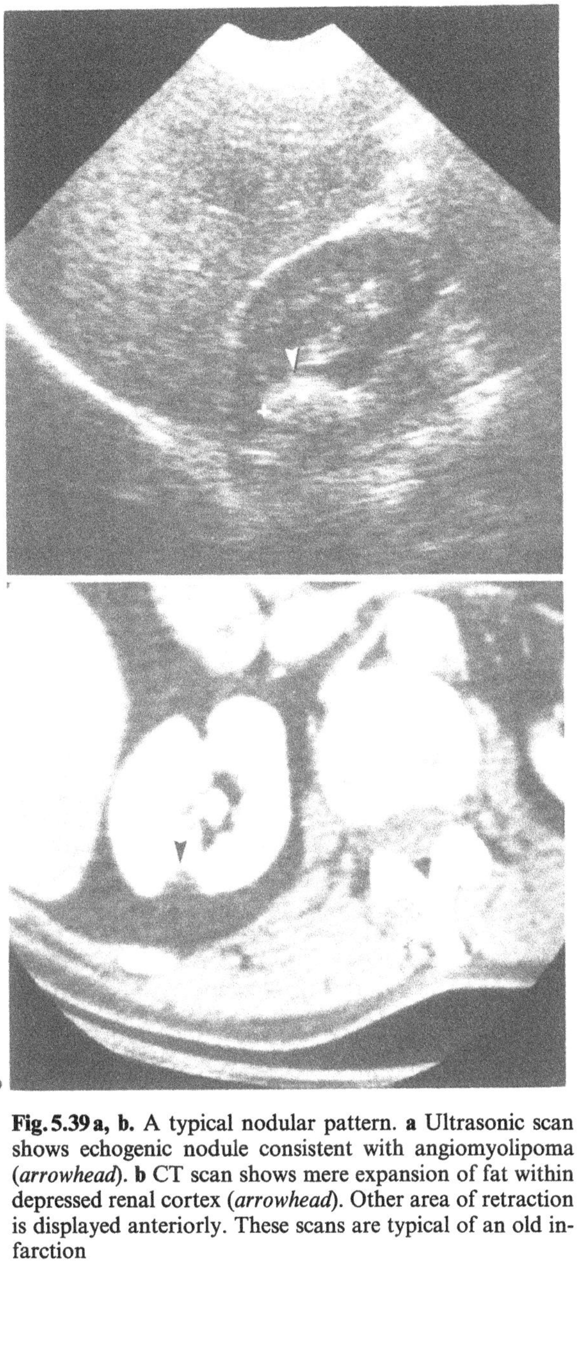

Fig. 5.39 a, b. A typical nodular pattern. **a** Ultrasonic scan shows echogenic nodule consistent with angiomyolipoma (*arrowhead*). **b** CT scan shows mere expansion of fat within depressed renal cortex (*arrowhead*). Other area of retraction is displayed anteriorly. These scans are typical of an old infarction

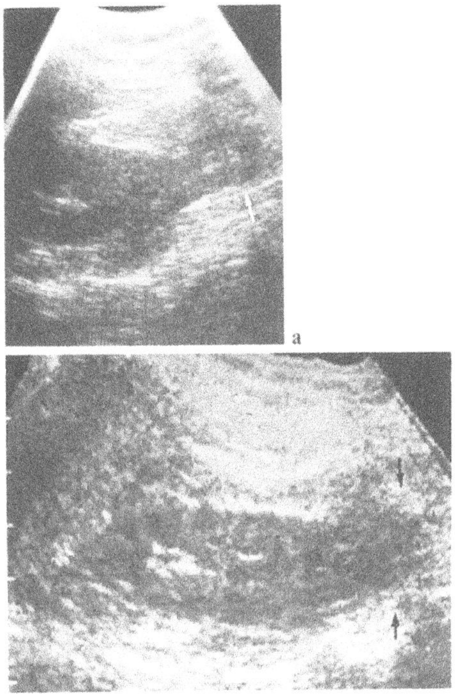

Fig. 5.40 a, b. Angiomyolipoma: unusual sonolucent pattern of pediculated tumor of lower pole (*arrow*). **a** Intercostal scan; **b** sagittal scan

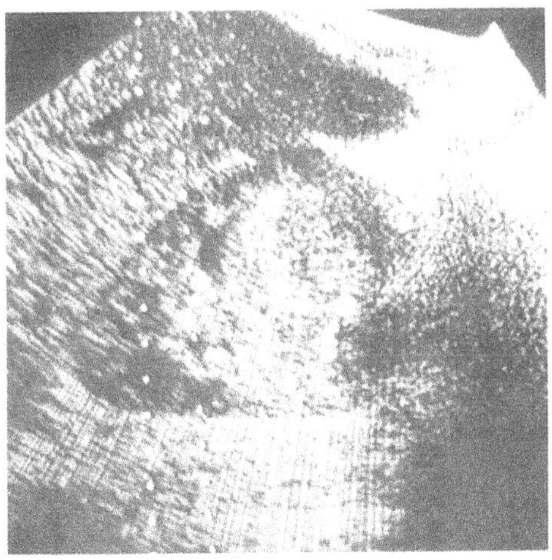

Fig. 5.41. Pattern similar to that in Fig. 5.38 in large adenoma (*arrow*). (Courtesy of M. Lafortune, Montréal)

5.3 Differential Diagnosis

Large Tumors (Over 10 cm in Diameter)

As we pointed out above in connection with large cysts and multilocular masses, the larger a tumor, the more difficult its origin is to establish. A mass in one of the upper quadrants, once its growth is sufficient to bring the mass and the abdominal walls into contact, can show the same pattern whether renal, hepatic, or splenic. Other intra- or retroperitoneal masses must also be considered (Figs. 5.42, 5.44).

It is possible to identify a mass as nonrenal once the image of the kidney itself is displayed, even deformed or flattened (Fig. 5.42). The possibility of exceptional pediculate renal tumors must nevertheless be kept in mind. As stated before, right masses, originating apparently from the kidney, may lack a line of separation from the liver: the diagnosis of a renal tumor then has to be weighed against that of a hepatic tumor. The same problem arises with adrenal tumors (see Chap. 11).

As seen from the last figures in this chapter, the old technique of manual scanning can be useful in the study of large masses, since the surface of their section extends beyond the field covered by real time machines. When dealing with large masses, CT is instrumental for a precise delineation. Angiography can be considered in order to study the anatomical origin of the tumoral blood supply.

Medium-Sized Tumors (4–10 cm in Diameter)

Medium-sized tumors are the easiest to evaluate. They do not usually bring about any problem of differential diagnosis – except for a few inflammatory processes, e.g., focal bacterial nephritis, which we shall study later. In any case, complementary procedures are necessary in order to assess the tumoral spread: they will also correct possible, but rare, diagnostic errors.

We have already discussed the diagnosis of necrotized tumors in connection with cysts (see Chap. 4). Cystic tumors have also been discussed above.

Small Tumors (Under 4 cm in Diameter)

Inflammatory processes are again one of the diagnostic possibilities to be discussed (see Chaps. 4, 7). But one of the first candidates for discussion must be a *pseudotumor*. Hypertrophy of the sinus margin and nonpathological cortical humps (see Chap. 1) give rather specific ultrasonic patterns. Regeneration nodules encountered in chronic pyelonephritis are usually accompanied by cortical atrophy, with local indentations. When such deformities are absent, a correct diagnosis is impossible without complementary procedures (see Fig. 5.45). Abnormal lobulation, or columnar hypertrophy are readily recognized.

Sonotransparent areas within the central zone can correspond to urothelial tumors and sinusal lipomatoses; echogenic foci within the pelvic lumen are urothelial tumors, blood clots, pus, and shadowfree lithiasis (exceptional). Such abnormalities are studied in detail by CT. The diagnosis of urothelial tumors are summarized in Table 5.2.

Table 5.2. Differential diagnosis of urothelial tumors

Central sonotransparent areas
urothelial tumors
sinusal lipomatosis
columnar hypertrophy
Intrapelvic echogenic foci
urothelial tumors
blood clots
pus
shadow-free calculi

In Chap. 9 we shall study in a synoptic way the differential diagnosis of renal masses. In any case, as we have seen, the diagnostic management is very stereotyped. After a primary ultrasonic diagnosis, it relies, if necessary, sometimes on IVU, mostly on CT scans, often on puncture, less often on angiograms. In fact, careful ultrasonic evaluation of small deformities and small masses is likely to lead to false-positive diagnoses rather than false-negative ones. In this context we advocate a military attitude. According to traditional military wisdom, the private wandering across the barracks yard is instructed thus: "If it doesn't move, sweep it or whitewash it. If it moves, salute it." Well our advice in the presence of a renal abnormal image which does not correspond, without any doubt, to a benign process is to use a CT broom, sometimes an angiographic brush, and to salute it with a needle. In most institutions, the diagnosis of renal tumors relies on the association of ultrasound with CT. Since CT permits one to check the contralateral renal function, IVU is often not carried out. Angiography is performed more in order to permit embolization rather than for diagnosis. Preoperative arterial topography can be demonstrated by intravenous digitized angiography.

Reliability

Several statistical studies have shown a rate of successful diagnosis of 96%–98% (PLAINFOSSE et al. 1980). Our own success rate in 1974, before the use of gray scale, was 89% (Table 5.3).

These different statistical results make it possible, in our opinion, to answer the question: Is sonography a reliable screening procedure for renal tumors? The answer is definitely yes, except for urothelial pelvic tumors. Multidirectional high-resolution scanning makes it possible to establish the normality of the renal parenchyma; the only risk is that of a few false-positive diagnoses, demanding complementary procedures, e.g., in the presence of a pseudotumor, as a columnar hypertrophy.

Table 5.3. Reliability of sonography in 133 masses (cysts excepted: see also Table 4.3, p. 70)

Successful diagnosis of cancer	119	
False-negative	1	(pseudocystic tumor)
False-positive	3	(cysts with hemorrhage)
"False" false-positive	10	

We term "false" false-positive inflammatory masses or columnar hypertrophy, considered as probably benign, but evaluated by complementary procedures as possible malignant masses

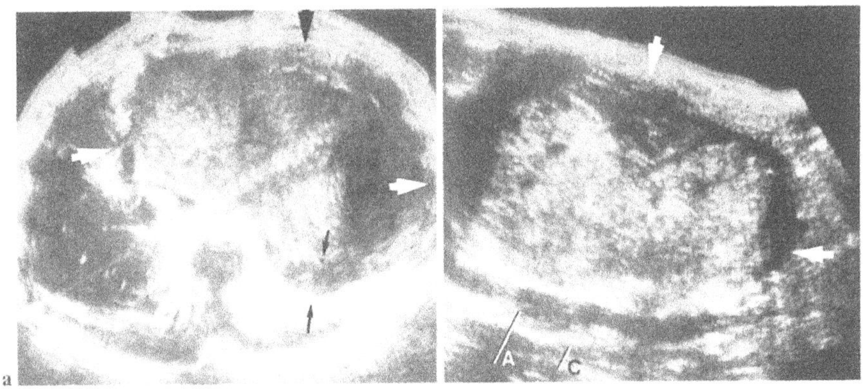

Fig. 5.42 a, b. Huge mass of the left upper quadrant (*broad arrows*). **a** Transverse scan: relation of the mass to the liver could lead to consideration of hepatoma. The left kidney (*small arrows*) is flattened. There is a cleavage plane between the mass and the kidney. **b** Coronal scan (left axillary scanning). Note the aorta (*A*) and vena cava (*C*). Angiography and surgery finally showed a retroperitoneal malignant mesenchymoma, arising from the perirenal tissues

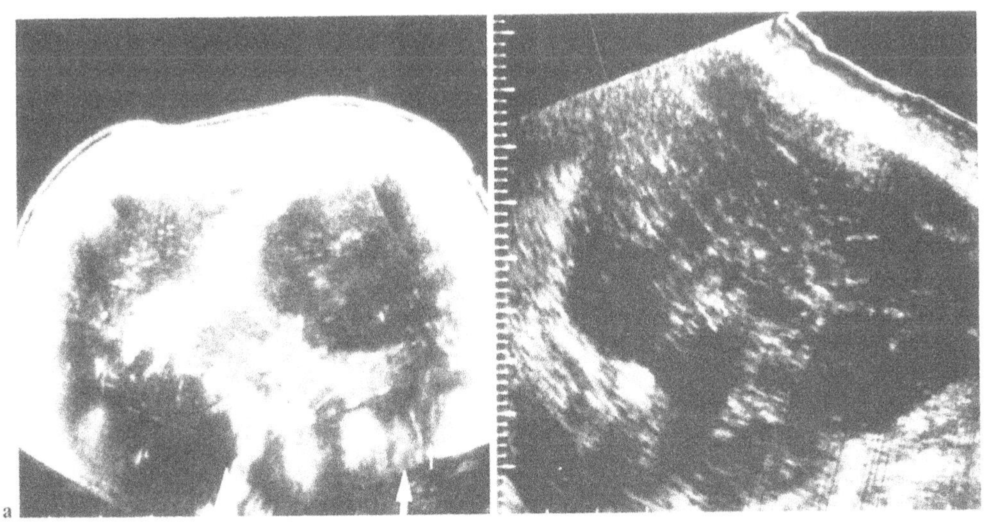

Fig. 5.43 a, b. Retroperitoneal nonrenal tumor. **a** Transverse scan. There are masses in the right lumbar fossa and the left upper quadrant. The left kidney (*broad arrow*) and spleen (*small arrow*) are distinct from the left mass: the other scan showed the right mass to be distinct from the right kidney. **b** Sagittal scan of the left mass. The final diagnosis was double localization of rhabdomyosarcoma

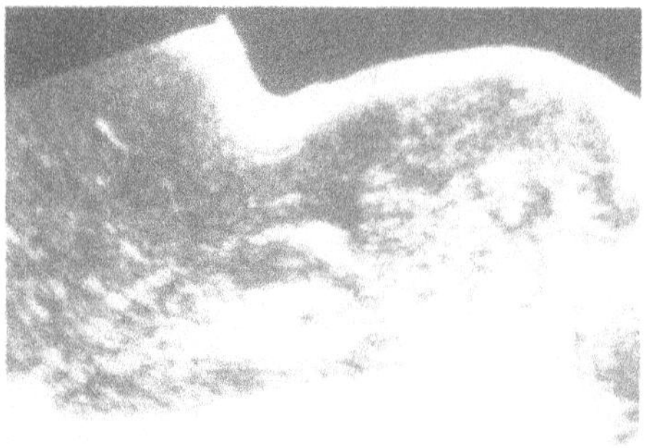

Fig. 5.44. Juxtarenal mass. Delineation of the mass from the kidney is sharp, thanks to the echogenicity of intact perirenal fat. The mass is hepatic (hepatocarcinoma)

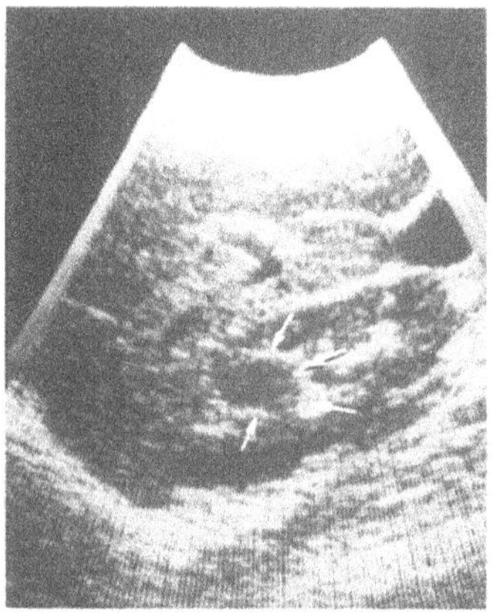

Fig. 5.45. Pseudotumor due to chronic pyelonephritis. The patient complained of pain thought to be of biliary origin. Intercostal scan of the right kidney shows a well-delineated nodule. Since the renal contours were smooth, chronic pyelonephritis was not considered. The nodule was thought to be tumoral. Surgery led to the correct diagnosis

6 Evaluation of Tumoral Spread: The Retroperitoneal Space

Once the diagnosis of a malignant renal tumor has been made, the tumor's spread must be evaluated. This demands the assessment of direct spread across the perirenal tissues, of lymphatic and venous spread in the retroperitoneal space, and of hematogenous spread, particularly to the liver.

The evaluation of the spread of renal tumors is also based on CT. However, after the ultrasonic diagnosis of tumor, a thorough ultrasonic evaluation of the tumoral extension can give reliable results particularly on sagittal sections, whereas CT only yields transverse scans.

6.1 Direct Spread

We have already mentioned, in Chap. 5, two signs of local extension:

1. Disappearance of the perirenal fat image, the reflective layer becoming thinner and distorted, before being directly involved (Figs. 5.13, 6.1)
2. Disappearance of the kidney's respiratory mobility

But with ultrasound it is very difficult to demonstrate an involvement of the paraspinal muscles, whereas this kind of abnormality is readily disclosed by CT scans.

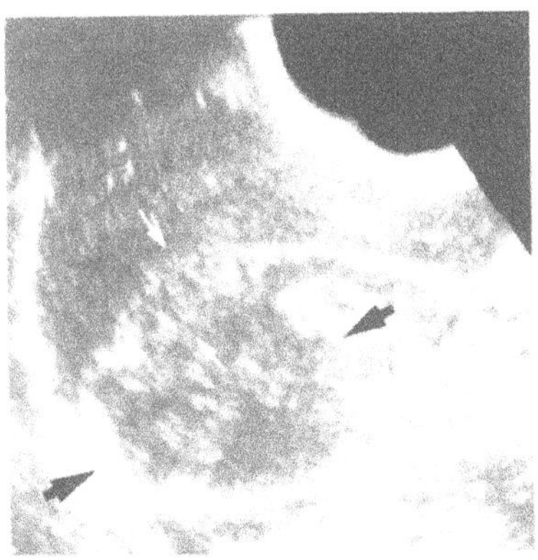

Fig. 6.1 Direct tumoral spread: tumor (*broad arrows*) has invaded the perirenal fat. The involved fatty area has a heterogeneous, sonolucent echotexture (*small arrows*)

6.2 Lymphatic Spread

Ultrasonic evaluation of the retroperitoneal compartment gives excellent results, provided intestinal gas does not interfere. This problem can usually be corrected by examining the patient in the lateral decubitus and in the standing position. Fluid filling of the stomach may also help.

A personal comparative study (DROUET 1983; DROUET et al. 1983) showed that, with regard to lymphomatous lymph nodes, ultrasound achieved almost as good a result as CT in the diagnosis of adenomegaly. In another study (MANIERES 1984) we checked on normal lymphographies and CT the criteria for adenomegaly. Lymph nodes over 15 mm in diameter on transverse sections must be considered pathological (30 mm adding together two perpendicular diameters). The maximum diameter of lymph nodes within the mesentery (see Fig. 6.10), rarely involved in renal carcinoma, and within the hepatoduodenal ligament, more often involved, is smaller (Fig. 6.2c).

Juxtahilar lymph nodes distort the renal vessels (Fig. 6.3) and are liable to push them forward. Other lymph nodes are displayed at a distance from the kidney, in the vicinity of the large vessels (Fig. 6.4). Yet other lymph nodes are retrocaval (Figs. 6.5, 6.6). Hypertrophy of the upper margin of the renal sinus may mimic such a retrocaval adenopathy (see Chap. 1, Fig. 1.30) if the examination is not thorough enough.

Enlarged juxtacaval lymph nodes can often be followed posterior to the ipsilateral renal vein, and even the contralateral vein (Fig. 6.6). Thus metastatic lymph nodes of renal carcinomas can extend to the contralateral side (Fig. 6.7), even sometimes involving the contralateral renal hilus (Fig. 6.8). Most of those metastatic lymph nodes have a polycyclic shape. Some of them, mimicking lymphomatous lymph nodes, give rise to a continuous pervascular cuff (Fig. 6.8).

Retroperitoneal lymph nodes push forward the mesenteric vessels (Fig. 6.8, 6.9) (the mesenteric vein sign – WEILL 1978) and even the splenic vein

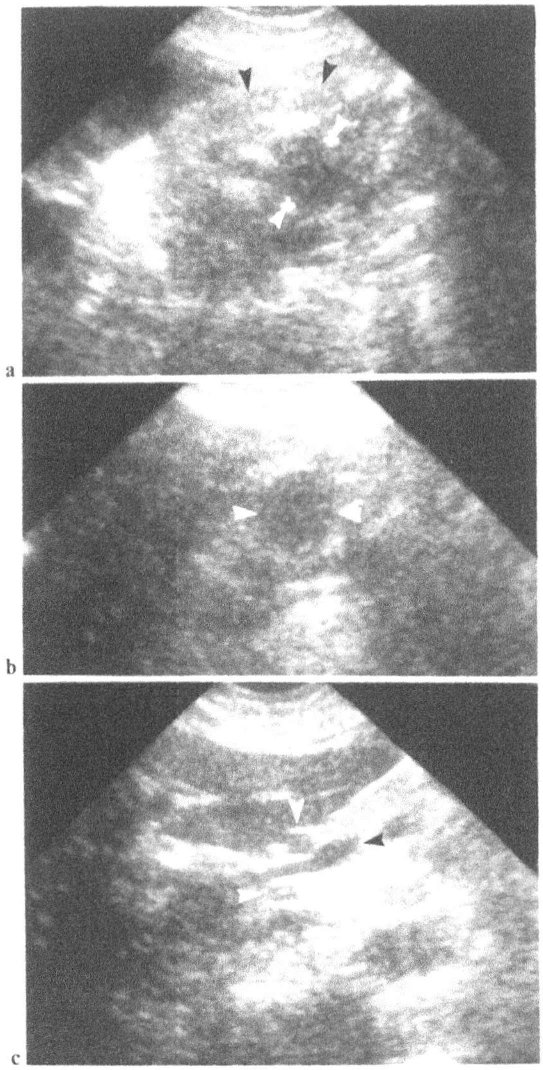

Fig. 6.2 a–c. Metastatic lymph nodes 1 year after left nephrectomy for renal cell carcinoma. **a** Transverse scan shows sonotransparent lymph node, 20 mm in diameter (*white arrowheads*), pushing the pancreas (*black arrowheads*) forward. **b** Sagittal section of lymph node. **c** Longitudinal section of the vena porta (*black arrowhead*) shows several lymph nodes (*white arrowheads*) within the hepatoduodenal ligament. The patient also had hepatic and splenic deposits (see Fig. 6.25)

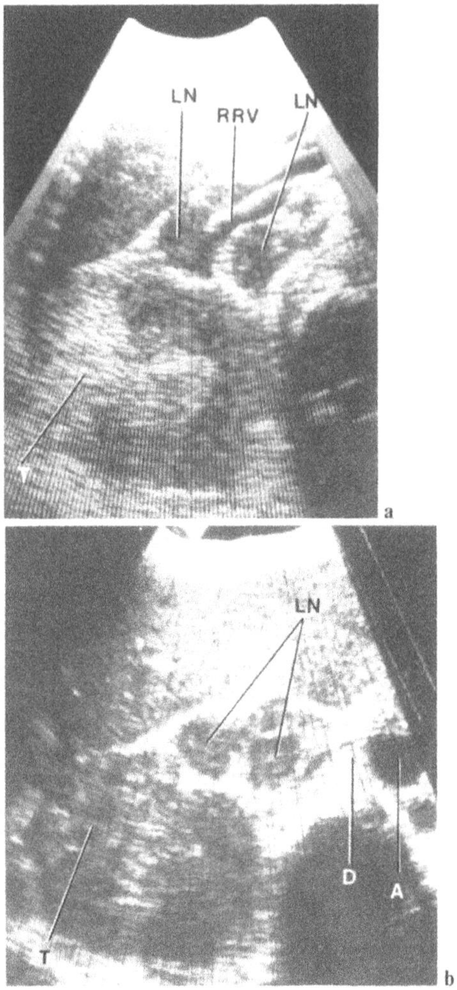

Fig. 6.3 a, b. Metastatic lymph nodes. **a** Real time transverse scan of right kidney shows external, echogenic renal cell carcinoma (*T*). Several lymph nodes (*LN*) are displayed in the vicinity of the right renal vein (*RRV*). Note the reflectivity of the lymph nodes, much higher than that of lymphomatous adenopathies. **b** Parallel, more cranial contact scan. *D*, right crus of diaphragm; *A*, aorta

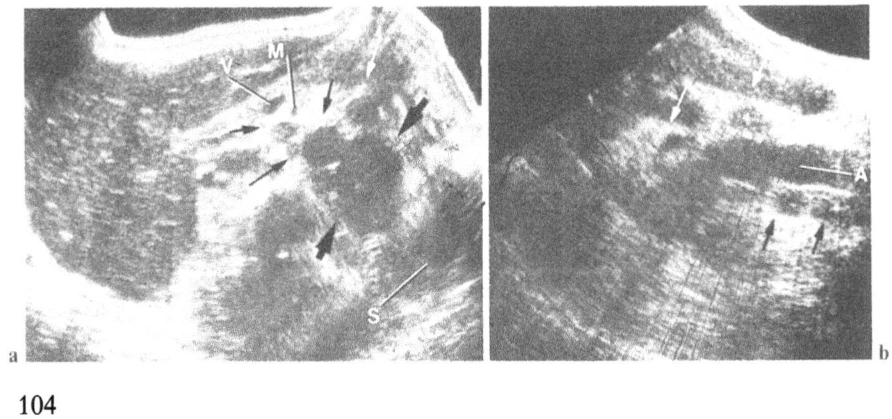

Fig. 6.4 a, b. Metastatic lymph nodes. **a** Transverse scan. Sonolucent tumoral mass of the left kidney upper pole (*broad arrows*) is shown between the spine and spleen (*S*). The group of lymph nodes (*small arrows*) located between the tumor and the pancreas (*V*, portal vein, *M*, SMA) gives rise to a multilocular pattern. **b** Sagittal section through the aorta (*A*) shows multiple pre- and retrovascular lymph nodes (*arrows*)

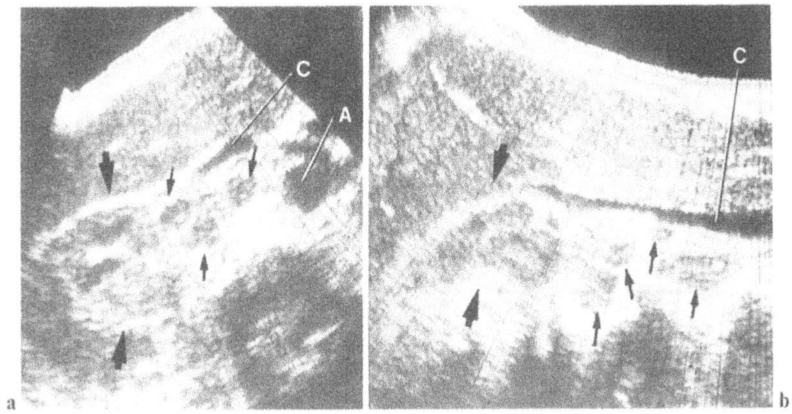

Fig. 6.5 a, b. Renal carcinoma with adenopathies. **a** Between right renal cell carcinoma (*broad arrows*) and aorta (*A*) transverse scan displays several metastatic lymph nodes (*arrows*). Cava (*C*) is pushed forward. **b** Sagittal scan through the cava shows retrovascular tumoral extension (*broad arrows*) and metastatic lymph nodes (*small arrows*)

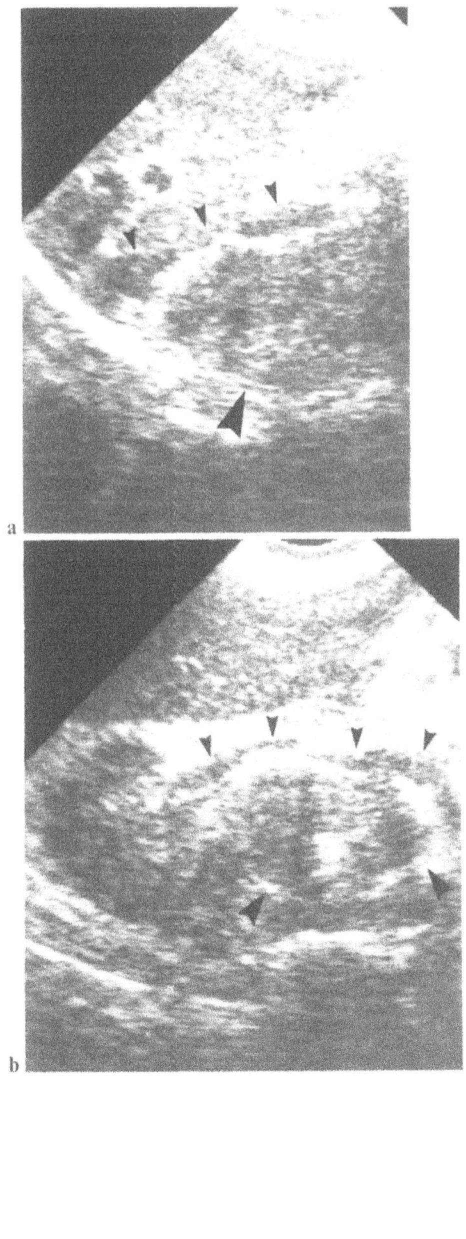

and pancreas, in one piece (Figs. 6.2, 6.8 d). Metastatic lymph nodes have smooth contours. Their echotexture is variable, as is their level of reflectivity. They may be frankly echogenic (Figs. 6.3, 6.5, 6.6); but most adenopathies are sonolucent (Figs. 6.2, 6.4, 6.7, 6.8) as in a lymphoma.

In small tumors, and when the ultrasonic study of the retroperitoneal space has been satisfactory, without intestinal acoustic shadowing, its results, whether positive or negative can be sufficient. But CT scans can add valuable information when the superficial location of the mass or its size are consistent with a spread beyond the limits of the renal area. Moreover, CT scans can display, better than ultrasound, an involvement of the most cranial abdominal lymph nodes, in the vicinity of the diaphragmatic crura. As we shall see later, CT is also instrumental in the study of tumoral spread to the renal vein: finally, after a positive ultrasonic diagnosis, CT represents a commendable step in the evaluation of renal carcinoma.

Fig. 6.6 a, b. Metastatic lymph nodes 1 year after left nephrectomy for renal cell carcinoma. **a** Sagittal scan shows a retrocaval mass (*broad arrowhead*). Cava is pushed forward and flattened (*small arrowheads*). **b** Transverse scan shows polycyclic lymph nodes (*broad arrowheads*) pushing forward right renal vein, cava, and left renal vein (*small arrowheads*)

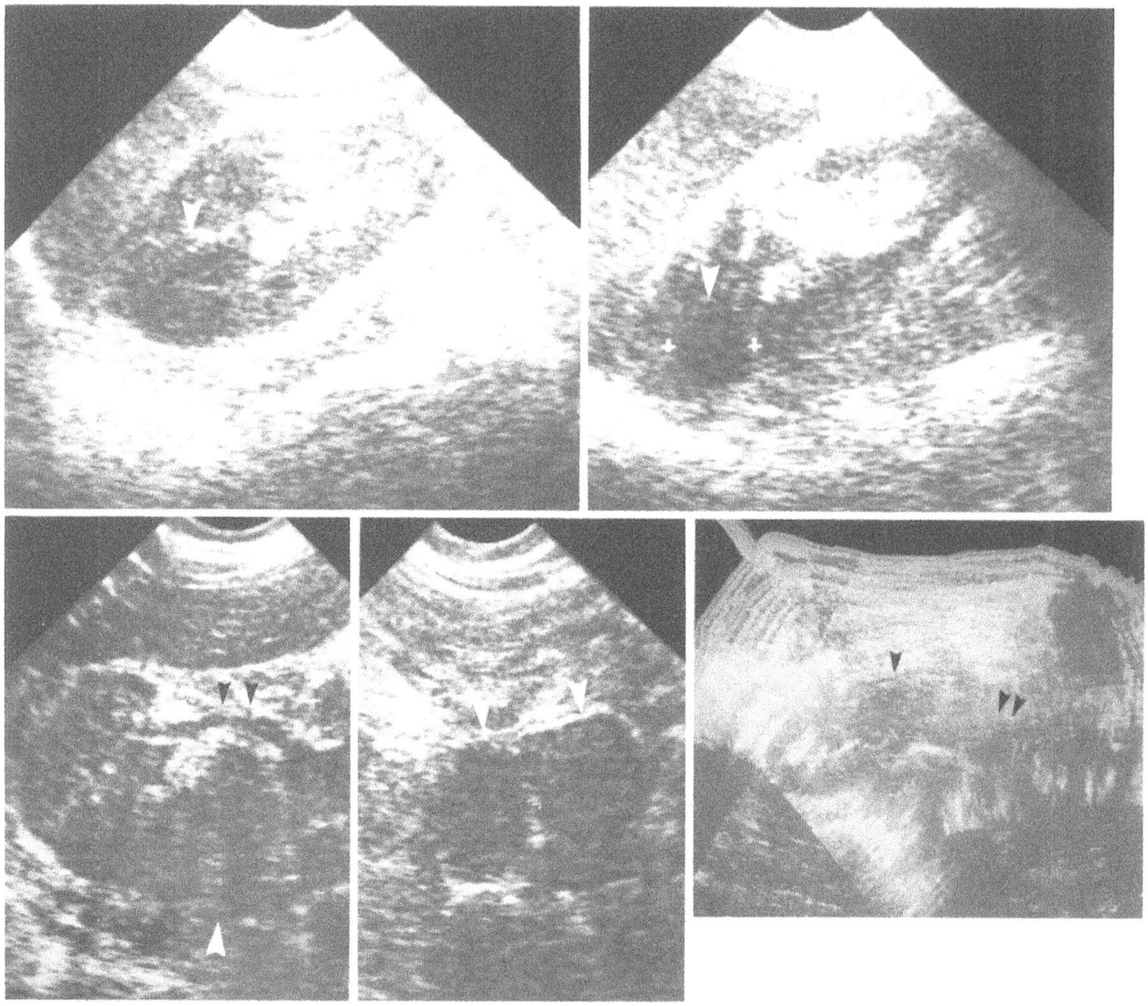

a, b

c–e

Fig. 6.7 a–e. Renal carcinoma with extensive adenopathies. **a, b** Two sections of right kidney show mass (*arrowheads*) in upper pole. **c** Transverse scan shows lymph nodes (*white arrowheads*) pushing forward renal vein (*black arrowheads*). **d** Transverse scan shows anterior to spine two large lymph nodes (*arrowheads*); one of them is located left of the medial sagittal plane. **e** Global transverse scan confirms that the lymph nodes (*arrowheads*) extend to hilus of left kidney (*double arrowhead*)

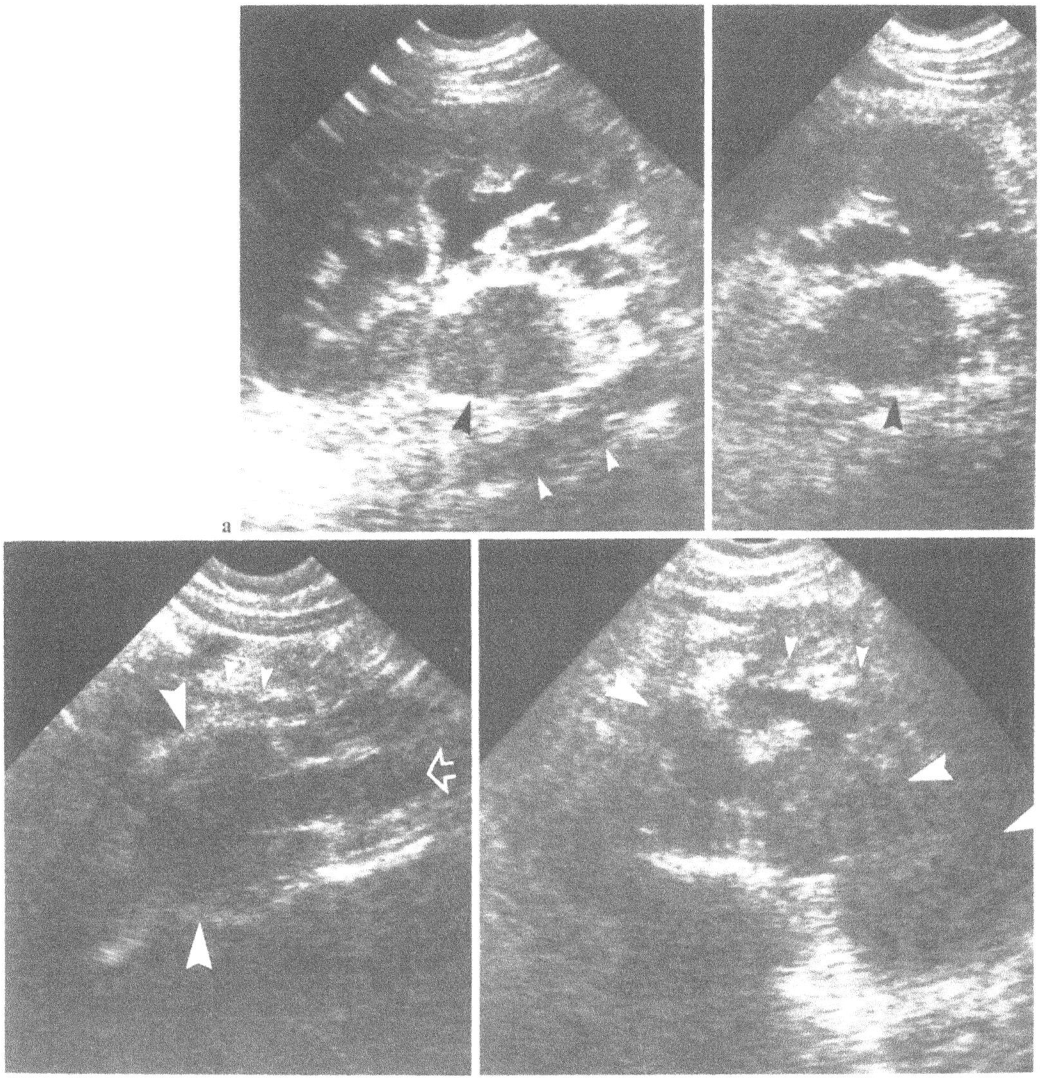

Fig. 6.8 a–d. Extensive metastatic lymph nodes 2 years after right nephrectomy for carcinoma. **a** Left coronal scan shows lymph nodes (*black arrowheads*) in the hilus of remaining left kidney. Note coronal section of the aorta (*white arrowheads*). **b** Transverse scan of the kidney and lymph node. **c** Sagittal scan through aorta (*open arrow*) shows ganglionic perivascular cuff (*broad arrowheads*). Note anterior displacement of mesenteric vessels (*small arrowhead*). **d** Transverse section of lymph nodes (*arrowheads*). Pancreas (*small arrowheads*) is pushed forward with splenic vein

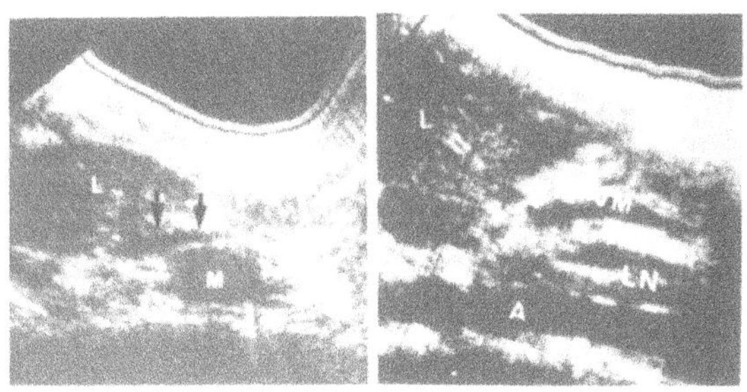

Fig. 6.9 a, b. Retroperitoneal lymph nodes: the mesenteric vein sign. **a** Sagittal scan shows ganglionar mass (*M*) pushing forward the SMV (*arrows*). *L*, liver. **b** Another case: preaortic lymph nodes (*LN*) push forward the SMV (*VM*). *A*, aorta; *L*, liver

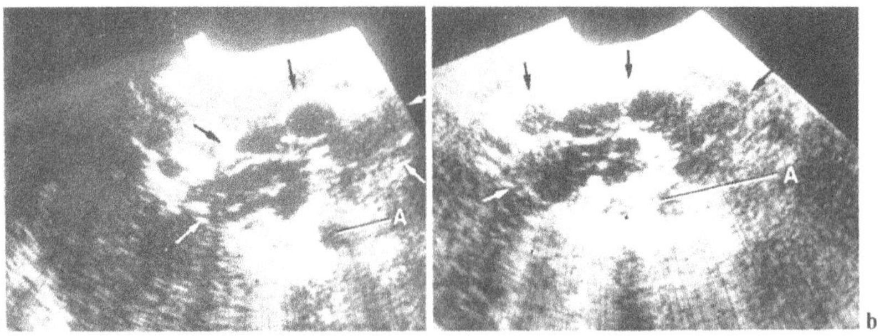

a b

Fig. 6.10 a, b. Polycyclic lymph nodes in the mesenter (*arrows*). Lymph nodes are centered by the mesenteric vessels. The two layers of ganglia, on both sides of the vessels, have been compared to a sandwich pattern. *A*, aorta

6.3 Intracaval Extension

The vena cava, with its specific respiratory kinetics, constitutes one of the constant elements displayed by sagittal and transverse real time scans. The disappearance of its respiratory expansion and the presence of echoes within the vascular lumen are relevant signs of venous obstruction (TAYLOR 1975). Transverse sections can show thrombosis of the renal vein (Figs. 6.11, 6.12). Finally, renal carcinomas involving the venous network give rise to three different patterns.

1. Images of diffuse thrombosis, as those we just saw above. They correspond to both a tumoral extension and a thrombosis above and/or below the tumoral growth, with no delineation between them. They are confirmed by Doppler studies.

2. Images of tumoral extension, with a mass bulging within the cava lumen, which widens (Figs. 6.13 b, 6.14, 6.15). The intraluminal growth is surrounded by blood, except where it reaches its maximal diameter. Transverse scans carried out at that level mimic a complete obstruction (Fig. 6.15 a–b). The tumoral growth can also widen the renal vein (Fig. 6.13 b). The blood flow, above or below, can remain free or come to a stop (Figs. 6.13 c). In most cases the associated thrombosis can be evaluated with precision (Fig. 6.15 c), taking into account the caval kinetics and the sonotransparence of the caval lumen. Thrombosis below the tumoral extension (i.e., topographically, above the kidneys) can induce an acute Budd-Chiari syndrome, with hepatomegaly and loss of the transparence of the lumen of the hepatic veins (WEILL 1981).

3. In the last pattern, tumoral foci adhering to the venous wall are encountered (Fig. 6.16; see also Figs. 6.18, 6.20).

Tumoral emboli are sometimes demonstrated within the lumen of the hepatic veins (Fig. 6.17). These patterns of caval involvement are also displayed in other malignant processes: malignant pheochromocytoma (Fig. 6.18), malignant melanoma (Figs. 6.19, 6.20), and choriocarcinoma (Fig. 6.21). A mere compression of the vein, due to precaval lymph nodes or to a prevascular tumoral bulging (Fig. 6.22) must not be confused with an obstruction.

When screening for small growths, the relief of the right renal artery, which bulges forward through the posterior venous wall during deep suspended respiration (Fig. 6.22) can constitute a pitfall.

An accessory but relevant sign of caval obstruction is the discovery of collateral channels, as for instance a dilated ovarian vein (EISENSCHER 1979). The various features of caval obstruction are summarized in Table 6.1.

Table 6.1. Caval obstruction

Patterns	Loss of kinetics
	Solid pattern of lumen
	Intraluminal growths
	Display of collateral channels
	"Silent" doppler
Pitfalls in diagnosis	Compression by tumor or lymph nodes
	Forward bulging of right renal artery
Etiology	Tumoral spread
	Primary thrombosis
	Thrombosis secondary to tumoral spread or compression
	Retroperitoneal fibrosis

CT scans, carried out in order to assess the retroperitoneal space, can also display intracaval growths; CT is reliable in the evaluation of the renal vein.

CT scans also make possible the evaluation of the caval wall: a thickened wall is a sign of direct tumoral involvement, whereas in thromboses the wall is not altered. Direct tumoral involvement of the venous wall is also often accompanied by an increase in density after contrast injection. This kind of information is better yielded by CT. But ultrasound shows much more precisely than CT the cranial extension of a tumor thrombus.

Conventional cavagraphy is performed if ultrasound and/or CT have shown an abnormal vena cava, particularly if radical surgery, with caval resection, is being considered. Failure of ultrasound or CT, or inconclusive results, also represent an indication for cavagraphy. But cavagraphy yields litte information regarding the cranial extension of thrombi. This is precisely the most important feature to be evaluated, since cranial extension may require surgery under heart-lung bypass. MRI will of course give excellent results when commonly available.

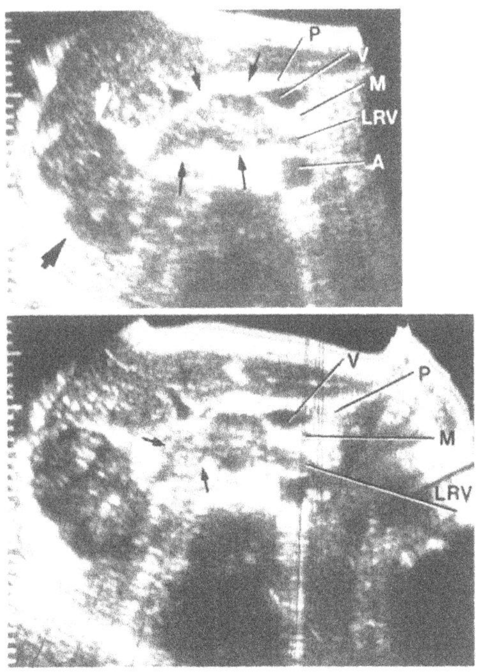

Fig. 6.11 a, b. Renal cell carcinoma. Venous involvement. **a** Transverse scan shows renal mass (*broad arrows*). Echotexture of venous lumen is solid in right renal vein and cava (*arrows*), and also in left renal vein (*LRV*). Pancreas (*P*) and splenic vein (*V*) are pushed forward. *M*, SMA, *A*, aorta. **b** Parallel scan

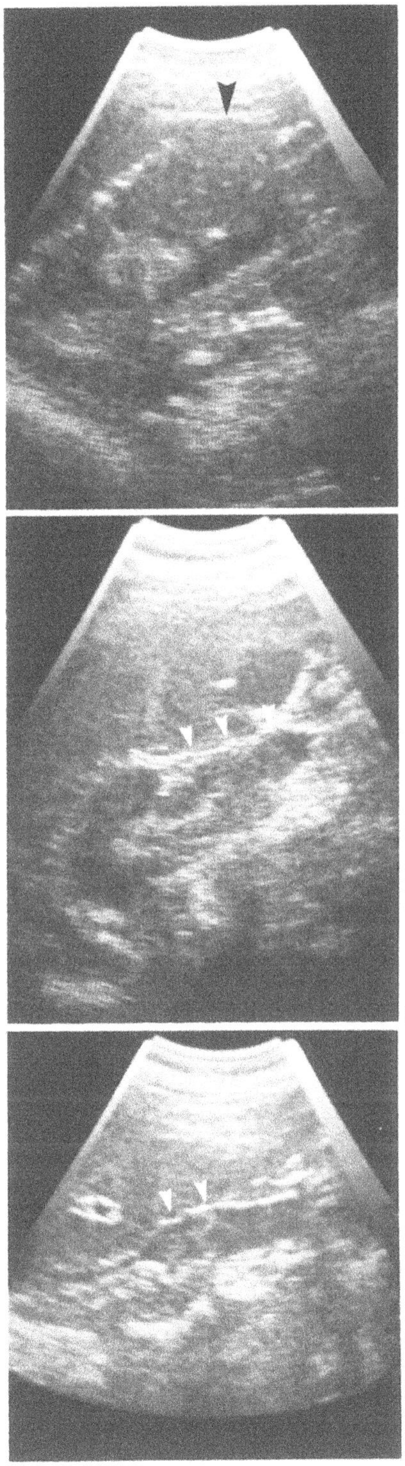

Fig. 6.12 a–c. Renal cell carcinoma with venous involvement. **a** Sagittal scan of right kidney show mass in lower pole (*arrowhead*). **b** Transverse scan shows right renal vein and IVC swollen and occupied by solid tissue. **c** Sagittal section of IVC shows intraluminal tumoral tissue (*arrowheads*). Distal to the tumoral involvement, behind the liver, IVC is free; caval lumen proximal to tumoral involvement is enlarged and has solid echotexture due to thrombosis

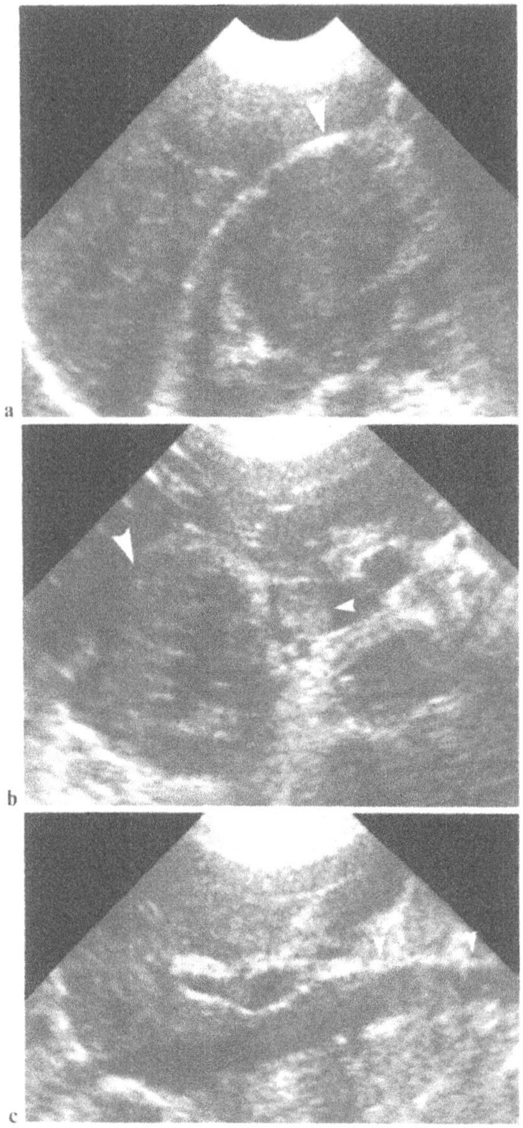

Fig. 6.13 a–c. Right renal cell carcinoma with venous involvement. **a** Sagittal scan of tumor in lower pole (*arrowhead*). **b** Transverse section of tumor (*broad arrowhead*) and IVC with endoluminal tumoral growth (*small arrowheads*). **c** Sagittal scan of invaded IVC (*arrowheads*)

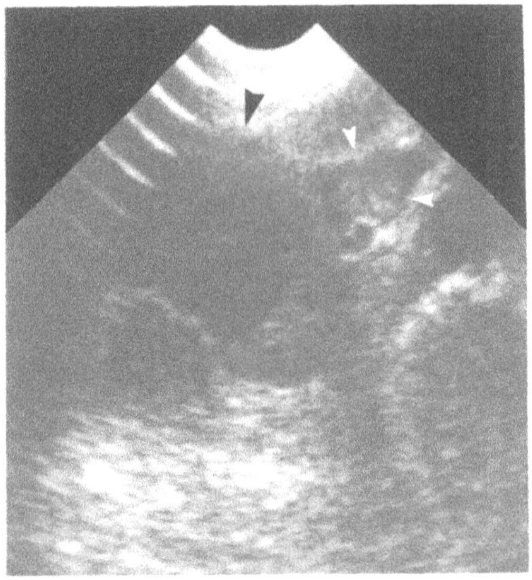

Fig. 6.14. Transverse scan of carcinoma (*black arrowhead*) and IVC with endoluminal tumoral growth (*white arrowheads*). Note section of right renal artery posterior to IVC

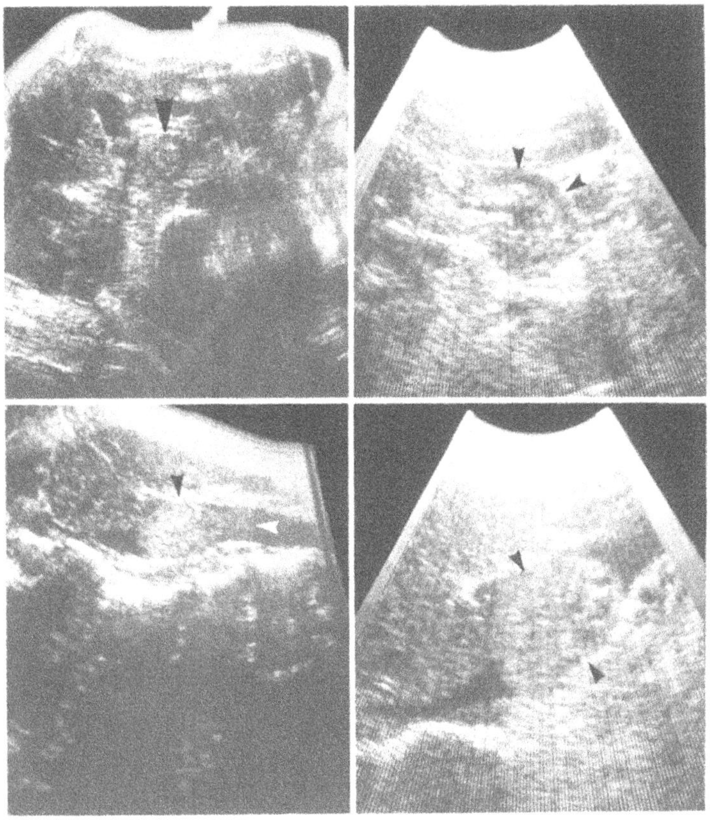

a, b

c, d

Fig. 6.15 a–d. Invaded vena cava. **a** Global transverse scan: right kidney is swollen. Tumoral mass has developed within IVC (*arrowhead*), whose lumen is almost completely obstructed. **b** Real time transverse scan also shows an enlarged and obstructed IVC. **c** Sagittal section: cava is enlarged by mass (*black arrowhead*); proximal to mass vein is thrombosed (*white arrowhead*). **d** Real time section of endoluminal mass

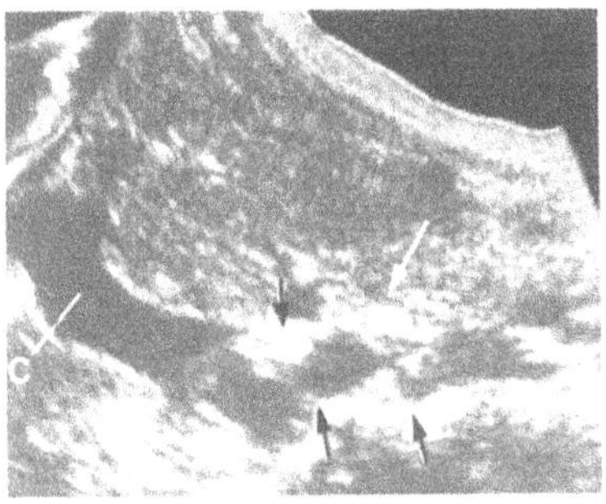

Fig. 6.16. Sagittal scan of cava (*C*) shows multiple parietal growths (*arrows*). Some of them are obstructing lumen (*white arrow*). Primary tumor is renal

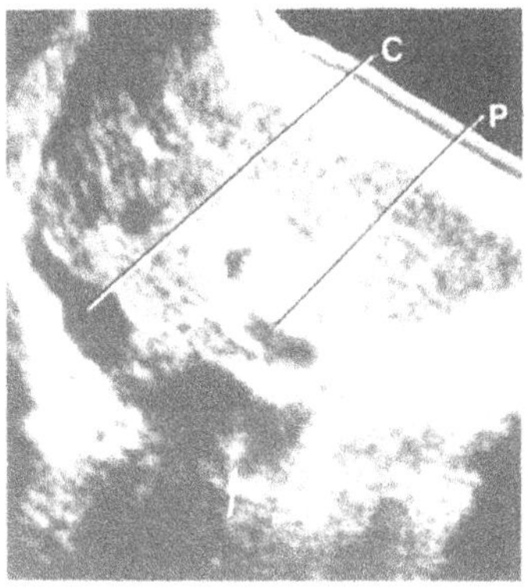

Fig. 6.18. Sagittal section of vena cava (*C*): multiple parietal growths (*arrows*) due to spread of malignant pheochromocytoma (*P*)

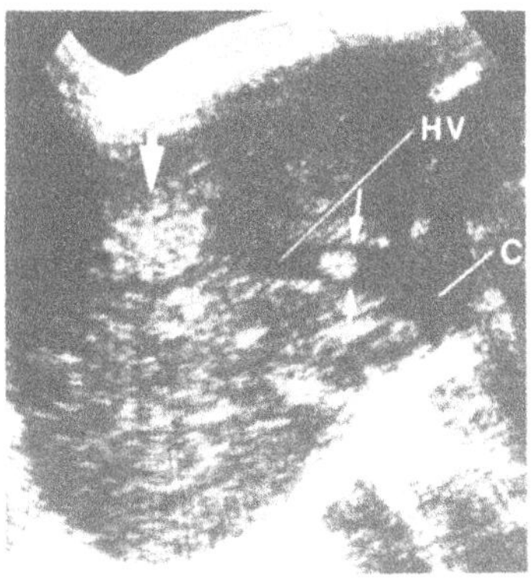

◂ **Fig. 6.17.** Hepatic deposits (*broad arrow*) of renal carcinoma; tumoral embolus (*small arrow*) within right hepatic vein (*HV*). *C*, vena cava

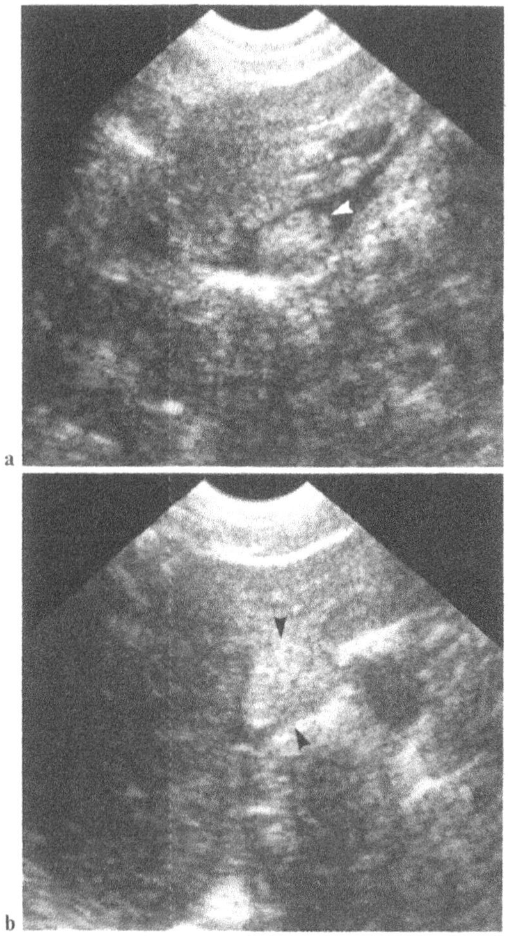

Fig. 6.19 a, b. Endoluminal mass (*arrowhead*) due to spread of melanosarcoma. **a** Sagittal scan; **b** transverse scan

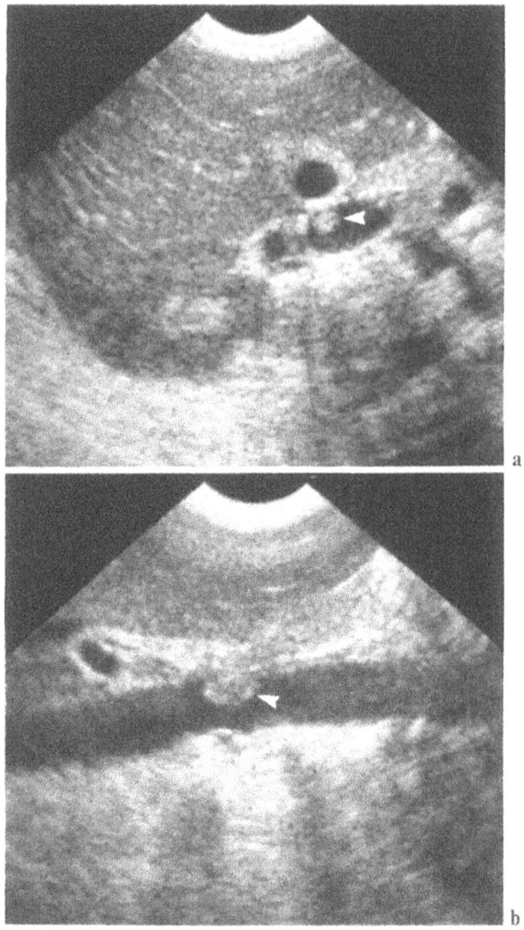

Fig. 6.21 a, b. Caval parietal growths (*arrowhead*) due to spread of choriocarcinoma. **a** Transverse scan: growths develop within the right renal vein and cava. **b** Sagittal scan

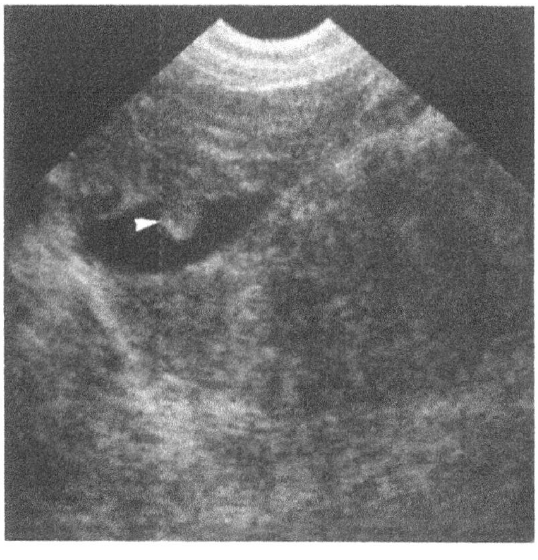

Fig. 6.20. Sagittal scan of vena cava: parietal growth (*arrowhead*) due to spread of melanosarcoma

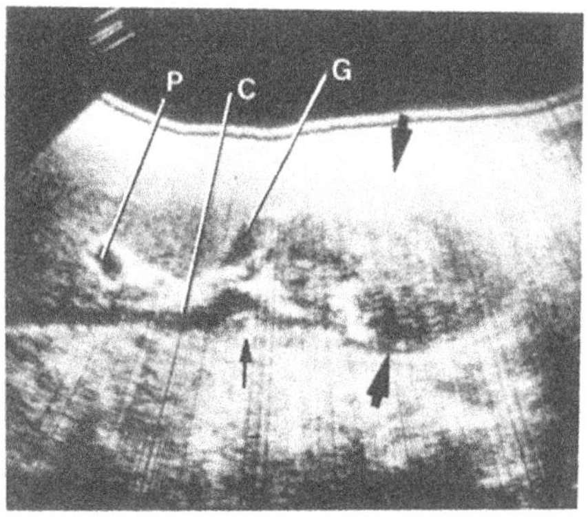

Fig. 6.22. Venous compression: a pitfall. Sagittal scan through vena cava (*C*) shows vessel flattened by tumor (*broad arrows*). Pseudogrowth (*small arrow*) corresponds to forward bulging of the right renal artery. *P*, portal vein; *G*, gallbladder

6.4 Metastatic Spread

A deposit (or another primary tumor) may be found in the contralateral kidney (see Chap. 5). The discovery of a renal abnormality does not dispense with a thorough contralateral examination. Multiple tumors can appear as the manifestation of a general disease, as tuberous sclerosis, or as Von Hippel-Lindau disease.

We have described elsewhere (WEILL 1978, 1980, 1982, 1984) the different echopatterns of liver metastases. They are summarized in Table 6.2 (see Figs. 6.23–6.25). Exceptionally, splenic metastases are demonstrated (Fig. 6.25 b, c). Several statistical studies (TAYLOR 1975; PIETRI et al. 1979) show the rate of successful ultrasonic diagnosis to be over 90%. A personal survey, before the era of high resolution real time, (PERRIGUEY 1980) was less optimistic, with a success rate of only 80%. In our experience, ultrasound is as sensitive as CT when screening for liver metastases.

Table 6.2. Echopatterns of liver metastases

Contour abnormalities	*Echotexture changes*	*Grouped images*
Hump sign	Nodules:	Sieve pattern
Edge sign	sonolucent	Hailstorm pattern
	reflective	Mottled pattern
	bull's-eye	
	sonotransparent (necrosis)	
	Increased reflectivity in fields	

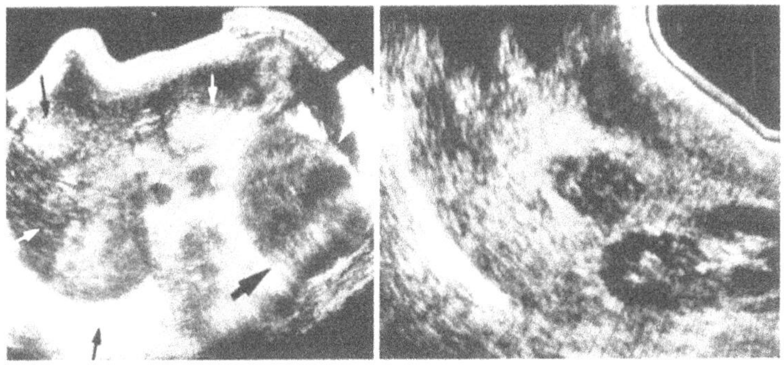

Fig. 6.23 a, b. Liver metastases. **a** Transverse scan shows left renal tumor (*broad arrows*). Multiple intrahepatic reflective nodules (*small arrows*) give rise to a "hailstorm" pattern. **b** Sagittal scan in another case shows areas of increased reflectivity and multiple sonolucent nodules (mottled pattern)

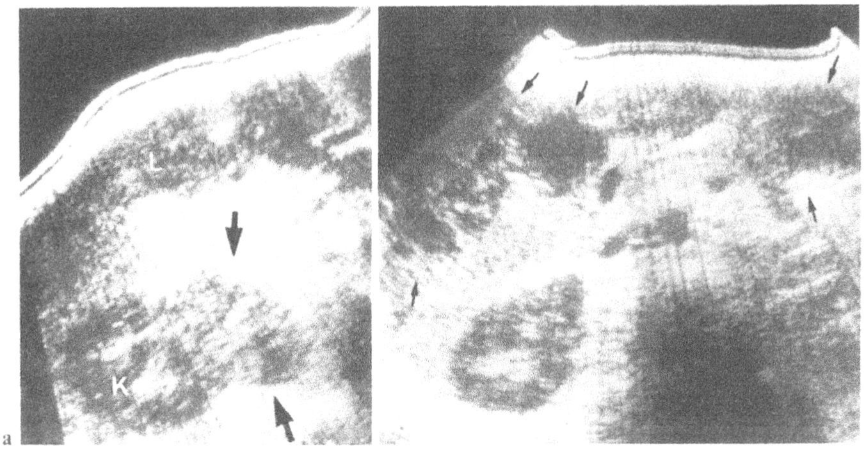

Fig. 6.24 a, b. Liver metastases. **a** Transverse section shows a tumoral mass (*arrows*) bulging out of the right renal hilus. *K*, kidney. **b** Parallel more cranial scan discloses multiple hepatic nodules (*arrows*)

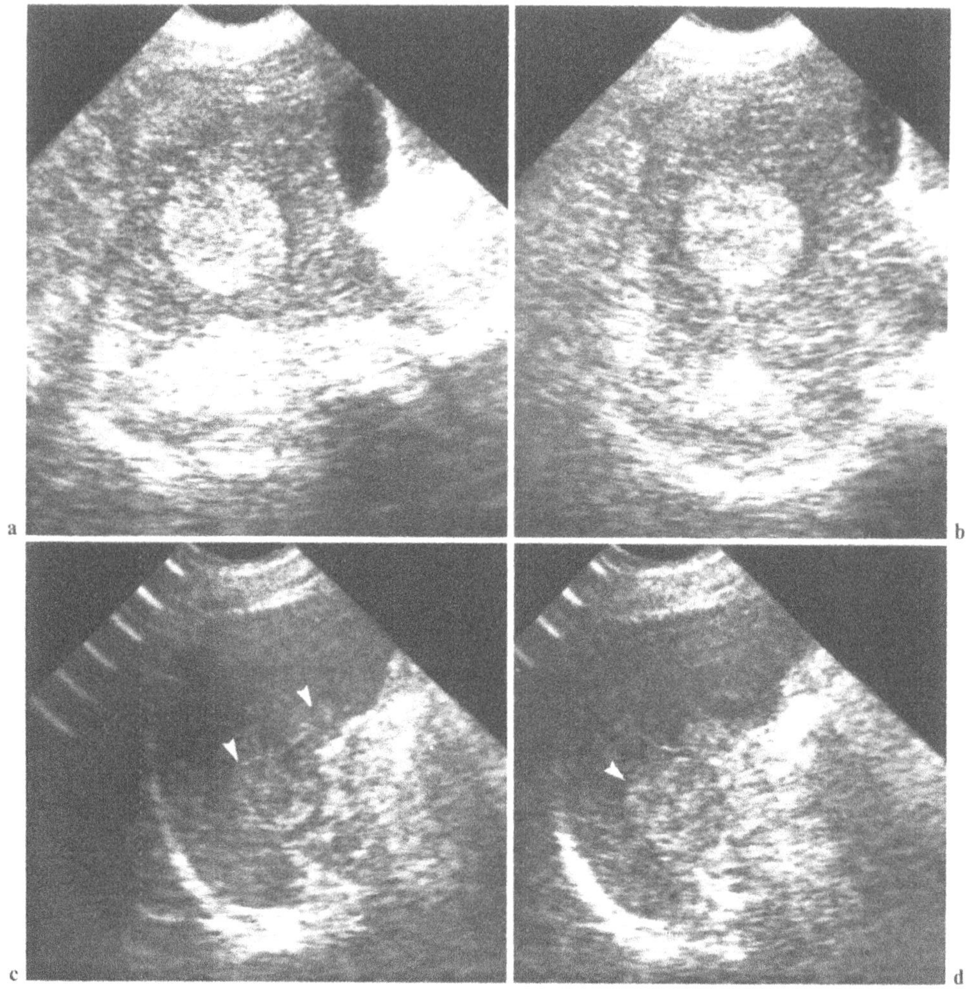

Fig. 6.25 a–d. Deposits of renal cell carcinoma (same patient as in Fig. 6.2). **a, b** Liver sections: echogenic nodules. **c, d** Splenic deposits (*arrowheads*)

6.5 Clinical and Radiological Policy

What we have stated above shows that ultrasound can clarify the extension of renal cell carcinoma in most cases. CT is useful to study the involvement of the juxtarenal compartments, fascias, and abdominal wall. It is also instrumental in the evaluation of the renal veins and invaluable in the case of failure of ultrasound in the assessment of lymph nodes, i.e., 5% of cases on the right side, and 10% of cases on the left side. Ultrasound and CT are now the two pillars of renal tumoral evaluation in the frame of modern radiology. If angiography is required preoperatively in order to obtain arterial cartography, it is possible to rely on intravenous digitized angiography.

Angiography is also considered when CT shows, in a large mass, a particularly marked tumoral vascularity, since in such cases angiography is also therapeutic, with the aim of embolization. Indications for cavagraphy have been discussed above.

6.6 Particular Cases

Urothelial Tumors

Urothelial tumors are also best documented by CT, despite the fact that such tumors do not, usually, develop beyond the renal capsule. But multiple urothelial localizations, at different levels of the urinary tract, are possible: a complete IVU study is mandatory. Ultrasonic scans of the bladder can help, as can cystoscopy.

Tumors in Children

The possibility of avoiding angiography is particularly valuable in children. In infants, especially newborns, it is nevertheless often impossible to obtain satisfactory ultrasonic images of the retroperitoneal space because of abundant intestinal gas. Posterior and coronal scanning will helps. CT proves by anterior approach helpful in such cases – not without other difficulties, due to the absence of fat.

Local Recurrences After Nephrectomy

After nephrectomy the renal area is occupied by the large bowel. Therefore only posterior or lateral scanning remains possible. The interpretation of that region becomes very difficult in the absence of fixed, constant anatomical elements. CT scans seem more clear and precise in the operated patient, the more so since the radiological study is carried out to look for parietal and retroperitoneal involvement rather than to look for a recurrent mass.

Other Retroperitoneal Abnormalities

We have already mentioned, in discussing the differential diagnosis of large renal tumors (see Chap. 5), tumors arising from retroperitoneal connective tissue, from the posterior muscles, or from nervous elements.

JACOBSON and REDMAN (1974), SANDERS et al. (1977), and FAGON et al. (1979) have depicted the ultrasonic pattern of retroperitoneal fibrosis. It gives rise to prevascular, more or less echogenic strips. COOPERBERG (1977) has encountered, in two cases of retroperitoneal fibrosis, images of sonolucent perivascular cuffs, similar to those induced by lymph nodes (Figs. 6.26, 6.27). Relevant associated signs are hydronephrosis (uni- or bilateral) and caval obstruction.

A Musical Conclusion. Once again in this chapter we have played five instruments: ultrasound, IVU, CT, arteriography, and cavagraphy. Records and concerts give us the opportunity of listening to Bach's toccatas either in the original organ version or in Leopold Stockowski's symphonic adaptations. Most will prefer the soloist's interpretation. In any case neither patients nor hospital managers wish to pay for the full orchestra if a soloist can do just as well – or still better. In this respect ultrasound plays second fiddle to none. But please do not forget what the lady answered the conductor who enquired what she most loved in Beethoven's symphonies. Her reply was: "The silences"!

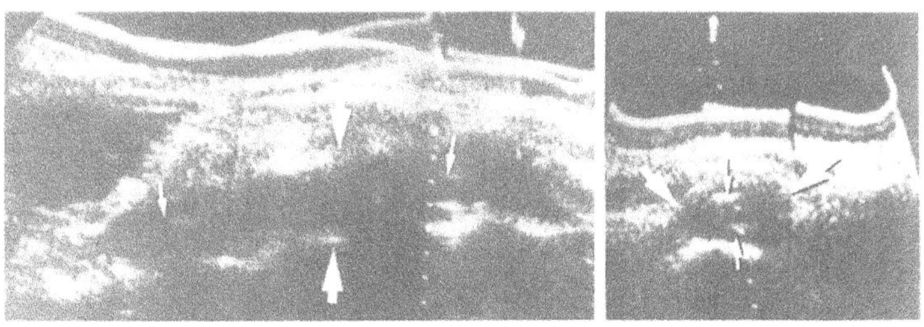

Fig. 6.26 a, b. Retroperitoneal fibrosis. **a** Sagittal scan shows an apparently enlarged aorta (*broad arrows*). In fact the aortic wall is more internal (*small arrows*). The image is due to a periaortic fibrotic cuff. The pattern is similar to that of the perivascular lymph nodes (see Figs. 6.7, 6.8) and not unlike an aortic aneurysm with a thrombopenic layer. **b** Transverse section. (Courtesy of Dr. Cooperberg, Vancouver)

a, b

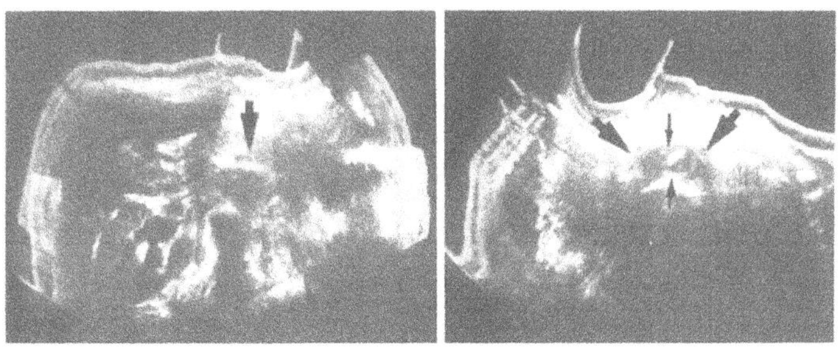

Fig. 6.27 a, b. Another case of retroperitoneal fibrosis with an identical pattern (*broad arrows* fibrotic cuff, *small arrows* aortic wall). (Courtesy of Dr. Cooperberg, Vancouver)

a, b

7 Infections and Inflammatory Processes

7.1 Abscesses

Bacterial

Acute. Acute abscesses, due either to a local process, lithiasis for instance, or to hematogenous bacterial seeding are usually accompanied by a specific clinical syndrome; as in the case of hepatic abscesses, the two best ultrasonic signs are, in our opinion (1) fever and (2) pain.

In fact there is an ultrasonic symptomatology, and it becames more clear as the process of collection progresses. The first abnormality is a nonspecific sonolucent local swelling (Fig. 7.1), with a semisolid echotexture. The process of collection brings about a liquid pattern. At this stage, the limit of the cavity may present an irregular pattern, with a thick, ill-defined wall. There may be necrotic debris (Fig. 7.2). Scattered echogenic foci and also echogenic foci located in the upper part of the collection correspond to gas bubbles, as demonstrated by CT.

Once the process of collection is complete, the pattern of the abscess can be quite similar to that of a simple cyst, with, however, less marked posterior reinforcement (Figs. 7.3, 7.4). A high-amplitude study can nevertheless show the liquid contents to be incompletely sonotransparent, with scattered or dependent echoes.

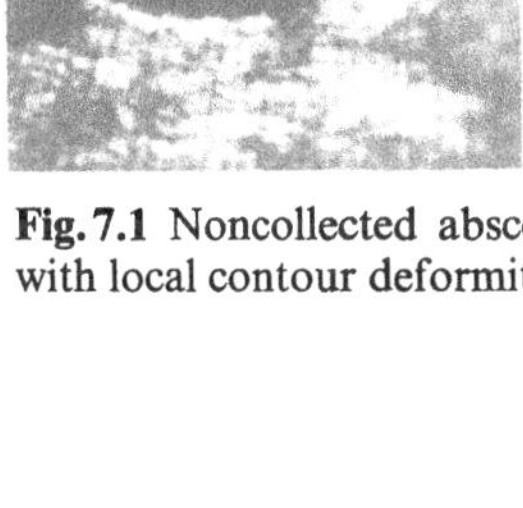

Fig. 7.1 Noncollected abscess: semisolid parenchymal area with local contour deformity (*arrows*)

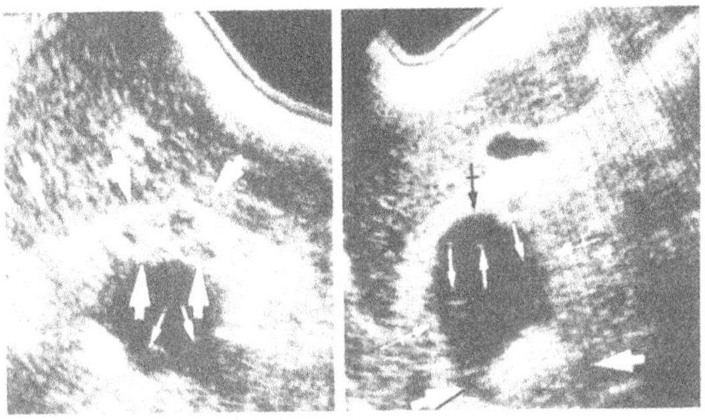

a, b

Fig. 7.2 a, b. Collected bacterial abscess. **a** Sagittal section: the abscess is surrounded by echogenic perirenal fat, partially involved (*arrows*). Note the floating debris (*arrows*). **b** Transverse section: the kidney (*broad arrows*) is flattened by an anterior abscess (*arrows*) with floating debris (*arrows*)

Abscesses can be multiple. A particular pattern is brought about by multiple small bacterial abscesses: they produce multiple adjacent sonolucent areas, rather well delineated (LEE 1980), disappearing under antibiotherapy.

Frank renal swelling is a reliable sign of primary upper urinary tract infection. Swelling is less marked in ascending infection (DINKEL et al. 1986).

Complications and Evolution. An abscess can spread to the perirenal and pararenal compartments, where pus collections will appear (Figs. 7.4, 7.5). Such collections give rise to echo-free areas, similar, when present, to those due to urinomas or hematomas, which we shall study in Chap. 10 (see Fig. 10.1).

Under antibiotic therapy, after spontaneous drainage into the collecting system, or after puncture and evacuation, the liquid pattern will disappear, to be replaced, owing to retraction of the cavity, by a reflective heterogeneous echopattern. The final evolution can lead to a reflective fibrous scar.

Particular Patterns. KRESSEL and FILLY (1978) showed that microbubbles can produce a solid pattern in abscesses. Larger amounts of gas will produce acoustic shadowing. The presence of gas is better documented by CT than by ultrasound.

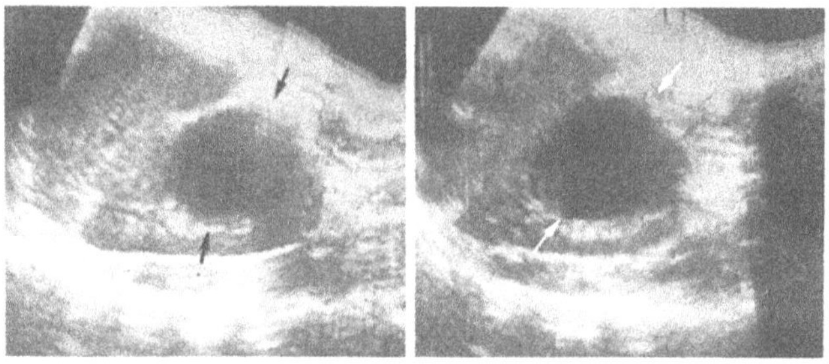

a, b

Fig. 7.3 a, b. Collected bacterial abscesses. Two parallel sagittal sections. The abscess is completely echo-free, but lacks posterior reinforcement

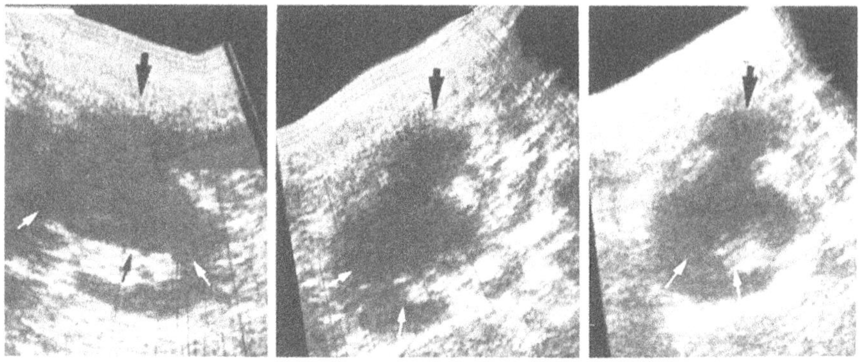

a–c

Fig. 7.4 a–c. Renal abscess. **a** Sagittal section with the patient in procubitus shows a posterior sonotransparent process, pressing on the central zone (*small arrows*). Note the extension to the posterior wall (*broad arrow*). **b, c** Transverse sections show extension of the lesion (*small arrows*) to the posterior pararenal compartment (*broad arrow*)

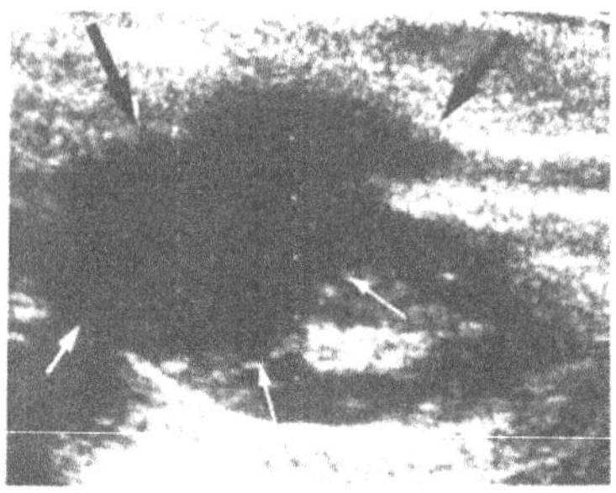

Fig. 7.5. Abscess: posterior sagittal section shows a large lesion within the renal upper pole (*small arrows*). The adjacent renal parenchyma is depressed. Note the purulent migration to the posterior wall through the posterior pararenal compartment. (Courtesy of Dr. M. Lafortune, Montreal)

Tuberculous

Tuberculous abscesses possess the same echopattern (Fig. 7.6) as bacterial abscesses. We shall study later the ultrasonic pattern of other tuberculous abnormalities.

Differential Diagnosis

In the case of noncollected abscesses, if only images are taken into account, any sonotransparent solid process could be considered, such as tumors and pseudotumors. But clinical symptoms of abscesses are rather specific. Knowledge of them will focus the diagnostic discussion to few hypotheses.

Xanthogranulomatous pyelonephritis gives rise to an anechoic renal enlargement (Von Kirk 1980). CT (Sagel et al. 1977) is not very specific, nor is IVU. Puncture will be considered if previous examinations yield non-relevant results. Abscesses under cicatrization can mimic any reflective process: tumors, sequelae of vascular lesions, or cortical scars due to chronic pyelonephritis. We shall study such abnormalities later.

In fact, the main discussions arise from collected abscesses, although these will only be considered if

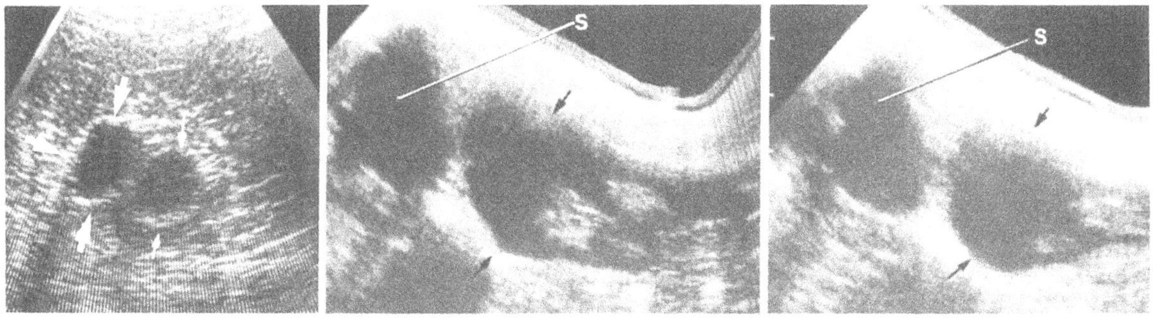

a–c

Fig. 7.6 a–c. Tuberculous abscesses. **a** Upper pole pseudocystic tuberculous abscess (*broad arrows*), still limited by perirenal fat, is in contact with the dilated pelvis (*small arrows*) (left intercostal scan). **b, c** Another case. **b** Sagittal scan shows swollen upper pole with echo-free area (*arrows*), lacking delineation. *S*, spleen. **c** Parallel more external scan

relevant clinical symptoms are also present, keeping in mind the possibility of fever and pain accompanying evolutive tumors. The association of clinical symptoms of infection with an ultrasonic pattern of renal fluid collection will lead to the discussion of an infected cyst, or an infected hydronephrosis on one of the pyelons of a duplicated kidney. Lastly, a necrotized tumor can exceptionally be considered. The diagnosis will be achieved by puncture. However, some morphological details are relevant: in abscesses, an IVU with early nephrotomograms may display a hyperdense rim. Necrotic tumors can also display a peripheral hyperdense rim, but with a less smooth and homogeneous character. Peripheral hyperdensity is lacking in infected cysts or in pyonephroses. Peripheral hyperhemia is still better displayed on contrast-enhanced CT scans. CT can also show regional edema, with for instance thickening of the fascias. CT can also demonstrate gas bubbles within the cavity, consistant with an infection. CT also makes possible precise topographic analysis of lesions, particularly in case of perirenal extension. It will therefore be carried out if clinical symptoms and relevant ultrasound images did not lead to immediate puncture. It will anyway be followed by puncture and drainage (Fig. 7.7).

a

b

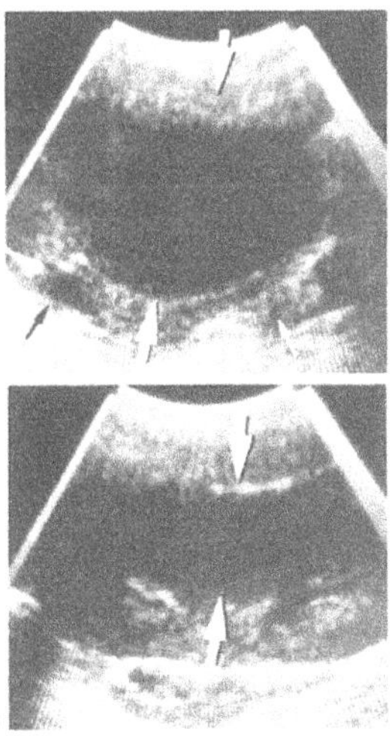

Fig. 7.7 a, b. Bacterial abscess: puncture. **a** Left intercostal scan discloses large subcapsular echo-free area (*broad arrows*), again lacking posterior reinforcement. The renal parenchyma (*small arrows*) is flattened. **b** Follow-up examination after puncture and evacuation of 70 ml pus. Collection (*arrows*) is not completely removed. Permanent drainage is still necessary

7.2 Bacterial Nephritides

Diffuse renal changes can appear in the course of *septicemia,* due to white cell infiltration. The size and echogenicity of the kidney can increase (Fig. 7.8). Plain nephromegaly is also encountered. In most cases those alterations disappear under antibiotherapy, without abscess formation.

A particular process requires close attention: *focal bacterial nephritis,* also termed *lobar nephronia,* whose features were described by the Yale group (Rosenfield 1979) and by Lee (1980). Clinical symptoms are similar to those of collecting abscesses. Sonography shows a local swelling as do abscesses before collection (Fig. 7.9). This focal mass is echo-poor and rather well delineated. Multiple masses are exceptional. Evolution under antibiotherapy is prolonged, usually without the appearance of a collected abscess. However, late collections have been reported. This particular infectious process, due to gram-negative bacteria, must be kept in mind: prolonged pain and hyperhemia, without immediate recession under antibiotherapy, associated with an ultrasonic pattern of mass could also be consistent with the diagnosis of malignant tumor. Other imaging modalities are not much more specific. Puncture can contribute to a precise diagnosis.

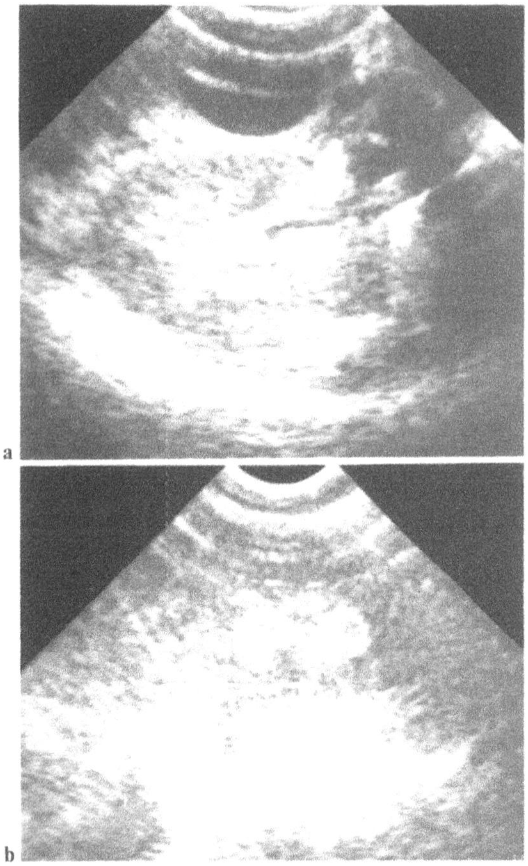

Fig. 7.8 a, b. Bacterial nephritis during septicemia: the parenchyma is diffusely echogenic. **a** Transverse scan; **b** coronal scan

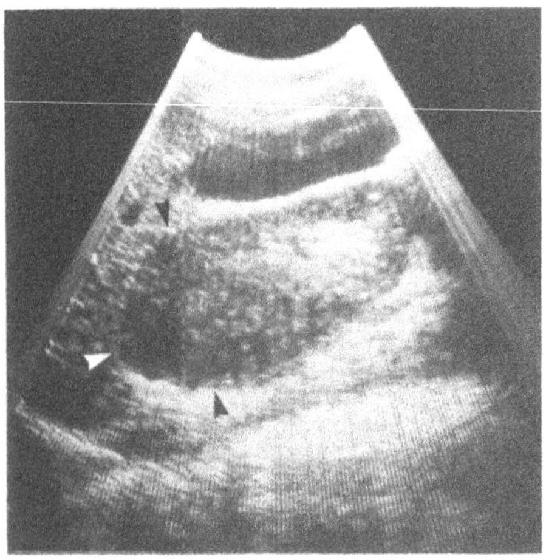

Fig. 7.9. Focal bacterial nephritis: sagittal scan shows swelling of the upper pole. Limit of central zone is altered without frank depression

Fig. 7.10. Pyonephrosis: General pattern is similar to that of ▶ hydronephrosis. Note, however, dependent echoes (*arrows*). There is major cortical atrophy

7.3 Pyonephrosis

Recently Infected Hydronephrosis

The pattern of recently infected hydronephrosis is similar to that of noninfected hydronephrosis unless high-amplitude scanning displays unclear contents, with scattered or dependent echoes (Fig. 7.10).

Older Pyonephrosis

In older infections, the walls of the collecting system are less sharply delineated. The liquid content is less sonotransparent (Figs. 7.11, 7.12). The parenchyma itself is subject to abnormalities. Such associated abnormalities lead to global changes of the renal pattern, with deformities and heterogeneities (Fig. 7.12). Cortical atrophy is usually present (Figs. 7.11–7.12).

7.4 Tuberculosis

Evolutive multifocal tuberculosis also gives rise to diffuse, heterogeneous pattern changes: the parenchymal and central architecture is altered. Cavities of liquid echopattern are seen, corresponding either to dilated minor or major calices, or to tuberculous collected abscesses (Figs. 7.13, 7.14; see also Fig. 7.6). When diffuse, the abnormalities are rather similar to those brought about by extensive, diffuse urothelial tumors.

The pattern of tuberculous pyonephrosis (Fig. 7.15) resembles that of bacterial pyonephrosis. The display of a renal tuberculous abscess requires a thorough analysis of the retroperitoneal compartments, and in particular that of the psoas muscle sheath, where a migrating abscess could exist. In later stages of renal tuberculosis, calcified foci give rise to reflective nodules with acoustic shadows and atrophy can occur (Fig. 7.15d and 7.16).

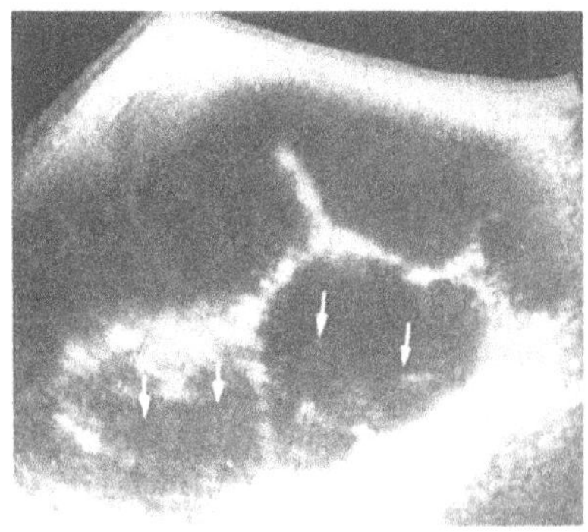

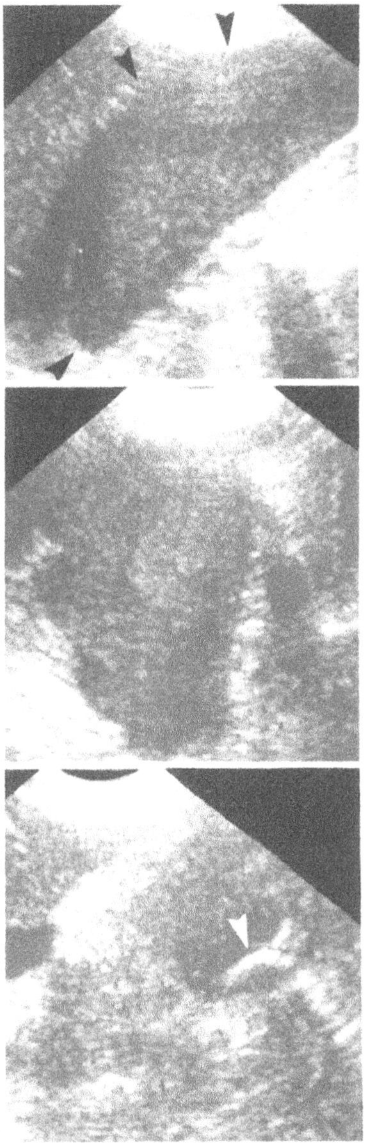

Fig. 7.11 a–c. Pyonephrosis. **a** Intercostal scan shows huge pelvic dilatation (*arrowheads*). Pelvic contents, purulent, are echogenic; **b** transverse scan; **c** parallel transverse scan shows stone (*arrowhead*)

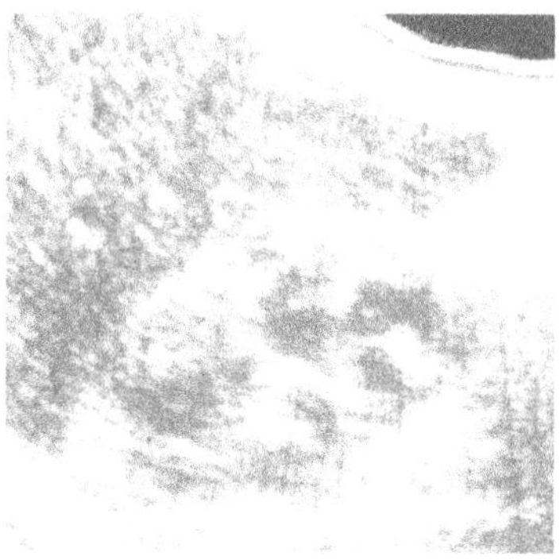

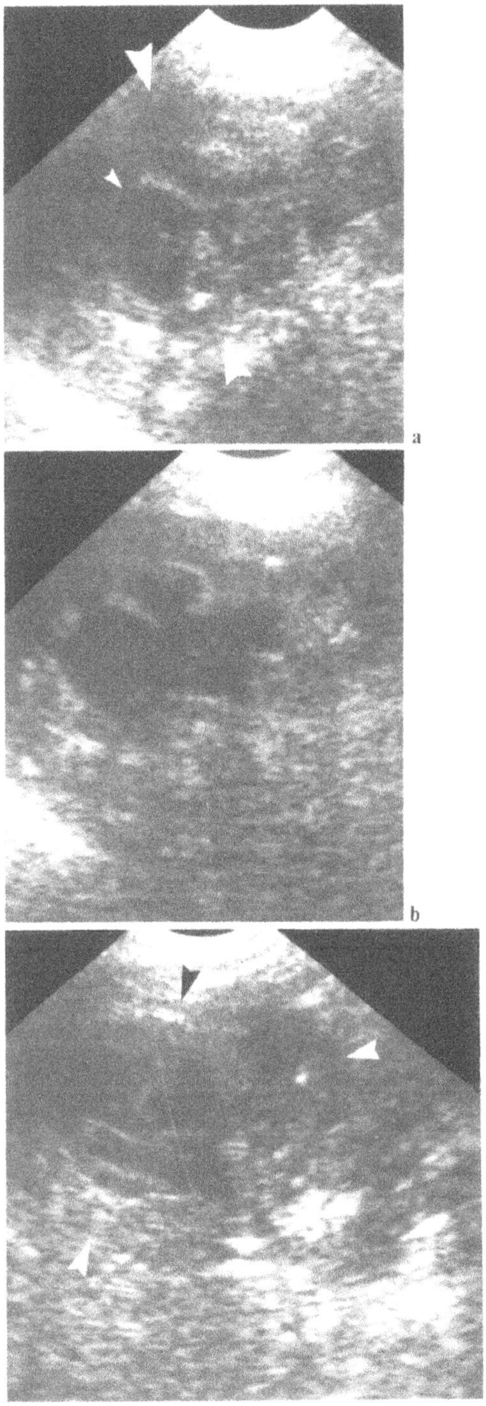

Fig. 7.13 a–c. Tuberculosis. **a** Coronal section of left kidney (*broad arrowheads*) shows diffuse changes. Defect (*small arrowhead*) is consistent with cavity. **b** Parallel scan in fact shows dilated collecting system. **c** Transverse scan of altered kidney (*arrowheads*)

◄ **Fig. 7.12.** Old pyonephrosis. Sagittal cut shows dilated calices; caliceal walls are thick. Contents are not completely echo-free

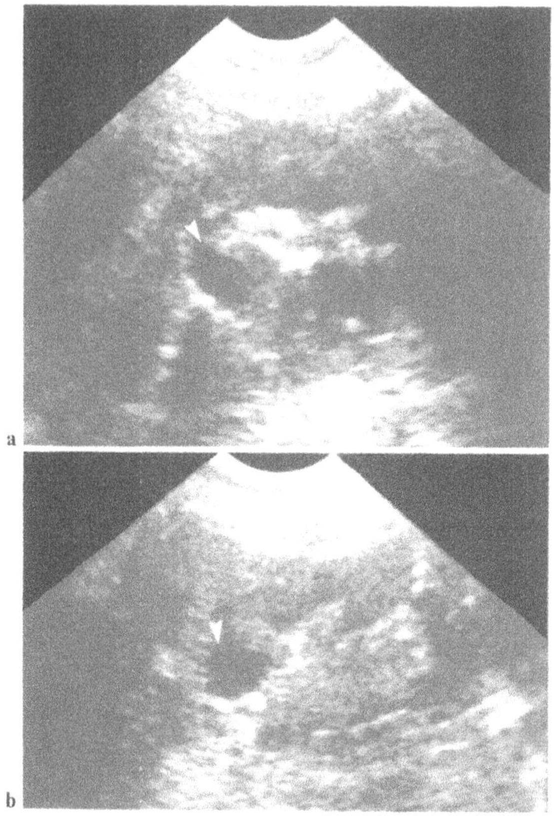

Fig. 7.14 a, b. Tuberculous cavity (*arrowheads*) which, on IVP, communicated with the collecting system (two parallel left coronal scans)

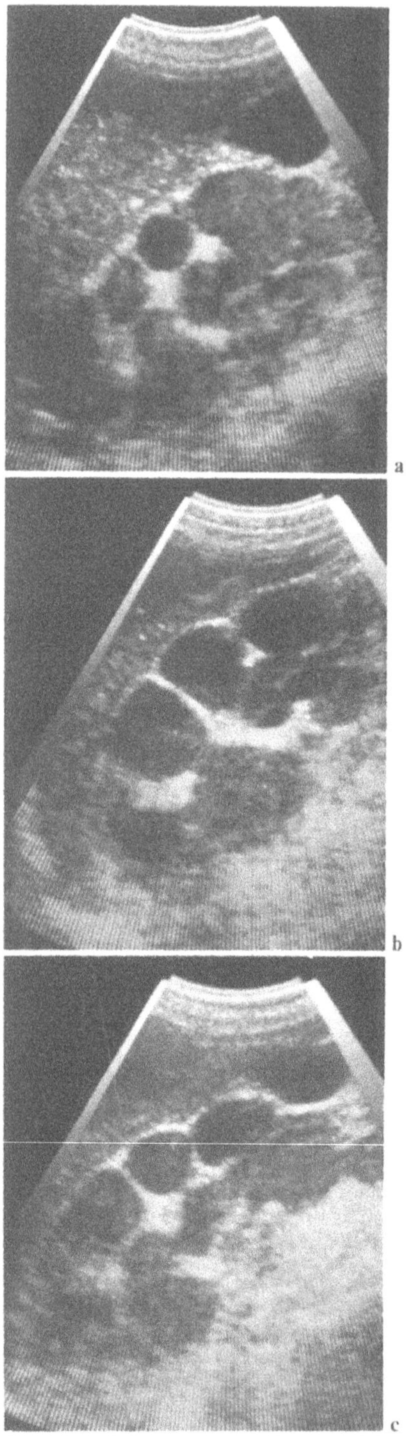

Fig. 7.15 a–c. Tuberculous pyonephrosis: several dilated areas show echogenic contents (three parallel sagittal scans of the right kidney)

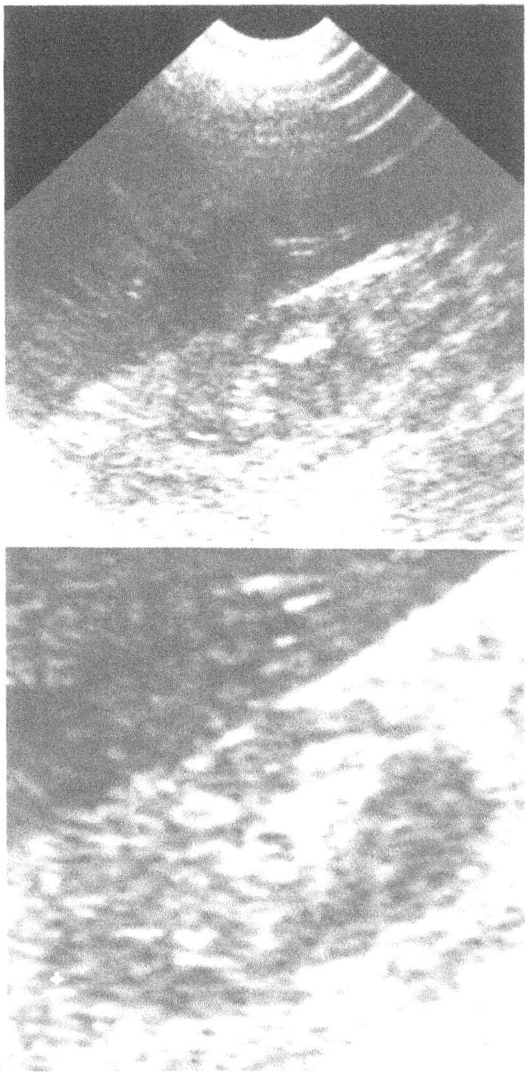

a b

Fig. 7.16 a, b. Old tuberculous pyonephrosis: scan shows asymmetrical atrophy, loss of differentiation, and calcified foci

7.5 Differential Diagnosis of Chronic Inflammatory Processes

In fact, all the ultrasonic patterns described above lack specificity. The images of diffuse tuberculosis, of old pyonephrosis, and of xanthogranulomatous pyelonephritis are rather similar (KIRK 1980). Who cares? In this field IVU remains an important diagnostic tool, with its own limitations.

It is more important not to confuse a diffuse urothelial tumor or a large renal cell carcinoma, comprising several foci of necrosis, with a mere inflammatory process. CT yields precise results in most cases. Sometimes angiography will be considered but the most specific procedure is, once again, guided puncture.

7.6 Chronic Pyelonephritis

Chronic pyelonephritis gives rise to the following abnormalities:

1. Superficial deformities with scalloping or atrophy of the cortex (Figs. 7.17–7.18). As stated in Chap. 1, cortical atrophy can be mimicked by a nonpathological anterior indentation.
2. Partial and localized alterations of the differentiation between the parenchyma and the central area (Fig. 7.19).
3. Caliceal dilatations (Fig. 7.17 b).
4. Local bulges due to regenerative pseudotumoral nodules, increasing the cortical deformities (see Fig. 5.45, p. 102).
5. A trend of decreasing renal size, partial or total (Figs. 7.17, 7.19, 7.20).

Stones can introduce acoustic shadows So does nephrocalcinosis.

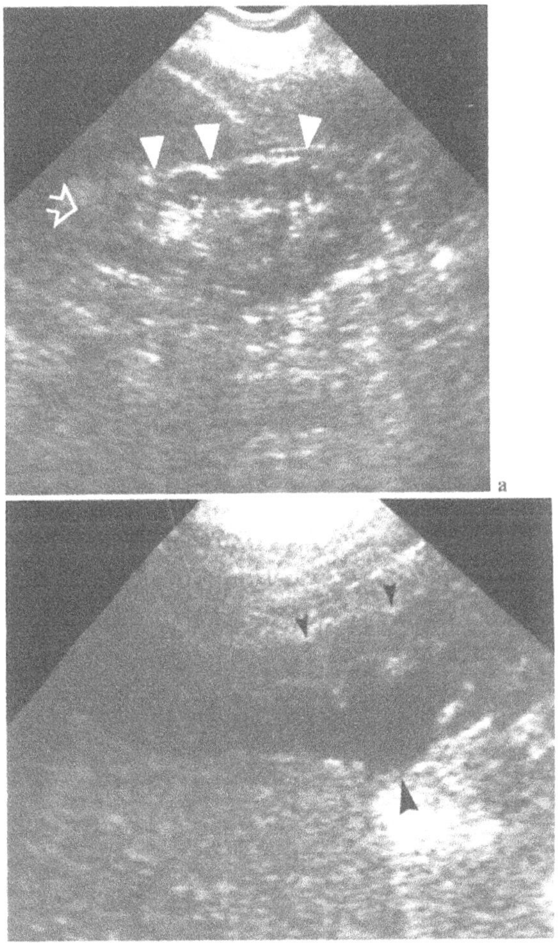

a b

Fig. 7.17 a, b. Chronic pyelonephritis. **a** Upper low pole cortical atrophy (*open arrow*). Scalloped contours (*arrowheads*). Note local loss of differentiation. **b** Another case: cortical atrophy with scalloping of contours (*small arrowheads*). Collecting system is dilated (*broad arrowhead*)

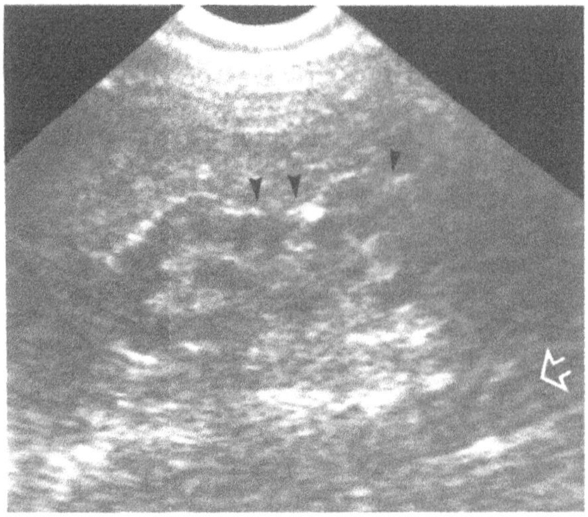

Fig. 7.18. Chronic pyelonephritis: coronal scan of the left kidney shows scalloping of contours (*arrowheads*). Note coronal section of the aorta (*open arrow*)

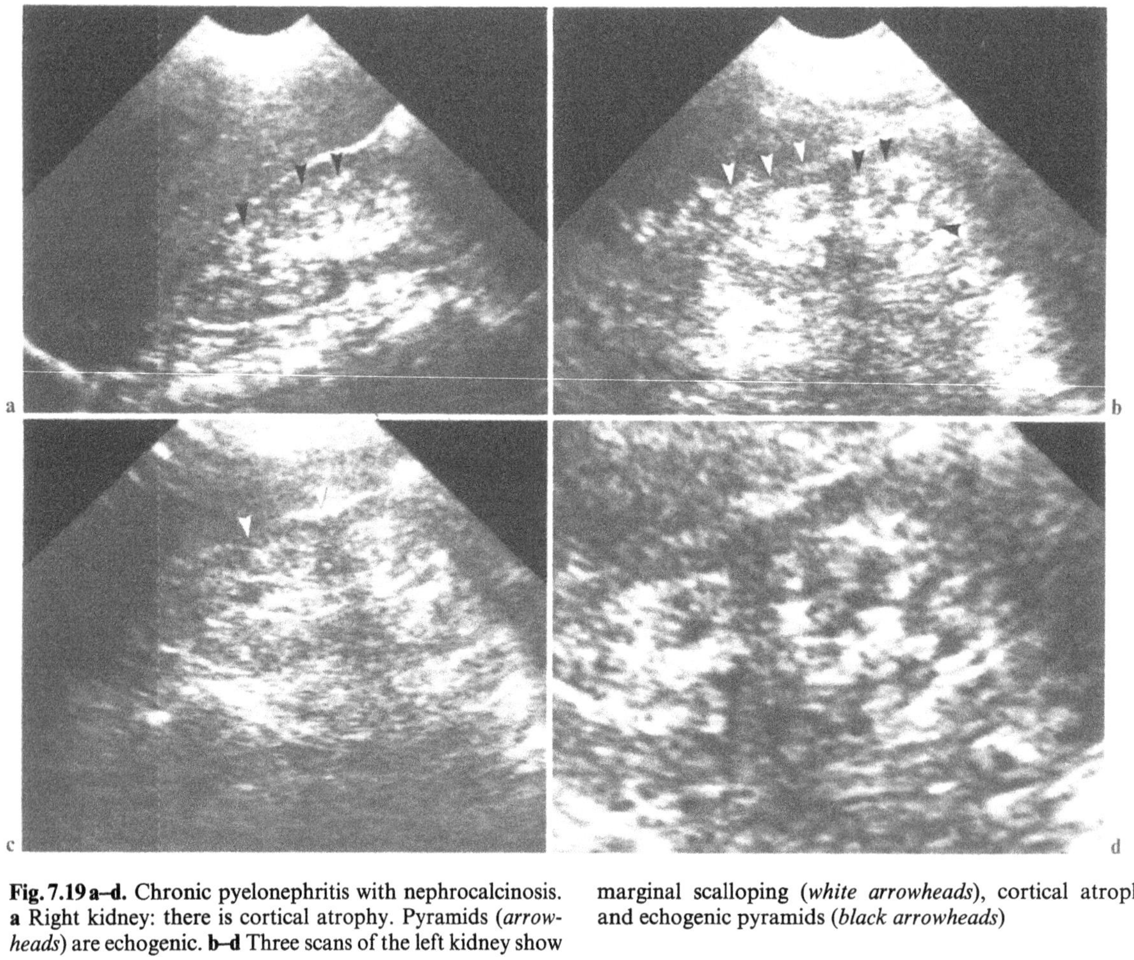

Fig. 7.19 a–d. Chronic pyelonephritis with nephrocalcinosis. **a** Right kidney: there is cortical atrophy. Pyramids (*arrowheads*) are echogenic. **b–d** Three scans of the left kidney show marginal scalloping (*white arrowheads*), cortical atrophy, and echogenic pyramids (*black arrowheads*)

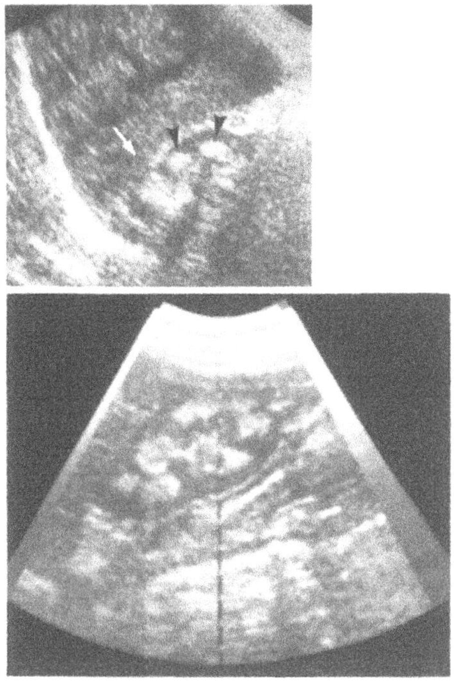

a b

Fig. 7.20. **a** Chronic pyelonephritis with nephrocalcinosis. Scan shows cortical atrophy (*arrow*) and echogenic pyramids (*arrowheads*). **b** Another case of nephrocalcinosis. (**b** Courtesy of Dr. Velay, Gray, France)

7.7 Nephrocalcinosis, Papillary Necrosis, and Cortical Necrosis

Nephrocalcinosis

Nephrocalcinosis brings about an intense medullary echogenicity, thus inversing the gradient of reflectivity within the renal parenchyma (Figs. 7.19, 7.20). The calcifications of nephrocalcinosis can induce shadowing (Fig. 7.20). Images similar to that of nephrocalcinosis, but without shadowing, are also encountered in sponge kidneys (Cacci-Ricci disease) and in caliceal diverticula.

Papillary Necrosis

Papillary necrosis induces juxtacaliceal cavities which, after complete necrosis, prolong frankly the minor calices. Sonograms then show a pattern of pseudohydronephrosis but without pelvic dilatation and with prolonged calices rather than dilated calices (Hoffmann 1982). Direct relationship to the pseudocalices with the arcuate artery in an important feature (see Chap. 3, Fig. 3.21 d).

Cortical Necrosis

Acute cortical necrosis brings about a subcapsular sonolucent rim (Selczek 1984).

7.8 Nephritides

Nephritides produce two kinds of morphological alterations: changes in renal size on one hand and changes in echotexture on the other hand.

Renal Size

In acute processes the renal size can remain unaltered. But often nephromegaly is encountered (see Chap. 8, Fig. 8.11). Conversely, chronic nephritides induce renal atrophy. The decrease in size can be dramatic in the latest stage of the disease.

Echotexture

In acute processes the renal parenchyma can become sonotransparent, markedly more sonotransparent that the neighboring liver or spleen, thus increasing the gradient of echogenicity which exists in the normal subject. But in most cases nephritides induce a frank increase in renal echogenicity, which is striking in comparison with the hepatic or splenic pattern (Figs. 7.21–7.24). The cortex tends to become as echogenic as the central zone. We term that loss of contrast "loss of cortical-central differentiation," or, more briefly "loss of differentiation." Some authors (Rosenfield 1978, 1979) attempted to analyze the morphological changes of the medulla and cortex in different nephropathies, in order to establish precise histological correlations. With our residents A. Belloir and P. Bagni we examined in 1982 a series of patients with nephrological complaints in whom a pathological diagnosis had been obtained by renal biopsy. We found the same variety of patterns, without any specificity, in all kinds of nephropathies. The same morphological features are shown in tubular nephritis, glomerular nephritis, lupic nephritis and diabetic sclerosis. Identical conclusions were formulated by Hricak et al. (1982). However, those authors found a correlation between atrophy and echogenicity on one hand, and the degree of sclerosis and renal insufficiency on the other hand.

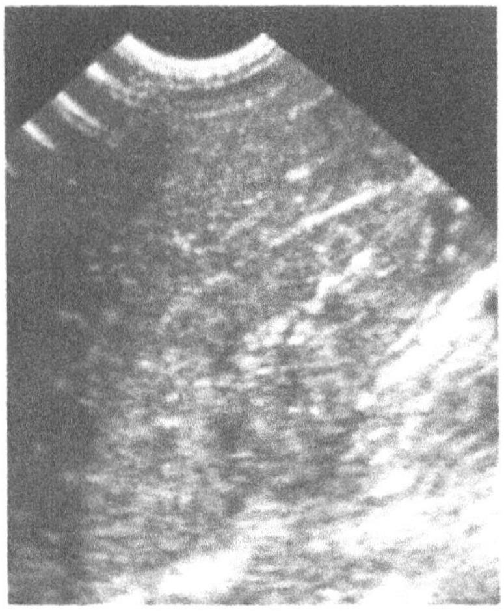

Fig. 7.21. Acute tubular nephritis. Diffuse echogenicity. Cortex has same echogenicity as liver. A few pyramids are still delineated

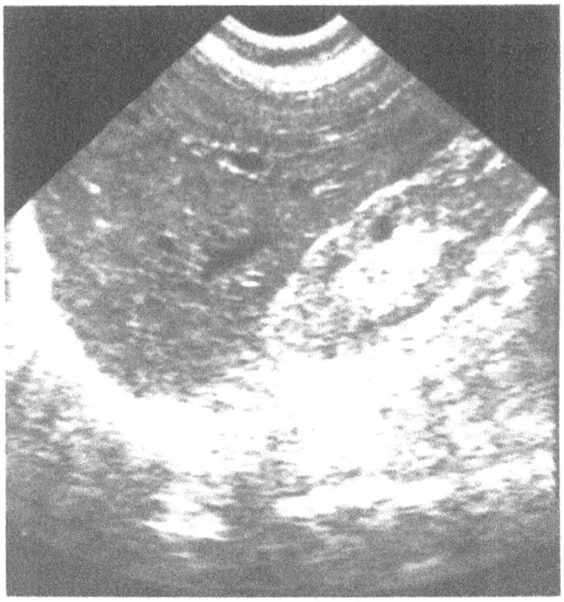

Fig. 7.23. Chronic glomerular nephritis. Kidney is atrophic and cortex is more echogenic than neighboring liver

a

b

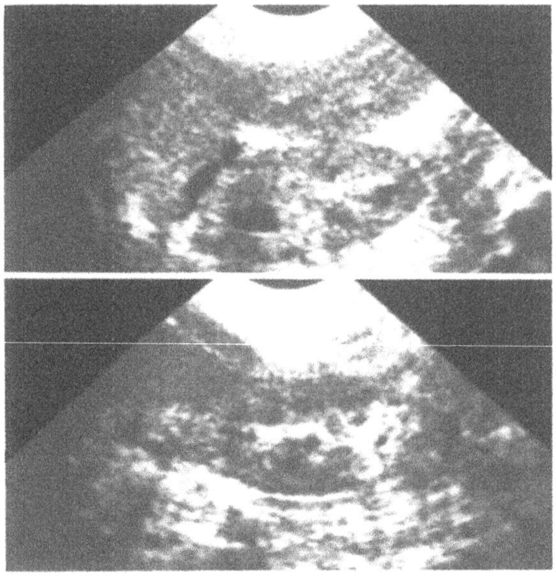

Fig. 7.22 a, b. Diabetic nephrosclerosis: both kidneys are small. Cortex is as echogenic as the liver. Pyramids are still sonotransparent. **a** Right kidney; **b** left kidney

a

b

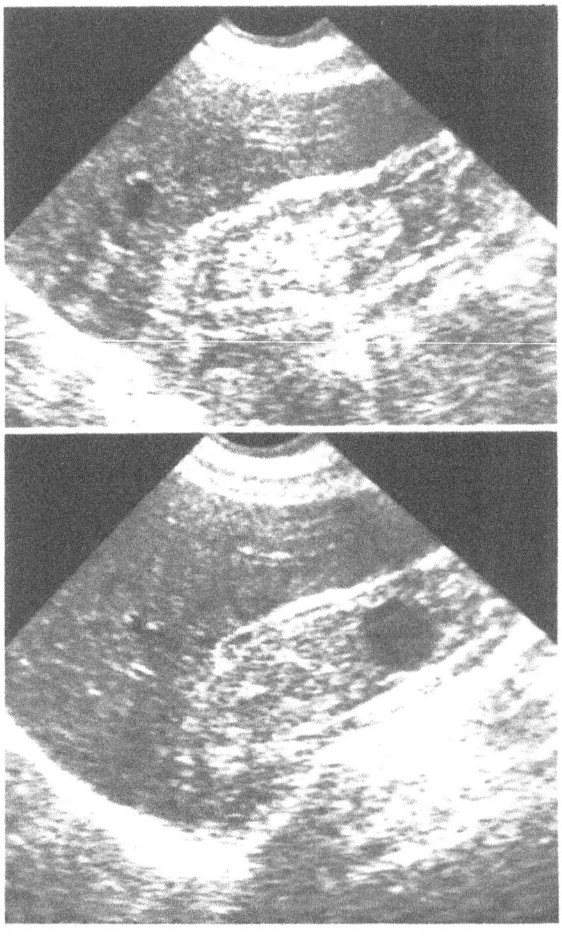

Fig. 7.24 a, b. Latest stage of chronic renal insufficiency. **a, b** Two sagittal scans of the right kidney show marked atrophy with hyperechogenicity. Note cyst in the lower pole

7.9 Postnephrectomy Abscesses

Once collected, abscesses in the lumbar fossa after nephrectomy possess a liquid echopattern (Fig. 7.25). The possibility of a solid echopattern due to gas bubbles must be kept in mind (KRESSEL and FILLY 1978). Differentiation with the colon is ensured by positional changes. In fact, since precise evaluation of the abdominal wall is required in this kind of process CT must be employed as the first procedure.

Forgotten surgical sponges give rise to marked acoustic shadowing (WEILL 1978). In such cases, scanning with a higher gain is likely to bring out several parallel linear reflections, due to folds of textile. When such intense acoustic shadows are observed, a follow-up examination after a few hours is mandatory, in order to avoid confusion with mere gas shadowing of colonic origin. In most countries, sponges are now readily demonstrated by X-rays.

Ultrasound and IVU in Chronic Inflammatory Processes

We have already emphasized the specificity of IVU in some inflammatory processes, such as tuberculosis. In fact, the significance of the rather unspecific ultrasonic patterns encountered in chronic inflammatory processes is quite different according to the clinical conditions of their display:

The discovery, during a screening abdominal examination, or in the context of anuria, of a primarily undetected diffuse renal disease will lead mostly to nonradiological examinations.

When discovered after an IVU, because of a nonfunctioning kidney, unspecific as it is, the chronic inflammatory pattern has the same pertinent value.

After demonstration of chronic pyelonephritis by IVU, ultrasound can be helpful in the diagnosis of early nephrocalcinosis or of non-opaque calculi. Ultrasonic demonstration of chronic pyelonephritis requires immediate ultrasonic evaluation of the lower urinary tract.

When an IVU has displayed images of tuberculosis, sonography will be considered only in the presence of a mass, which could be due to a caseous abscess, either intra- or extrarenal. Conversely, there is no indication for IVU after the ultrasonic diagnosis of abscesses or of nephritides.

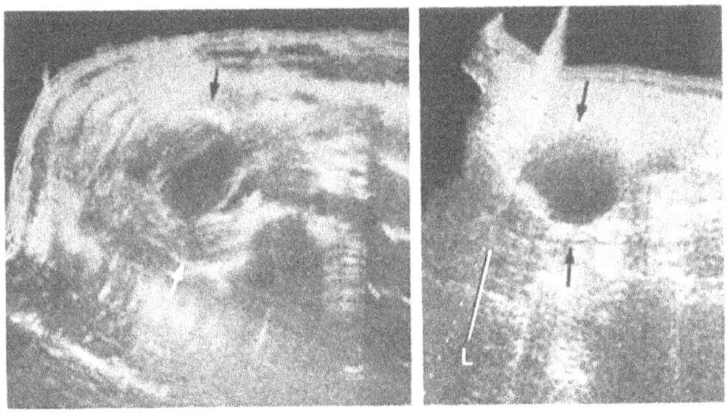

a b

Fig. 7.25 a, b. Postnephrectomy abscess (*arrows*). **a** Transverse scan; **b** posterior sagittal scan. *L*, liver

8 Hunchbacks, Dwarfs, and Giants

Renal anomalies can be encountered and diagnosed during screening abdominal examinations. But in most cases the anomaly has been diagnosed with an IVU. Ultrasound is not then of any interest.

We shall merely recall ptosis of the right kidney, often interpreted at physical examination as a tumoral process. Ultrasonic examination with the patient in decubitus and in the erect position readily shows that the "mass" corresponds to a normal kidney, located frankly below the last rib, and bulging through the abdominal wall.

8.1 Horseshoe Kidneys

A horseshoe kidney is considered when a medial abdominal mass is found (Fig. 8.1). Real time makes it possible to demonstrate a continuity between the mass and the lateral paraspinal part of the kidneys. The double obliquity of the renal crescent makes it difficult to obtain global sections of the abnormal kidney (Figs. 8.2, 8.3). It is important to demonstrate that continuity since usually there is no pyelovascular central area in the medial, symphyseal part of abnormal kidneys: their central part could be confused with a tumoral mass. Indeed, the section pattern of the central part of a horseshoe kidney can mimic a mass, whether retroperitoneal or digestive. Is it necessary to carry out an IVU once horseshoe kidneys have been identified on ultrasonic scans? Not in our opinion, if there are no clinical symptoms and no ultrasonic parenchymal abnormalities.

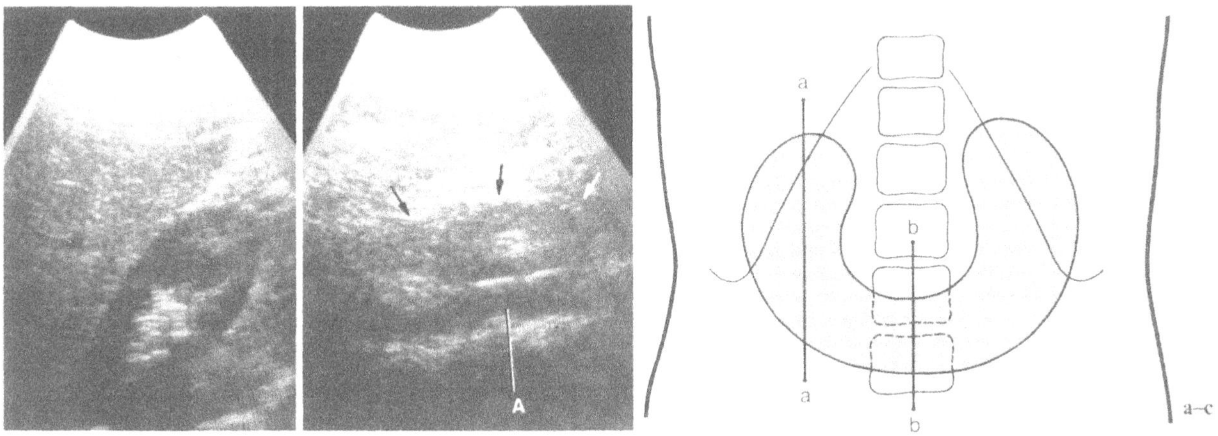

Fig. 8.1 a–c. Horseshoe kidney. **a** Normal appearance of the right kidney (right sagittal scan). Note however depression of central zone in lower pole. **b** Medial sagittal scan displays a mass (*arrows*) with a renal pattern in front of the aorta. **c** Scanning planes used in **a** and **b**

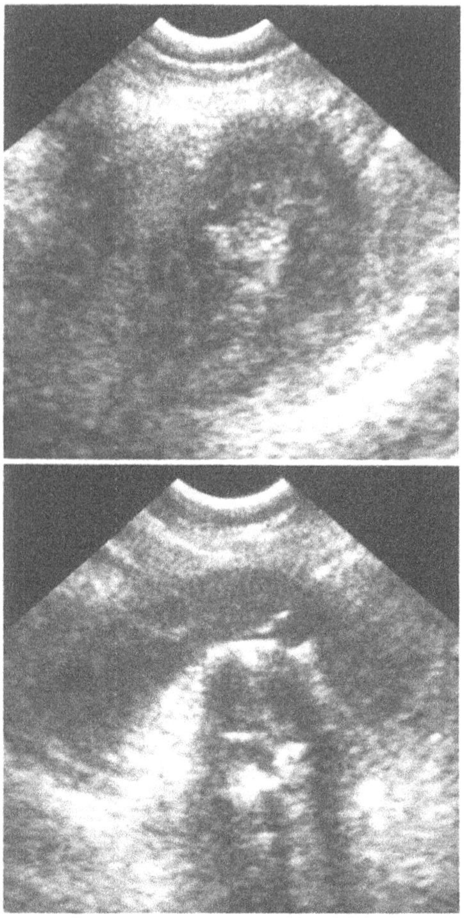

Fig. 8.2a, b. Horseshoe kidney. **a** Right intercostal scan shows an apparently misshaped kidney. **b** Transverse scan shows horseshoe pattern

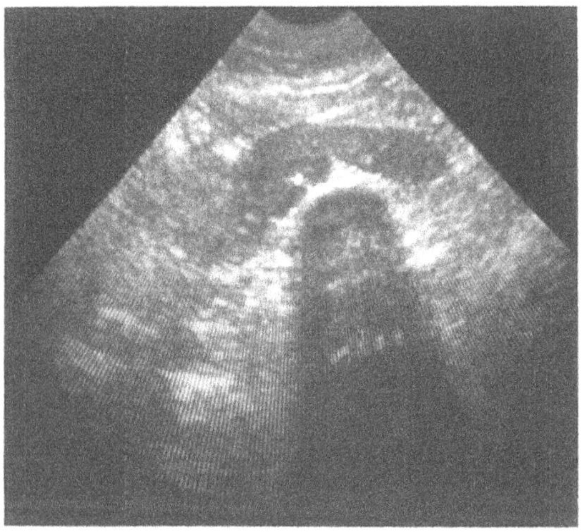

Fig. 8.3. Horseshoe kidney: transverse scan of the medial parenchymal bridge

8.2 Miscellaneous Anomalies

Unilateral fused kidneys, malrotated kidneys, or lobulated kidneys (Fig. 8.4) can be misinterpreted as being due to an inflammatory process (chronic pyelonephritis) or a tumor: IVU will permit a more accurate diagnosis; some tumoral patterns can require CT scanning.

In *duplicate or supernumerary kidneys,* the increased renal size and the separation of the reflective zone into two distinct areas can be relevant. On the other hand, separation of the reflective central zone into the distinct areas totally lacks specificity when encountered alone, without an increased renal length: it usually accompanies mere columnar hypertrophy (see Chap. 1) but careful oblique scans can display the duplicated cavities. In duplicate or supernumerary kidneys the narrower symphysis could be confused with the cortical atrophy of chronic pyelonephritis. In such cases only, doubtful images displayed on ultrasonic scans will be checked by an IVU.

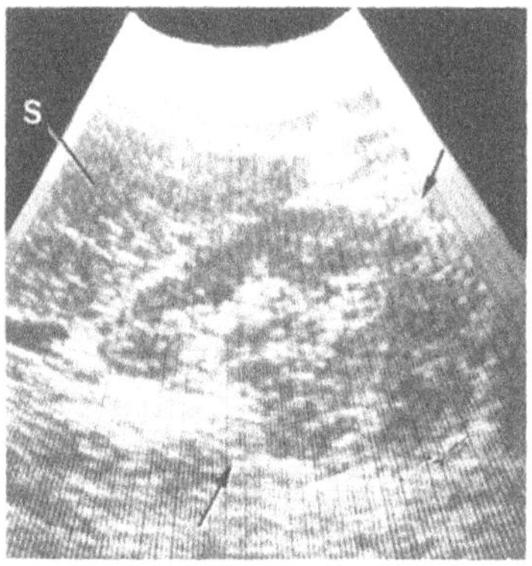

Fig. 8.4. Dysplastic kidney

8.3 Absence of Kidney; Ectopic Kidneys

In *congenital aplasia,* the lumbar fossa is empty while the single contralateral kidney is enlarged due to compensatory hyperplasia (Fig. 8.5). An *ectopic kidney must* be looked for, especially if there is no hypertrophy. Most ectopic kidneys are located in the pelvis (Fig. 8.6). Demonstrating them is not always easy because of intestinal gas getting in the way. A full bladder will help. IVU can be carried out in cases of renal aplasia. Conversely, ultrasound will necessarily follow the urographic disclosure of a nonfunctioning or absent kidney.

Renal aplasia can be very difficult to diagnose on ultrasonic scans. The colon moves into the anatomical depression whose normal renal occupant is absent, and colonic images may mimic a renal hypoplasia.

Finally when the abscence of one kidney is considered, the most relevant complementary procedures are scintigraphy and/or contrast-enhanced CT.

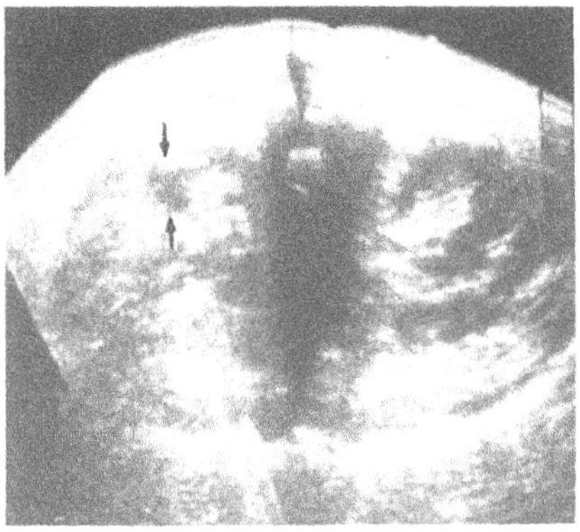

Fig. 8.5. Aplasia. Transverse scan with the patient in the prone position shows a large right kidney. On the left side no renal image is displayed. A small oval area (*arrows*) corresponds to the colon occupying the lumbar fossa. Ultrasonic diagnosis between aplasia and severe hypoplasia is in fact impossible

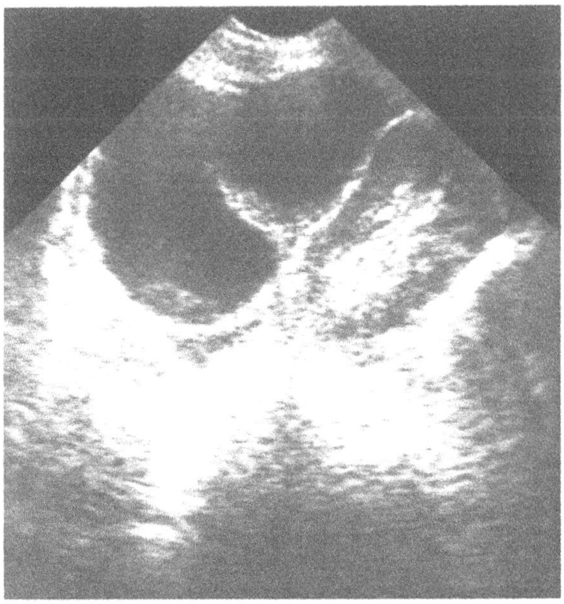

Fig. 8.6. Pelvic ectopic kidney. Transverse suprapubic scan shows the left kidney posterior to urinary bladder and associated ovarian cyst

8.4 Renal Hypoplasia

A decent hypoplastic kidney, surrounded by a thick layer of perirenal fat, gives very clear images. Congenital hypoplastic kidneys and ischemic kidneys possess smooth contours (Fig. 8.7). Whereas in terminal chronic pyelonephritis the contours of the small kidney are irregular (Fig. 8.8). In segmental aglomerular anomalies, there is cortical deformity (Fig. 8.9). We mentioned in the previous chapter that diffuse nephropathies induce renal atrophy and hyperechogenicity (see Figs. 7.23, 7.24). As mentioned above, these ultrasonic abnormalities will be considered and discussed only when discovered during a screening abdominal examination, in the context of anuia, or following the urographic disclosure of a nonfunctioning kidney.

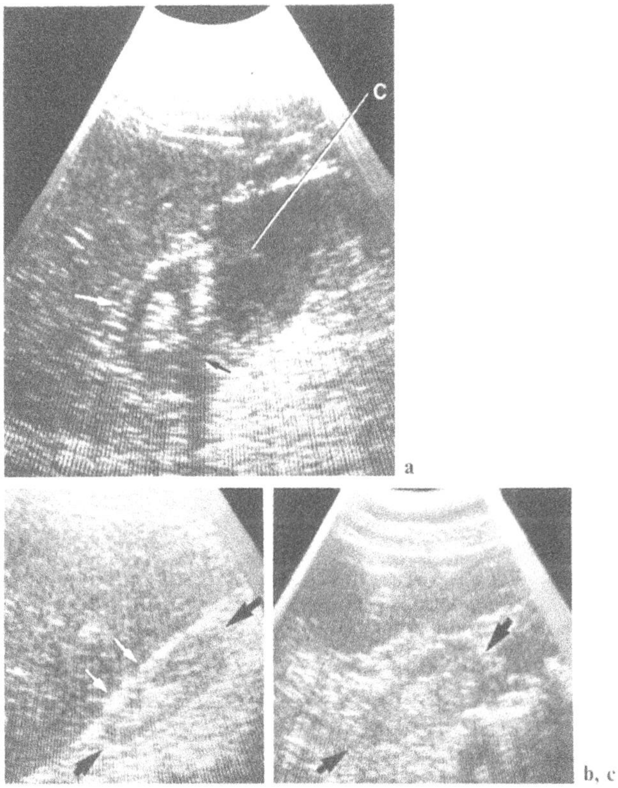

Fig. 8.7 a–c. Atrophy. **a** First case: congenital hypoplasia. Intercostal scan displays a strikingly small kidney (*arrows*). The renal axis is anteroposterior. Parenchymal-central differentiation remains normal. Parenchymal thickness is harmonious. The echo-free area (*C*) corresponds to the colon in the anterior pararenal space. **b** Another case: ischemic hypoplasia. An intercostal scan shows a small kidney (*broad arrows*). The medial part and upper pole are more atrophied (*small arrows*) than the lower pole. The anterior contour of the retracted parenchyma is irregular and heterogeneous (*C*). **c** Another case: similar scanning direction. Parenchymal atrophy is diffuse. Parenchymal-central differentiation is attenuated due to parenchymal heterogeneities

a

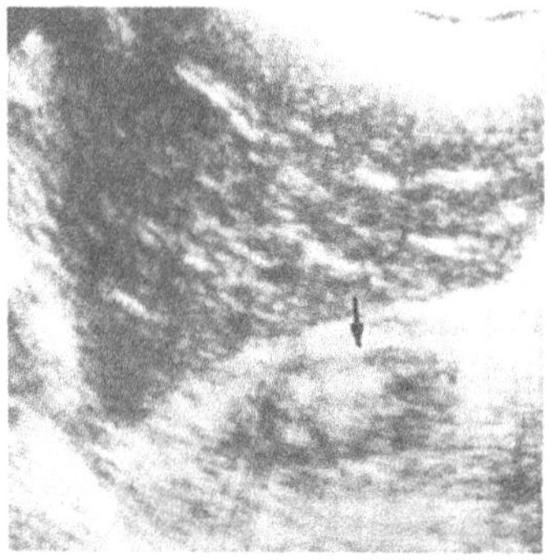

b

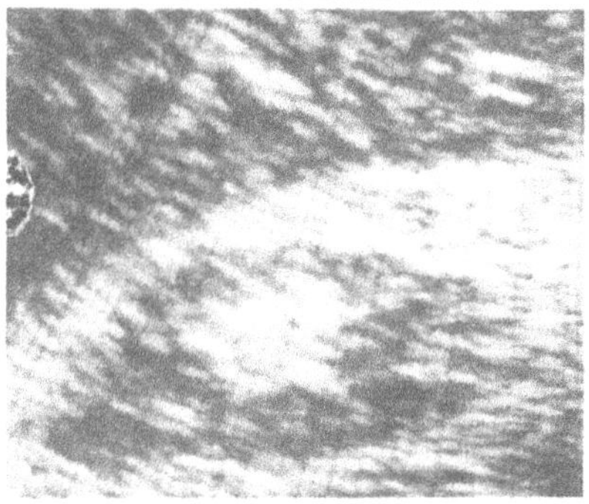

Fig. 8.8 a, b. Atrophy: last stage of chronic pyelonephritis; thin scalloped cortex (*arrow*)

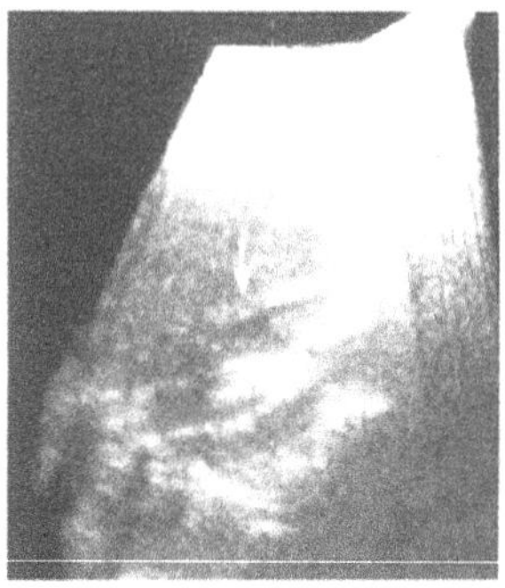

Fig. 8.9. Segmental aglomerular dysplasia. Anterior contour of the right kidney is irregular (*arrow*) (intercostal scan)

8.5 Nephromegaly

Enlarged kidneys may possess a normal echotexture; they can lose their parenchymal-central differentiation because of an increase of parenchymal reflectivity; enlarged kidneys can also possess a heterogeneous or even a nodular echopattern. These abnormalities may be uni- or bilateral. Alterations of renal echotexture in several diffuse processes have been studied by ROSENFIELD (1979 a, b). However, such diffuse echotexture changes lack specificity.

Nephromegaly with Normal Differentiation

We shall simply enumerate in Table 8.1 the possible etiologies of this kind of kidney enlargement, in which the parenchyma remains more sonotransparent than the central zone. Parenchymal transparency can be increased.

Table 8.1. Nephromegaly with normal echotexture

Chronic processes	Compensatory hyperplasia Diffuse metastatic infiltration Malakoplakia (Fig. 8.10a)
Acute processes	Acute nephritides (Fig. 8.11) Renal vein thrombosis

Malakoplakia is one of the causes of such nephromegalies. It is however, multifocal in 75% of the cases (HARTMANN et al. 180). There exists then, instead of a mere nephromegaly, a multinodular pattern similar to that encountered in some multiple bacterial foci and in multinodular lymphomatous involvement.

In *renal vein thrombosis,* sonography shows transparent nephromegaly (ROSENFIELD 1980). It may also display associated images of vena cava thrombosis. Doppler studies are of help and will lead to digitized angiography or CT. Clinical symptoms, the patient's history, or other ultrasonic findings represent the main diagnostic features in *amylosis* (chronic infection) or in *lymphomas* (lymph nodes, splenomegaly, etc.). If the various elements are absent or inconclusive, renal biopsy must be considered.

Nephromegaly with Loss of Parenchymal-Central Differentiation

A hyperechogenic echopattern is encountered in *amylosis* (SPRAMANYAN 1983), in pathological processes characterized by cellular infiltration, and in certain cases of *malakoplakia*: in the only case we have encountered, the parenchymal reflectivity was increased on one side (Fig. 8.10 b), but not on the other (Fig. 8.10 a). The pattern of the latter was more similar to the original description by LAMB and AYERS (1977). The different patterns of

Table 8.2. Malakoplakia

Nephromegaly with normal echotexture
Nephromegaly with loss of the differentiation between the parenchyma and reflective central area
Multinodular pattern

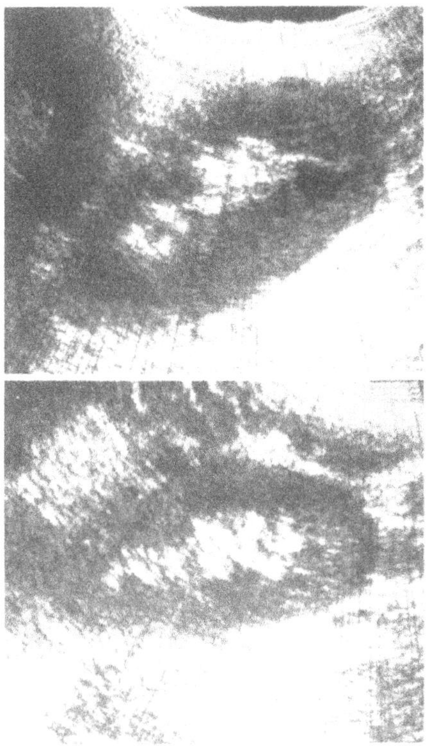

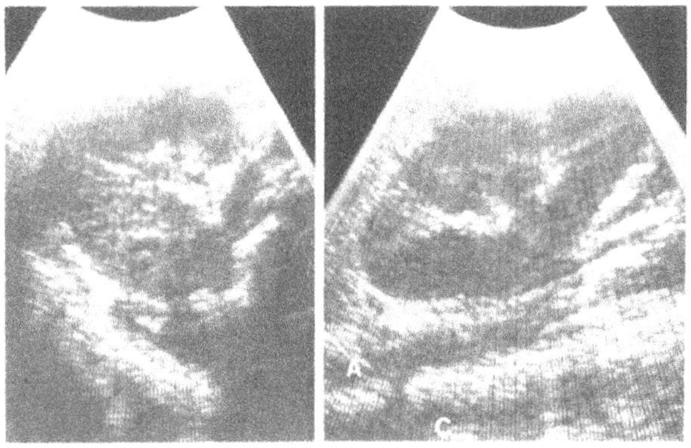

Fig. 8.11 a, b. Nephromegaly: acute glomerulonephritis in an 8-year-old child. **a** Transverse scan: renal width is 10 cm. **b** Left coronal scan: diffuse swelling of the kidney. The cortex is sonolucent (*A*, *C* coronal sections of aorta and vena cava)

◄ **Fig. 8.10 a, b.** Nephromegaly: malakoplakia. **a** Right kidney. Sagittal scan in the supine position. Parenchymal echogenicity is normal. Posterior parenchyma is more enlarged than anterior. **b** Left kidney. Renal enlargement is harmonious. Parenchymal echogenicity is diffusely increased

malakoplakia are summarized in Table 8.2. An increased reflectivity has also been reported in glomerulonephritis or lupus nephritis (ROSENFIELD et al. 1978, 1979 a, b).

Heterogeneous Nephromegaly

In our experience this type of echopattern is encountered in *lymphomatous infiltration* and in diffuse *tumoral processes* (renal cell carcinoma, Wilm's tumor, sarcoma, or urothelial carcinoma). In such cases the shape of the swollen kidney is usually altered.

Multinodular Nephromegaly

Multiplebacterial abscesses and *malakoplakia* were studied above. We shall not deal again with multicystic processes. A pseudopolycystic pattern has been reported by KAUDE and LACY (1978) in some *lymphomatous processes*. We have already described the sonolucent, almost liquid echopattern of lymphomatous retroperitoneal lymph nodes (see Chap. 6). A similar echotexture is seen in intrarenal nodules of similar origin (Figs. 8.12, 8.13). It can also be seen in cases of leukemic infiltration of the kidneys. Two signs should enable one to avoid confusing this multinodular pattern with that of a true polycystic process:

1. Abscence of thin proper walls, which are frequently demonstrated between two adjacent true cysts
2. Presence of a few scattered echoes on high-amplitude scans.

Another feature is the evolutive pattern of this multinodular process and the presence of general clinical symptoms, which are absent in a common polycystic disease as long as the renal function is not impaired.

The different ultrasonic echopatterns of lymphomatous renal localizations are grouped in Table 8.3.

Table 8.3. Ultrasonic patterns of renal lymphomatous localizations

- Simple nephromegaly
- Nephromegaly with loss of differentiation (Hyperechogenic nephromegaly)
- Multinodular nephromegaly

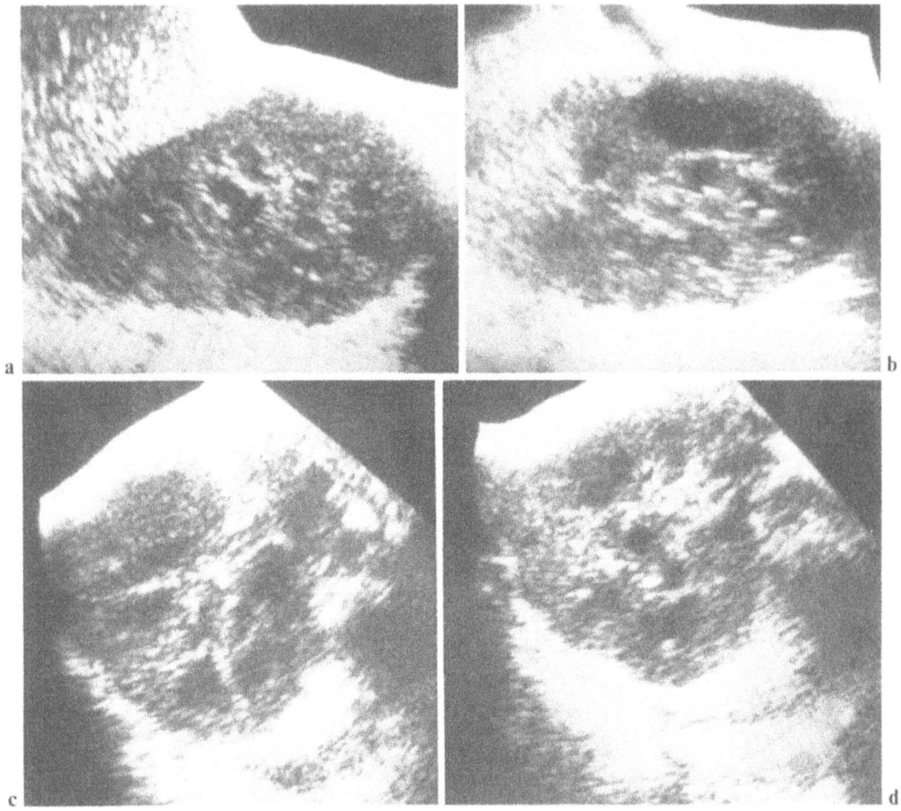

Fig. 8.12 a–d. Renal involvement by lymphoma. **a** Sagittal scan shows massively enlarged right kidney. Cystic-like areas are shown. **b** Sagittal scan of the left kidney shows a similar pattern. **c** Transverse scan of the right kidney: multiple echo-free areas are shown again. They are not adjacent and lack posterior reinforcement. **d** Parallel section. Cystic-like areas do not correspond to cysts, but to lymphomatous nodules

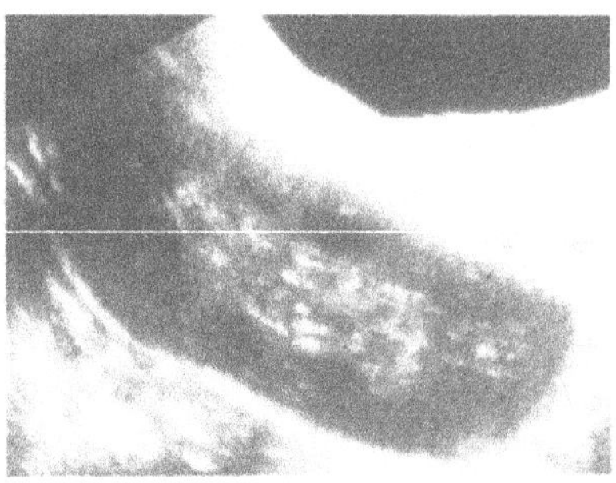

Fig. 8.13. Follow-up examination (left kidney, sagittal posterior scanning) after 10 days' chemotherapy (see Fig. 8.12). Renal size is normal again

8.6 Abnormalities of Vascular Origin

Renal Vein Thrombosis

The ultrasonic pattern of renal vein thrombosis has been studied in clinical and experimental conditions (ROSENFIELD et al. 1980). As mentioned above, acute venous thrombosis produces sonotransparent nephromegaly. Renal atrophy appears later on; the cortex becomes echogenic, inducing a loss of differentiation. Doppler studies of renal veins are rather easy.

Renal Artery Occlusion

In this field of vascular pathology, experimental studies have also made it possible to depict with precision the ultrasonic features (SPIES et al. 1984). In the first stage cortical echogenicity is increased. This is correlated by a clinical observation of ERWIN, who reported (1982) a case of renal infarct appearing as an echogenic mass. In the second stage, after a few days, the altered zone becomes sonotransparent and atrophic. We have already encountered this pattern of renal atrophy of ischemic origin when studying atrophic kidneys. A localized cortical depression can indicate old infarcts (GOLDBERG 1979) (see Fig. 5.39 b). Arterial Doppler studies are much more difficult than venous Doppler. Often only the hilar blood flow can be observed.

8.7 The Transplanted Kidney

Most sonographers will never deal directly with renal transplants (unless they need one themselves, an eventuality we do not wish them). This section will therefore be short.

Rejection

In the case of acute rejection, the kidney becomes swollen (LEOPOLD 1970; BARTRUM et al. 1974). The pyramids are unusually large and sonolucent. This causes a sharp contrast between the cortex and the pyramids, which are particularly well delineated (Fig. 8.14) (BARTRUM 1976; PETREK et al. 1977). In some cases the parenchymal echogenicity is globally increased, resulting in the loss of parenchymal-central differentiation.

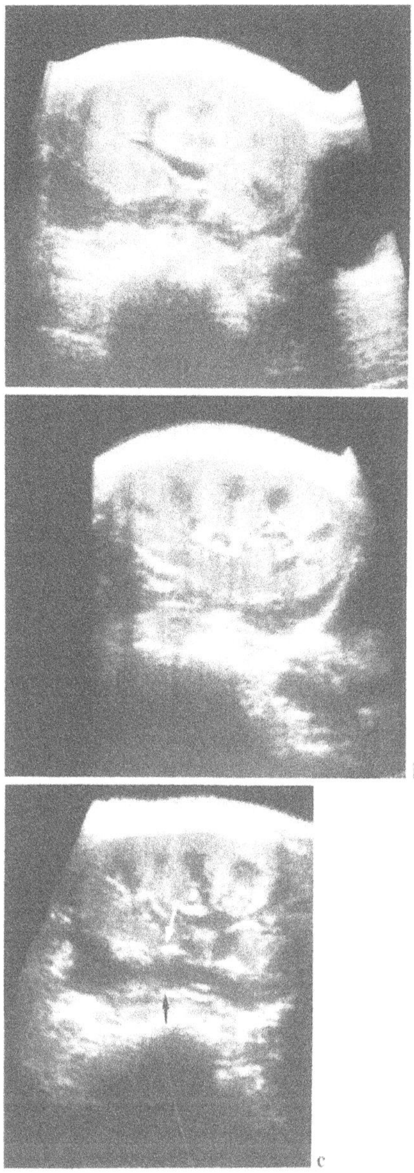

Fig. 8.14 a–c. Rejection of transplanted kidney. **a, b** Sections at 5 MHz. **c** Section at 2.6 MHz. Renal size is increased. The cortex is hyperechogenic. The pyramids are sonotransparent and enlarged. Note small lymphocele (*arrows*)

Conversely, the renal parenchyma can be sonotransparent, whereas the delineation between the medulla and cortex becomes ill defined (Fig. 8.15). FRIED et al. (1983) propose objective criteria of rejection: they measured the following index:

$$\frac{\text{pyramid width} \times \text{pyramid length}}{\text{cortical thickness}} = 4.6$$

The value of this ratio increases up to 7.50 during rejection.

HRICAK et al. (1982) reported another objective symptom of rejection: the central zone can become less echogenic. Due to reduction in size and fragmentation it can finally appear as a cluster of small echogenic islets (Figs. 8.16, 8.17). The importance of those morphological changes can reliably indicate the intensity of the process of rejection. Thanks to improved resolution, the latest machines are able to demonstrate another abnormality during acute rejection: due to edema, the pelvic wall becomes thicker (BIRNHOLZ 1985). Areas of infarction and hemorrhage can produce a heterogeneous echotexture (CONRAD 1979) (Figs. 8.18, 8.19). Spontaneous rupture of the transplanted kidney can occur, with morphological alterations resembling those of renal trauma (see Chap. 10). *Acute tubular nephritis*, which, besides rejection, represents a frequent and dramatic complication of renal transplantation, has no sonographic expression. Hemorrhage and infarctions can bring about parenchymal heterogeneities (CONRAD et al. 1978). Last but not least, Dopplerography displays very specific abnormalities in case of rejection (RIFKIN et al. 1985; TAYLOR, 1985; RIGSBY et al. 1986): the frequency spectrum of the diastolic flow disappears (Figs. 8.19 c, d).

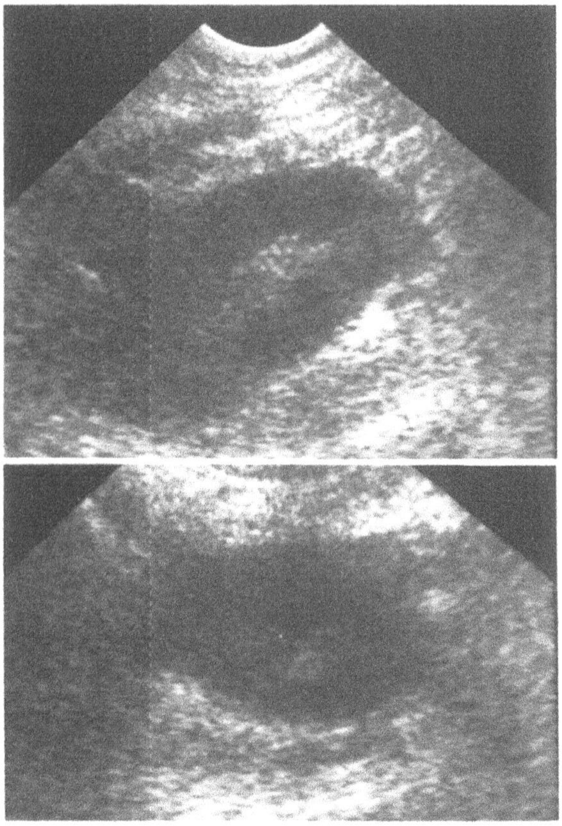

Fig. 8.15 a, b. Rejection. Renal size is normal. Echotexture is unusually transparent, with loss of differentiation

Arterial Thrombosis

Conventional ultrasound is of no help in diagnosing this condition. Doppler studies of the blood flow in the transplanted artery and arcuate arteries are very promising (PLAINFOSSE 1979), (see Fig. 8.19e, g). Arterial digitized angiography is valuable in evaluating the vascularization of the transplanted kidney with small amounts of contrast medium.

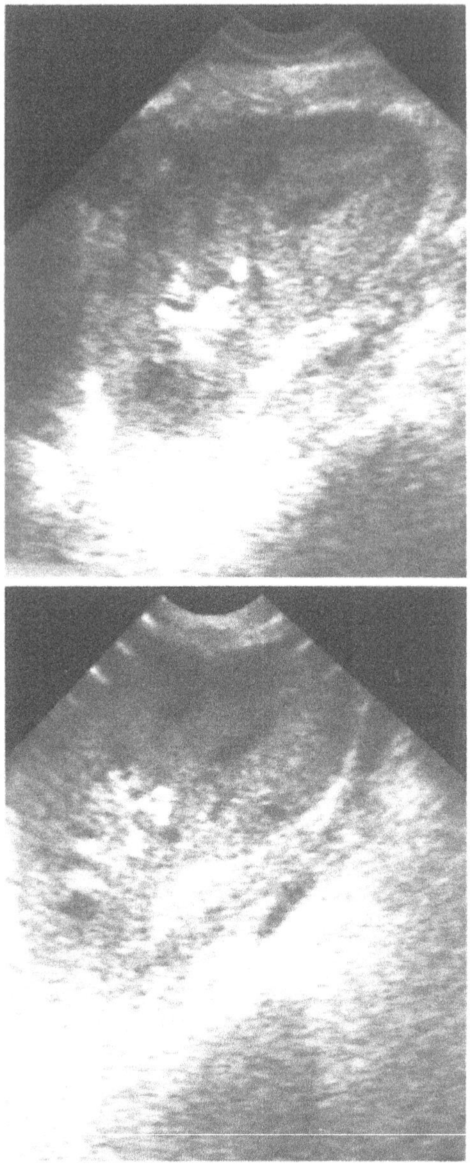

Fig. 8.16 a, b. Rejection: "vanishing" central zone. Note the thin lymphocele in **b**

Renal Vein Thrombosis

Renal vein thrombosis is accompanied by global swelling of the kidney – quite an unspecific sign in the field of post-transplantation abnormalities. Once again Doppler and digitized angiography will be of help.

Hydronephrosis

The pattern of hydronephrosis is similar to that already described in Chap. 3 (Figs. 8.20, 8.21). There are several causes of dilatation of the collecting system (ROSENFIELD et al. 1977):

1. Pelvis stenosis due either to surgery or to the cicatrization process (Fig. 8.22)
2. Stenosis due to local necrosis
3. Lithiasis (LEAPMAN et al. 1976)
4. Compression by an extrarenal collection.

Ultrasonic display of a hydronephrosis can be followed by puncture, with anterograde opacification.

If present, lithiasis appears, as we saw in Chap. 4, as an intrapelvic zone of reflection, with acoustic shadowing.

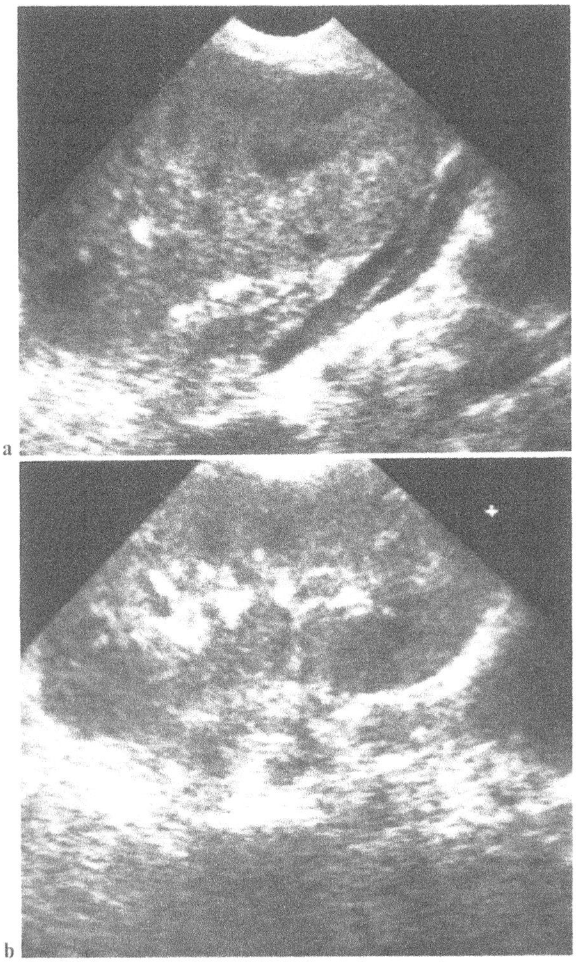

a b

Fig. 8.17 a, b. Rejection: "vanishing" pattern of central zone. Note the double lymphocele liquid strip in **a**

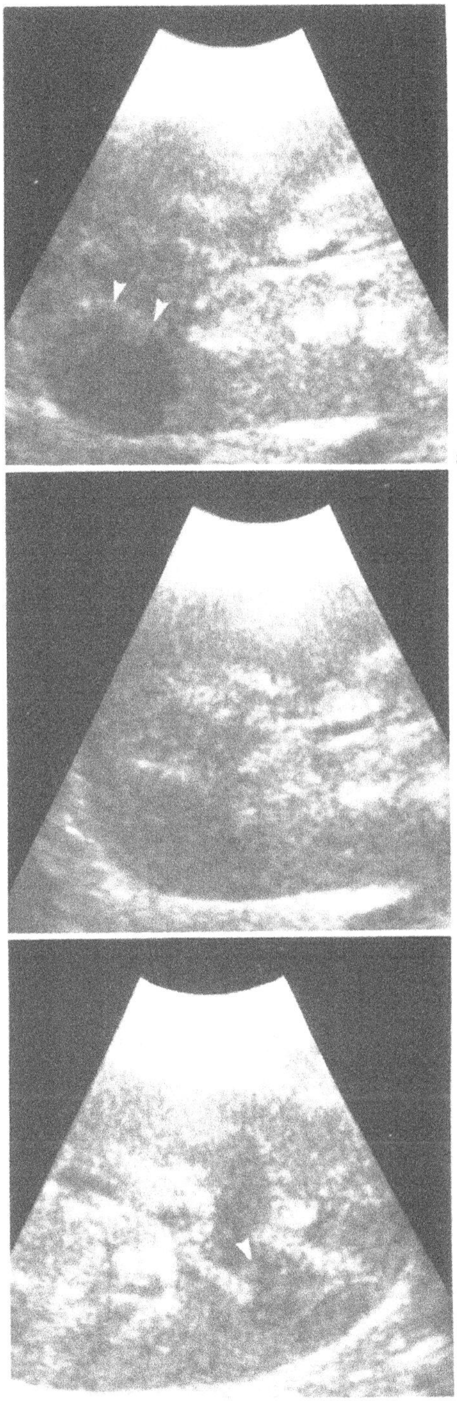

a b c

Fig. 8.18 a–c. Rejection. Three scans at 7.5 MHz show parenchymal heterogeneities (*arrowheads*)

Liquid Collections

Juxtarenal collections can correspond to lymphoceles (Fig. 8.23) (MORLEY et al. 1975), to hematomas (Fig. 8.24), to urinomas (SPIGOS et al. 1977), and to abscesses. Scattered echoes may be encountered in any kind of collection – in our experience, even in lymphoceles. A thin crescent of fluid proximal to the kidney is so common that it should not be interpreted as pathological (Fig. 8.17 a). Abundant collections will be punctured and drained.

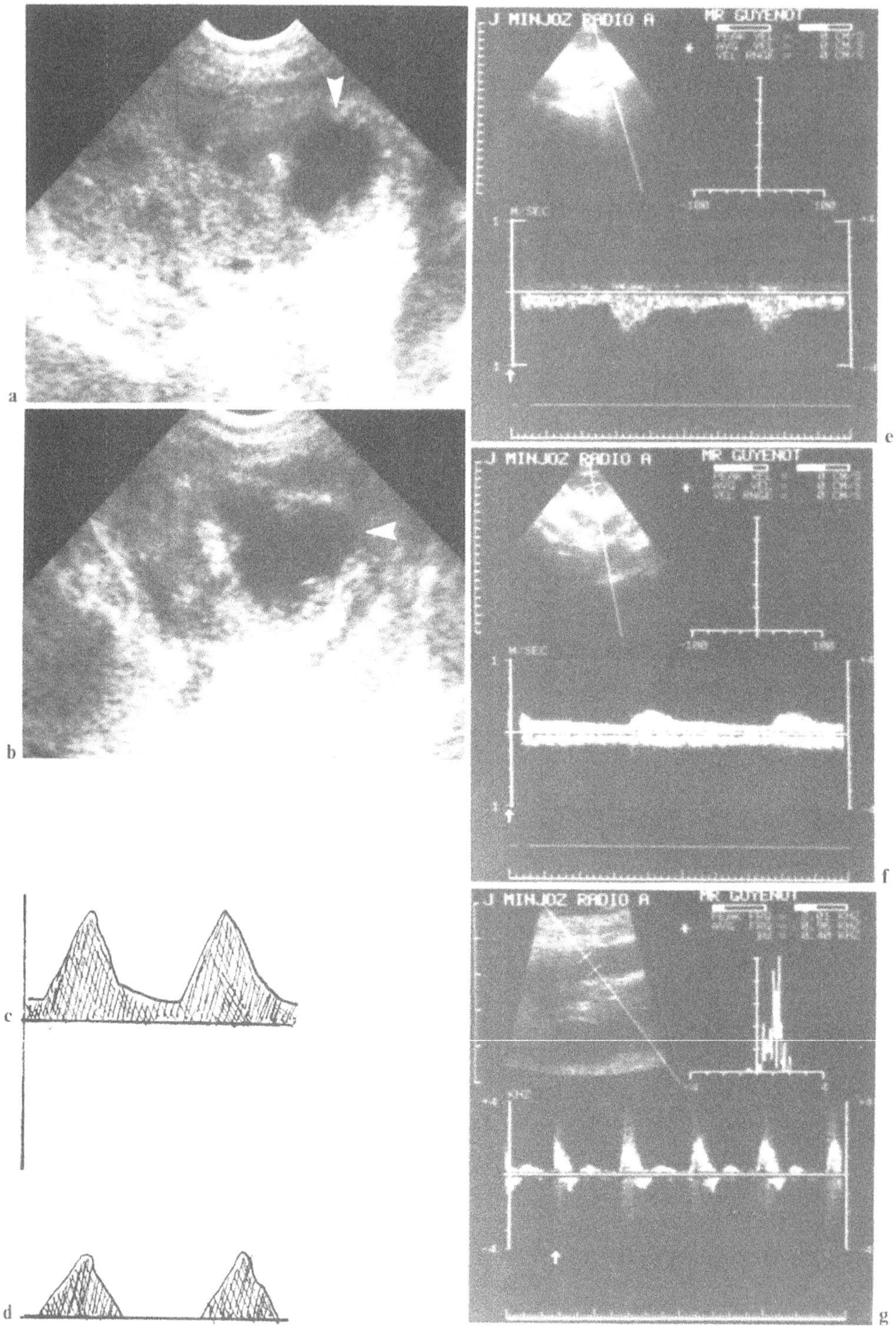

Fig. 8.19 a–g. Rejection morphologic changes. **a** Sagittal scan of a transplanted kidney. **b** Transverse scan: necrotized area in the lower pole (*arrowhead*) could lead to spontaneous rupture. **c, d** Doppler studies; **c** normal renal flow; **d** loss of diastolic flow. **e, f** Doppler study of tranplanted kidney. **e** Blood velocity in hilar artery. **f** Blood velocity in arcuate artery. **g** Blood velocity in femoral artery: note diastolic flow in visceral artery (**e**) and reverted diastolic flow in muscular artery (**g**)

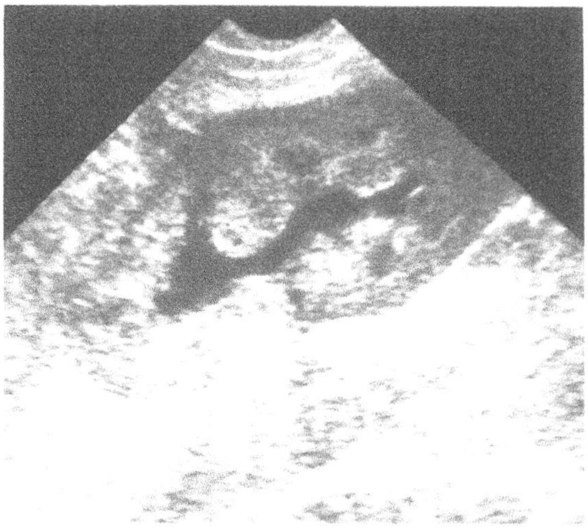

Fig. 8.20. Transplanted kidney: slight dilatation of the collecting system

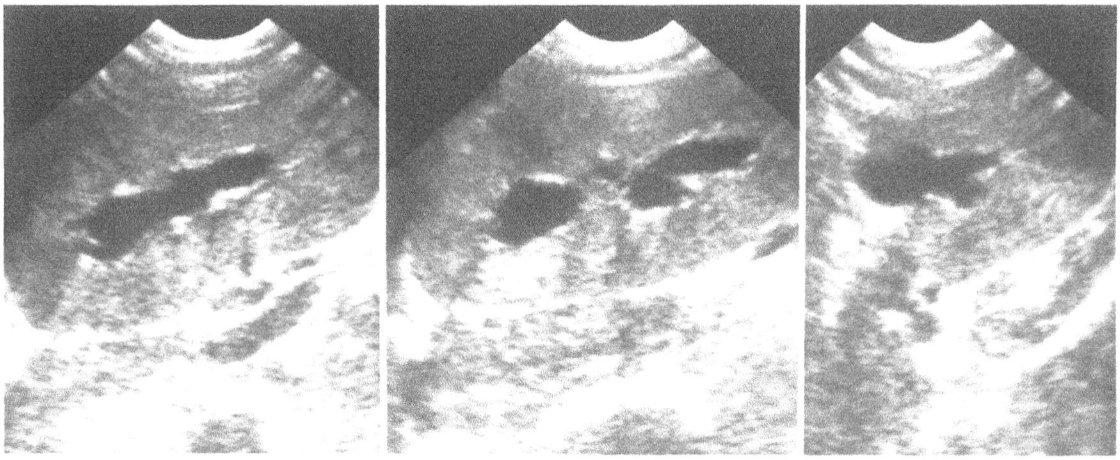

a–c

Fig. 8.21 a–c. Transplanted kidney: beginning hydronephrosis. **a, b** Sagittal scans; **c** transverse scan

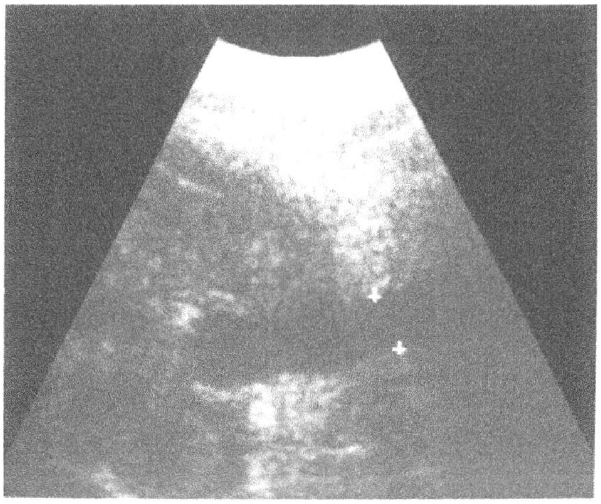

Fig. 8.22. Transplanted kidney: ureteral dilatation (diameter, 9 mm) above anastomotic stenosis

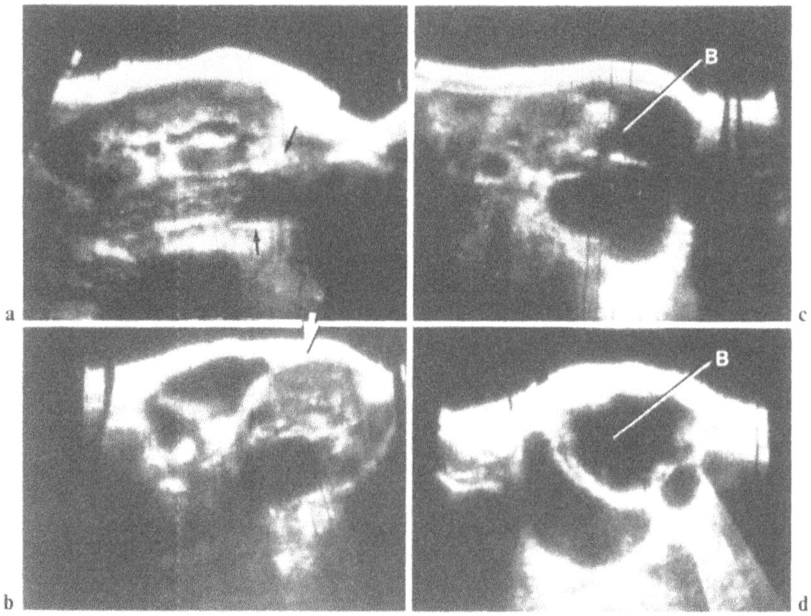

Fig. 8.23 a–d. Transplanted kidney: extensive lymphocele. **a** Sagittal scan: a small collection (*arrows*) is displayed at the level of posterior aspect of lower pole. **b** Transverse scan shows kidney (*broad arrow*) surrounded by multilocular liquid collection. **c** Medial sagittal section shows lymphocele extending behing the bladder (*B*). **d** Transverse section at level of the pubis

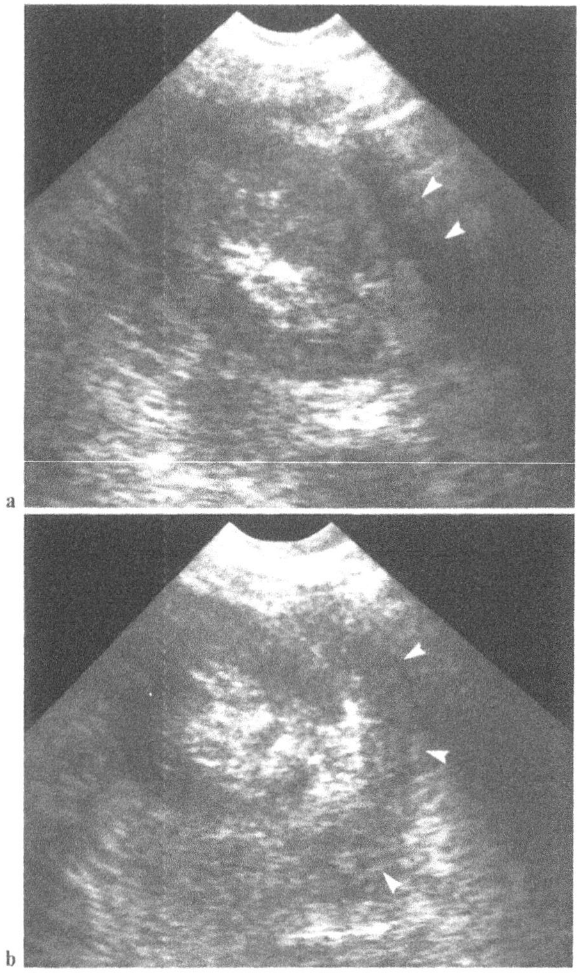

Fig. 8.24 a, b. Transplanted kidney: perirenal hematoma (*arrowheads*). **a** Sagittal scan; **b** transverse scan

Cancerization

Development of a carcinoma in the transplanted kidney can be observed in patients undergoing immunosuppressive therapy (Fig. 8.25). We have already mentioned in Chap. 4 that carcinomas arise with unusual frequency in chronically dialyzed patients.

8.8 Ultrasound in Renal Failure – Anuria

After studying so many miscellaneous abnormalities, we must stress the interest of ultrasound in renal failure. In a few minutes, ultrasonic scans may show, in the anuric patient, bladder retention, signs of dysectasia, or prostatic hypertrophy (see Chap. 12). Ultrasound may also demonstrate dilatation of the collecting system above a lower urinary tract obstruction (Fig. 8.26), a diffuse renal pathological process (Fig. 8.27), or a renal hypoplasia or aplasia. In the case of hydronephrosis, ultrasonic imaging can constitute a first step before ultrasonically guided puncture opacifation, and drainage (Fig. 8.28). Pulsed Doppler studies of arterial and venous blood velocities will still enhance ultrasound's efficiency in the field of renal failure.

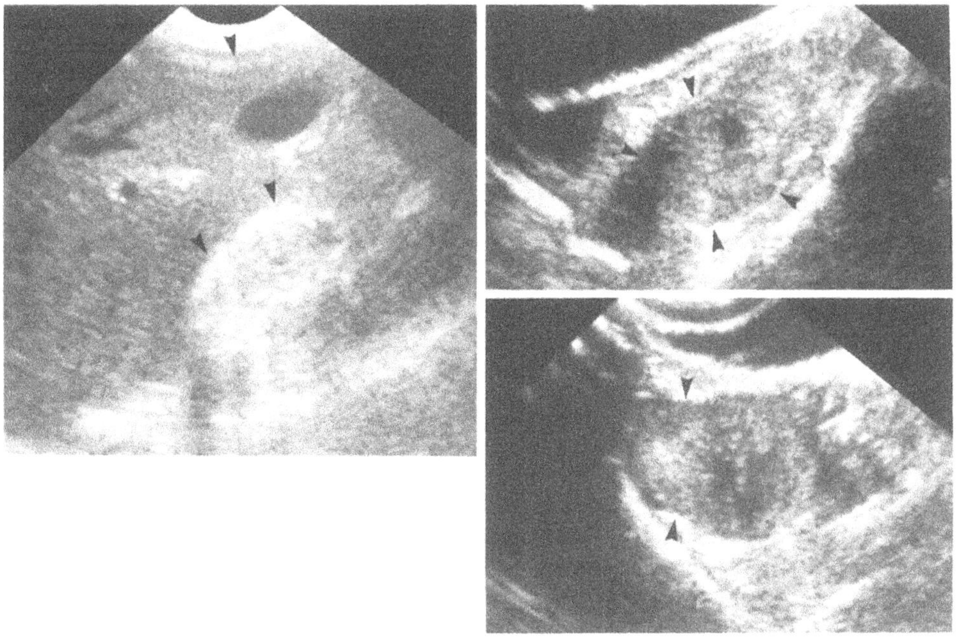

Fig. 8.25 a–c. Carcinoma developing in a transplanted kidney after 1 year. **a** Sagittal scan of the autonomous right kidney still in place (*double arrowheads*). **b** Sagittal scan of the transplant: the upper pole is swollen (*arrowheads*). A slight gradient of echogenicity exists between the tumor and the adjacent tissue. **c** Transverse scan

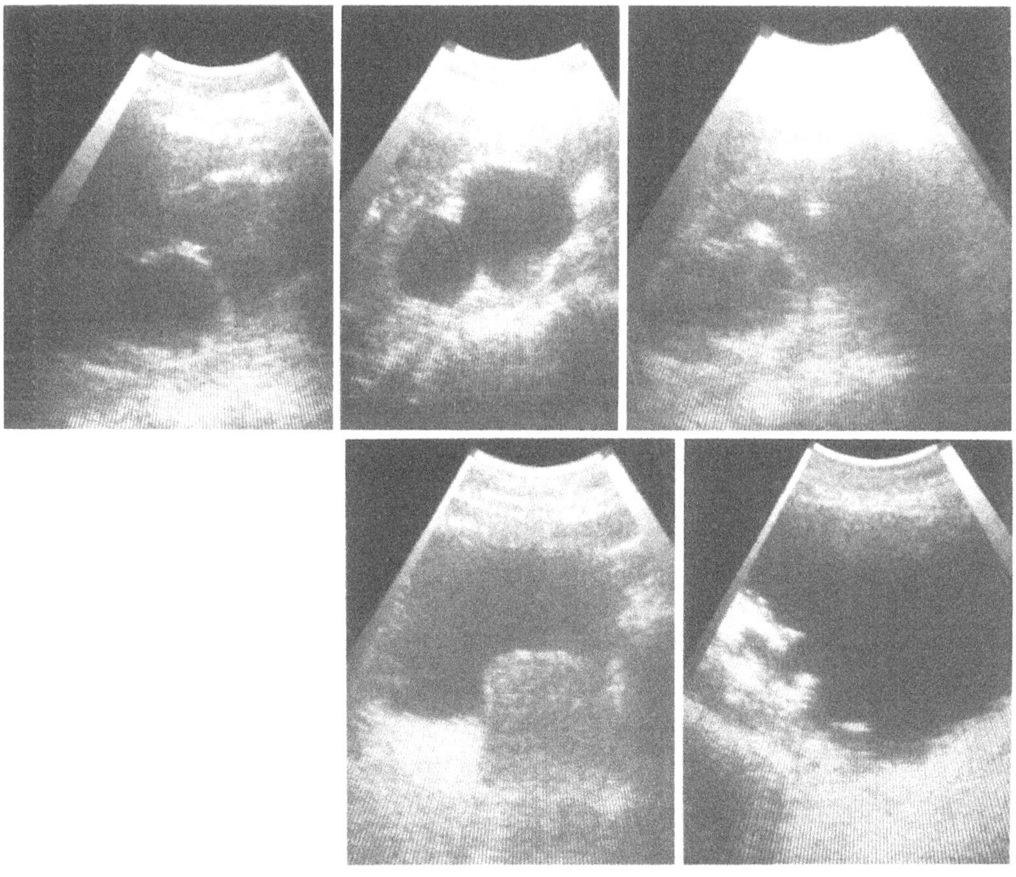

Fig. 8.26 a–e. "Anuria"-uremia. **a–c** Renal scans (**a, b** right kidney; **c** left kidney) show bilateral hydronephrosis. **d** Sagittal suprapubic scan shows hypertrophied prostate. **e** Section of the urinary bladder shows parietal alterations due to dysectasia. This is not true anuria, but bladder retention with significant renal distension

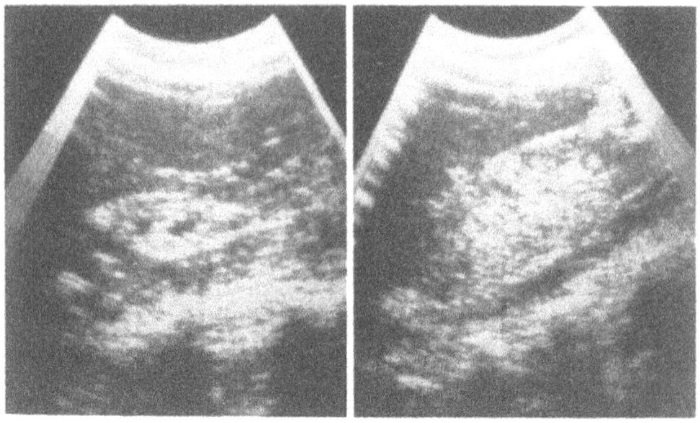

a b

Fig. 8.27 a, b. Anuria. **a** Right kidney is small; parenchyma is hyperechogenic. **b** Left kidney is less atrophied but also hyperechogenic. Collecting system is not dilated. Anuria is due to terminal stage of chronic glomerulonephritis

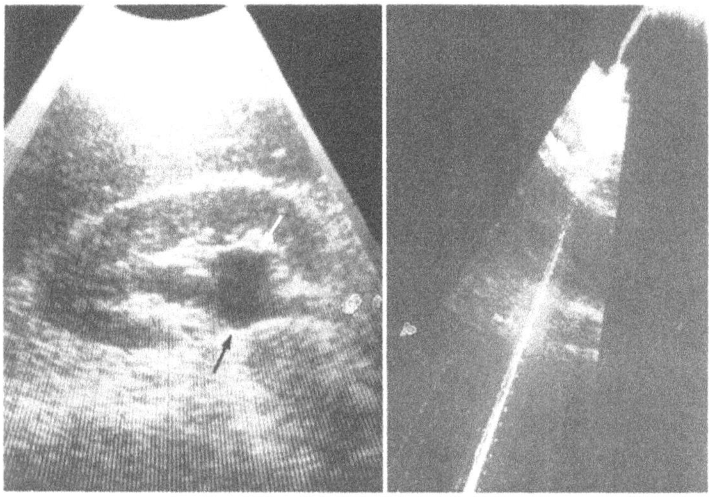

a b

Fig. 8.28 a, b. Anuria. Bilateral moderate hydronephrosis. **a** Intercostal section of the right kidney shows dilated pelvis (*arrows*). **b** Puncture in the prone position

9 Ultrasonic Differential Diagnosis and Diagnostic Policies: Synopsis

This synoptic study relies mainly on tables and algorythmic charts (Tables 9.1 to 9.12).

If a liquid collection is asymptomatic, with an echopattern suggesting a simple cyst, no complementary procedure is necessary except a follow-up examination 4 months later. Finally, following are the cysts which should be punctured: atypical cysts, cysts in young people, symptomatic cysts, and evolutive cysts if follow-up examinations showed any morphological change.

Table 9.1. Diagnosis of intrarenal frank liquid collections (see also Table 4.2)

Simple cysts
Caliceal dilatation
Pelvic dilatation
Hydronephrosis on one of the pyelons of a duplicated kidney
Collected bacterial abscess
Collected tuberculous abscess
Young hydatic cyst
Subcapsular extension of pancreatic fluid collection (exceptional)
Giant arterial aneurysm (exceptional)
Cystic tumors

Table 9.2. Diagnosis of incompletely sonotransparent collections (see also Table 4.1: 'Atypical pseudocysts' and 'Calcified "cysts"')

Infected cyst
Hemorrhagic cyst
Abscess
Tuberculous abscess
Infected dilated calix
Infected dilated pelvis
Necrotized tumor

Associated clinical symptoms must lead to an IVU: the collection may correspond to a sentinel cyst or to hydronephrosis on one of the pyelons of a duplicated kidney. Some of these images will also lead to a puncture after having ruled out the possibility of echinococcosis. Moreover, in order to avoid any hazard, it is advisable to have at hand, during puncture, hypersaline serum.

Any collection presenting a pattern other than that of a common simple cyst should be punctured. Discovery of hemorrhagic contents or a positive cytology will lead to complementary CT (and angiography in some cases) (Table 9.4).

Table 9.3. Cysts

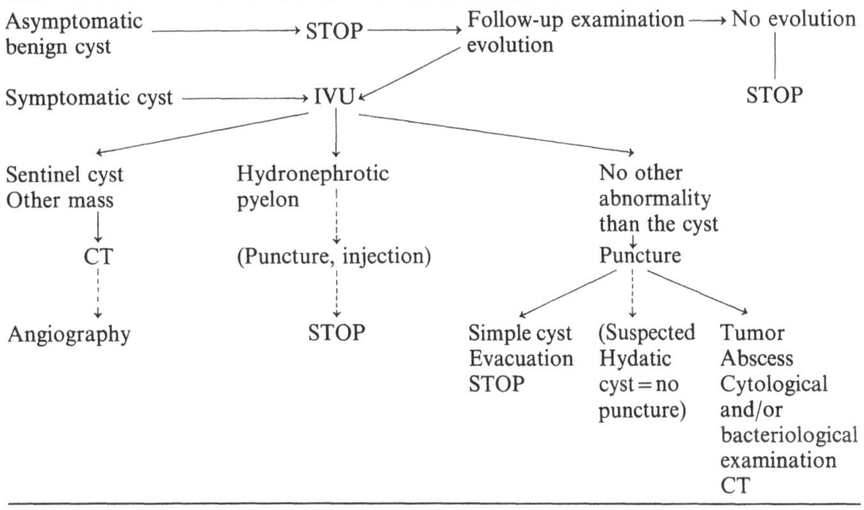

Table 9.4. Atypical cysts (and also cysts in young patients and symptomatic cysts

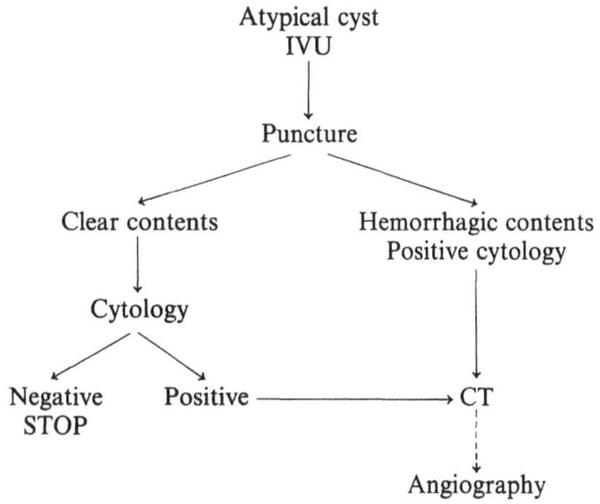

The diagnostic gamut of multiple renal collections, already presented in Chap. 4, is presented again in Table 9.5.

Any solid mass must be considered as a possible malignant tumor. IVU with early nephrotomograms is now replaced by CT for the diagnosis of pseudotumors. If an angiomyolipoma is considered, CT will show a region of fat density. If an angioma is considered, contrast-enhanced CT will establish the diagnosis.

Congratulations if you managed to take in the algorithm of Table 9.9. We have not yet succeeded. The best algorithm is in your brain, if you are a good clinician and you possess a minimum of common sense (a feature very rarely displayed on CT scans of the brain, even with high resolution).

As already mentioned in Chap. 5, the algorithm of tumors is tending to become simpler, since it relies more and more on the association of ultrasound and CT.

The last algorithms (Tables 9.10–9.12) show again that the uroradiologist's outfit is rather poor (even if expensive!). The following list of commandments was given personally to Saint Roentgen on Mount Sinai:

- Carry out as few examinations as possible
- The least invasive
- The least expensive
- STOP as soon as possible.

Finally despite its apparently high cost, CT is probably the best way of fulfilling this religious duty.

Table 9.5. Diagnosis of multiple renal collections

Extrarenal collections	Multiple hepatic cysts
	Multiple splenic cysts
	Septated ascites
	Multilocular ovarian cyst
	Cystic lymphangioma (retroperitoneal, suprarenal)
	Malignant mesenchymoma
Intrarenal collections	Multiple benign cysts
	Polycystic disease
	Multiple echinococcal cysts
	Hydronephrosis
	Benign cysts associated with other abnormalities:
	Cyst + hydrocalices
	Cyst + hydronephrosis
	Cyst + pseudocystic tumor
	Multiple abscesses
	Multiple tuberculous abscesses
	Tuberculous abscesses associated with dilated calices
	Lymphomatous nodules (pseudo-liquid)
	Tumor with multiple necrotized cavities
	Multicystic tumor

Table 9.6. Diagnostic policy in large liquid collections

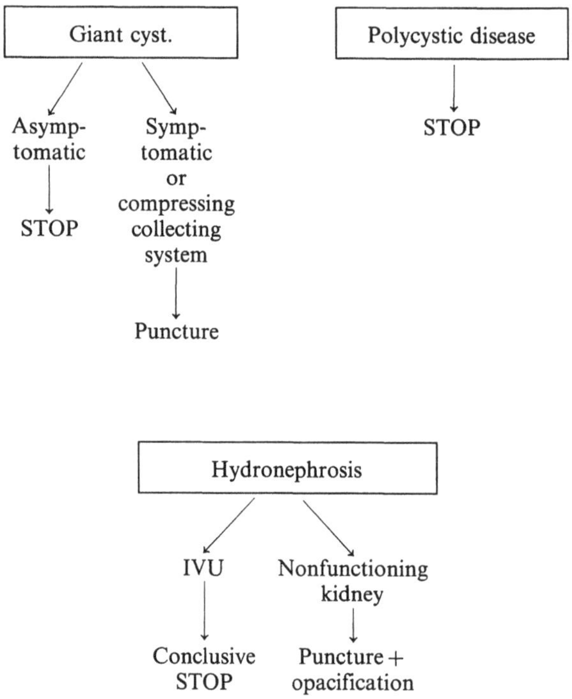

Table 9.7. Diagnosis of sonolucent solid masses

Pseudotumor	Sinus lipomatosis
Malignant tumor (types 1 and 5)	Lymphomatous nodules
Benign tumor (exceptional)	Infarction
Noncollected abscess	

Table 9.8. Diagnosis of echogenic masses

Malignant tumor (types 2 and 3)
Benign tumor (hamartoma, angioma, angiomyolipoma)
Abscess due to anaerobic germs (microbubbles)
Abscess under cicatrization
Mature hydatic cyst
Scar of renal infarct
Partially thrombosed renal artery aneurysm
Recent infarction

Table 9.9. Algorithm of ultrasonic images of renal pseudotumors

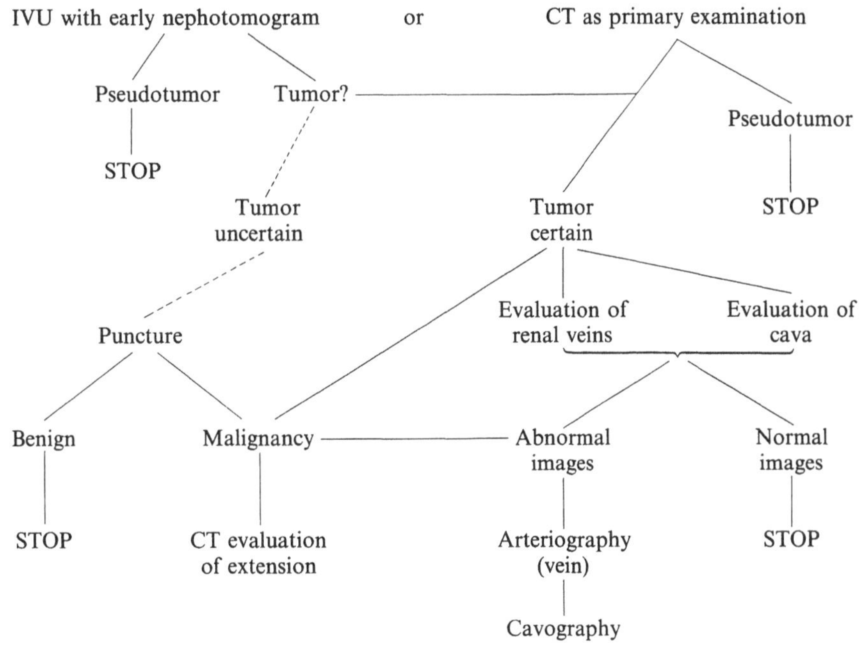

Table 9.10. Algorithm for large solid masses

Clearly renal	*Renal origin unclear*
(IVU)	(IVU)
CT (evaluation of spread)	CT
Arteriography (embolization)	Angiography
	STOP

Table 9.11. Nonfunctioning kidney

Liquid pattern	Hydronephrosis Polycystic disease Necrotized tumor (exceptional)
Solid pattern	*Small kidney* Old chronic pyelonephritis Renal artery occlusion *Hyperechogenic kidneys of normal size* Recent ischemia, nephritis *Enlarged kidney* Renal vein thrombosis Malignant tumor *No kidney* Congenital aplasia

Table 9.12. Algorithm for nonfunctioning kidney, according to results of sonography

- *Hydronephrosis* → Puncture + opacification
- *Tumor* → CT (Angiography)
- *Aplasia?* CT (Angiography)
- *Hypoplasia* Doppler *Angiography*
  - → Renal artery occlusion → STOP
  - → Normal arterial flow
    - → congenital → STOP
    - → old chronic pyelonephritis → retrograde cystography?
- *Renal vein thrombosis?* Doppler → CT or digitized angiography → renal phlebography

10 Renal Trauma and Juxtarenal Collections, Traumatic and Nontraumatic

10.1 Examination Procedure of Traumatized Patients

Traumatized patients are difficult to move: positioning in lateral decubitus or in the standing position is often out of the question. This makes it hardly possible to achieve completely intercostal and posterior scanning. A small positional trick will make things easier: the patient can be moved laterally, while remaining in decubitus, in order to shift the thorax over the edge of the bed. Lateral and posterior approaches of the intercostal region and lumbar fossa then become possible even in the supine position.

10.2 Renal Lesions

Contusion

Renal contusions give slight echotexture changes of two kinds: (a) sonolucent areas (Fig. 10.1) and (b) heterogeneous areas, with reflective zones, leading to loss of parenchymal-central differentiation (Figs. 10.1 b and 10.2, see also Fig. 10.6 b) (WEILL et al. 1973 a, b). These changes can be associated with local swelling.

Renal Wounds and Fractures – Intrarenal Hematomas

This kind of traumatic lesions brings about changes in the shape of the organ, which can be partially or totally swollen, and changes in its echotexture: echogenic areas of contusion can be associated with intrarenal hematomas, which are, in most cases, sonotransparent (Figs. 10.3 b and 10.5). Subcapsular hematomas can also be displayed. (Figs. 10.3 b, 10.6 b). Thin subcapsular hematomas do not depress the renal parenchyma. Larger hematomas give rise to a concave deformity. Large or multiple hematomas (Figs. 10.3–10.5) contribute to a general pattern of extreme heterogeneity. Perirenal hematomas are also often encountered.

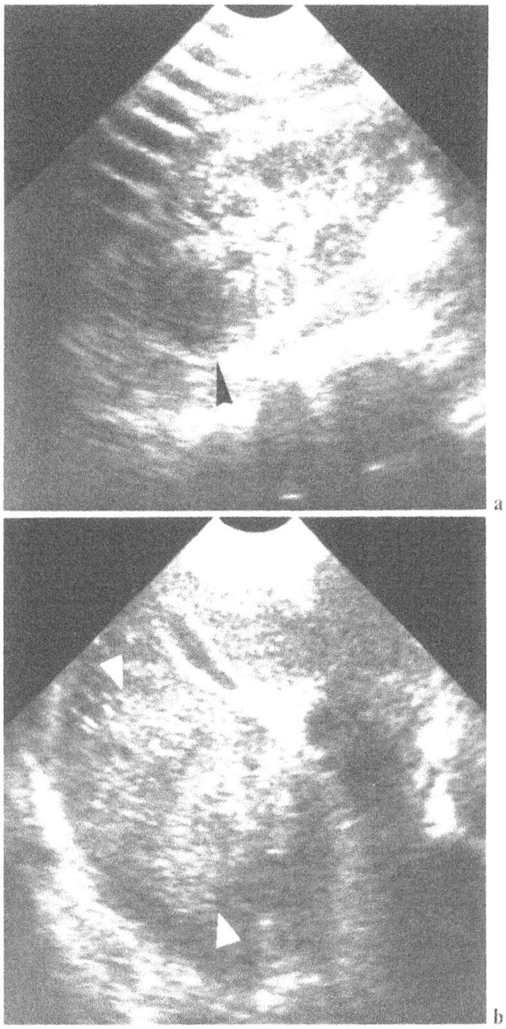

Fig. 10.1 a, b. Renal contusion. **a** Sagittal scan: hyper- and hypoechoic cortex hematoma in upper pole (*arrowhead*). **b** Transverse scan of liver: associated liver contusion (*arrowheads*). Some echogenic hematomas have a pattern similar to that of the renal parenchyma or perirenal fat and are therefore difficult to display without CT

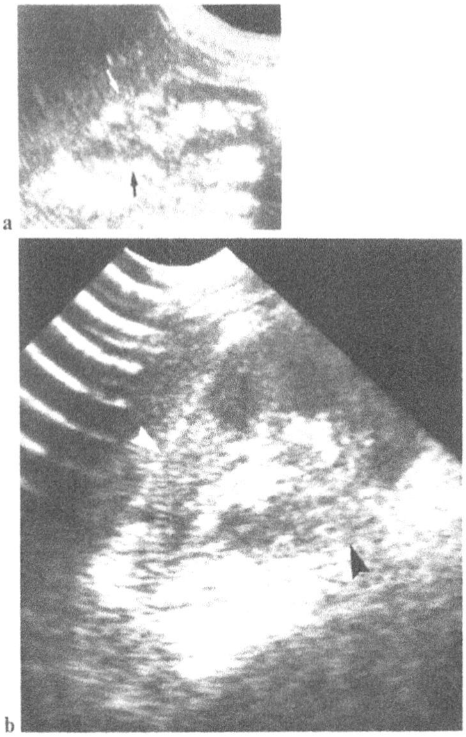

a

b

◄**Fig. 10.2 a, b.** Renal contusion: echogenicity is increased in altered areas. **a** Contusion and tears in the upper pole of the right kidney produce a heterogeneous pattern with loss of parenchymal-central differentiation. **b** Contusion of the renal upper pole produces echogenic areas (*arrowheads*) with loss of differentiation

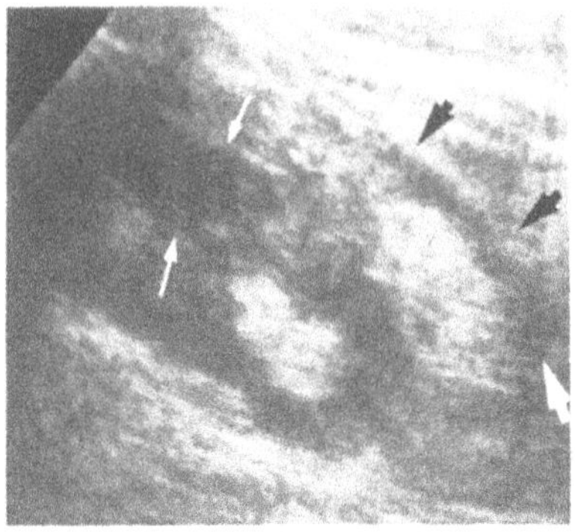

Fig. 10.4. Renal trauma: hematomas. Sonolucent area (*small arrows*) corresponds to intrarenal hematoma in left renal upper pole. The other feature is a sonolucent strip (*broad arrows*), due to hematoma, bordering the external contour of perirenal fat

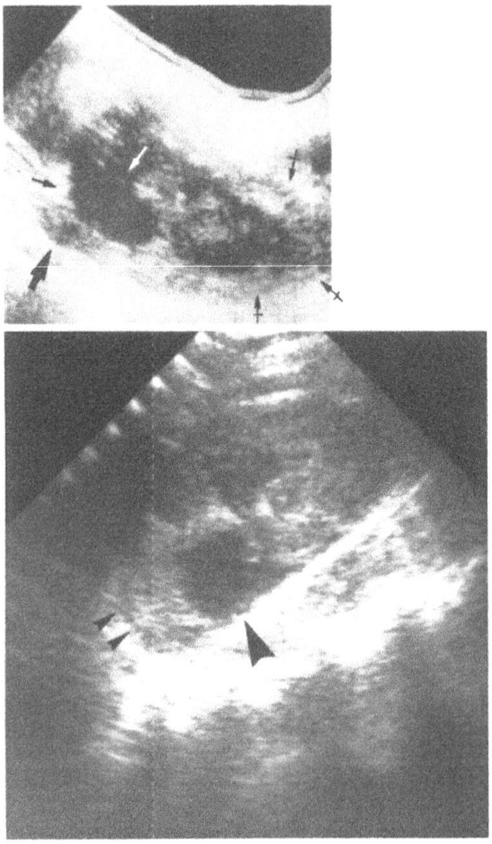

a

b

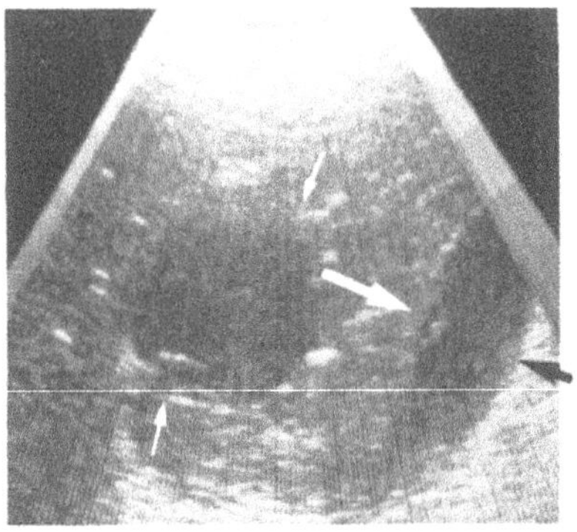

Fig. 10.5. Traumatic hematomas: an intercostal scan shows intrarenal hematoma (*small arrows*) and subcapsular hematoma (*large arrows*) depressing the parenchyma

◄**Fig. 10.3. a** Renal fracture with subcapsular hematoma. Sagittal scan of left kidney. Sonotransparent area (*small arrows*) corresponds to subcapsular hematoma. The general pattern of the renal tissue is altered. A small sonolucent zone in the lower pole indicates intrarenal hematoma. Note the decreased echogenicity of the perirenal fat associated with zones of heterogeneity (*broad arrow*), due to bleeding. **b** Another case. Hyperechogenic cortex. Thin subcapsular hematoma (*double arrowhead*) and intraparenchymal hematoma (*arrowhead*) in upper pole

10.3 Juxtarenal Abnormalities

Hematomas

Small hematomas, appearing as thin sonolucent strips (Figs. 10.6–10.8), are usually located in the perirenal space. Such small hematomas are often encountered following renal biopsies (WEILL 1973 a, b).

Hematomas are liable to occupy a much larger part of the perirenal space. They can also fuse and expand into the anterior or posterior pararenal spaces (Figs. 10.4, 10.9, 10.10).

Usually perirenal hematomas do not alter the convex shape of the renal contour. Contrarywise, large subcapsular hematomas depress the renal parenchyma, whose contour becomes concave (Fig. 10.5). Some juxtarenal hematomas are particularly abundant (Figs. 10.9, 10.10).

The association of renal lesions with juxtarenal hematomas gives rise to complex heterogeneous mass images (Fig. 10.11). In most cases free fresh blood is moderately echogenic. Recent hematomas are usually transparent, whereas older hematomas, with blood clots, are echogenic (features which are quite different from those displayed by CT since recent hematomas have higher *H* values). But we must underline that those ultrasonic characters are far from being constant. Recent blood clots are sometimes echogenic.

Despite the retroperitoneal location of the kidney, renal traumatic lesions can be accompanied by a hemoperitoneum. As in all other cases of abdominal emergency, renal trauma requires a thorough ultrasonic analysis of all peritoneal recesses. In the recumbent patient small quantities of free blood accumulate in Douglas' sac (Fig. 10.12 a). The evaluation of the lower urinary tract can disclose intravesical blood (Fig. 10.12 b, c).

If the patient is not operated on, follow-up examinations may show a regression of ultrasonic abnormalities, especially of hematomas.

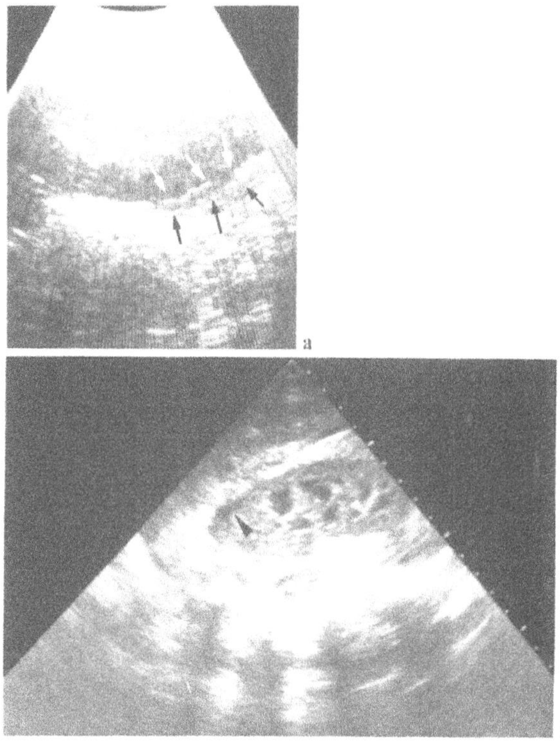

Fig. 10.6. a Thin perirenal hematoma (*arrows*) after biopsy. **b** Thin subcapsular hematoma (*arrowhead*). Note loss of cortex-medullary differentiation due to diffuse hyperechogenicity

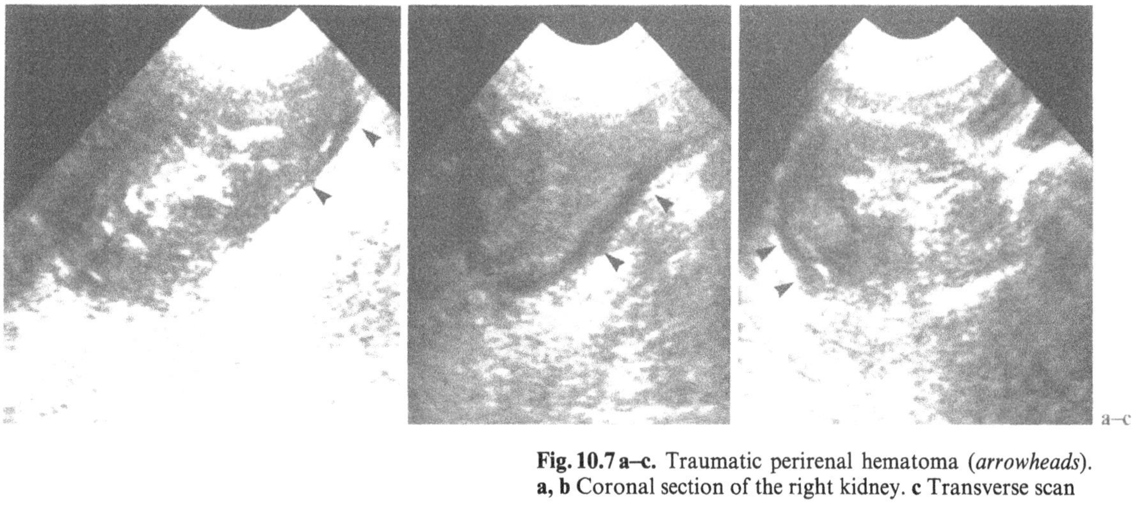

Fig. 10.7 a–c. Traumatic perirenal hematoma (*arrowheads*). **a, b** Coronal section of the right kidney. **c** Transverse scan

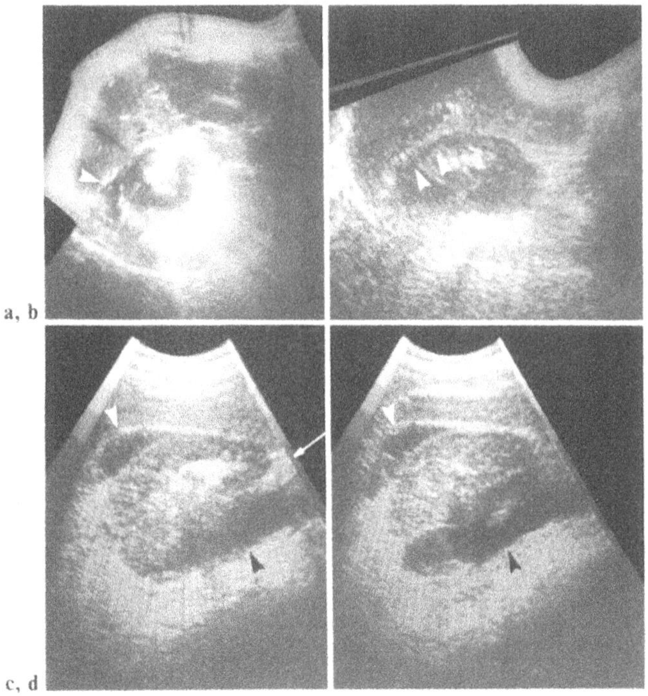

Fig. 10.8a–d. Traumatic hematomas. **a** Transverse scan shows perirenal hematoma (*arrowheads*). **b** Sagittal scan discloses a thin subcapsular hematoma (*arrowheads*). **c, d** Two parallel intercostal scans show two distinct hematomas. First image (*white arrowhead*) could lead to discussion either of subcapsular hematoma or of perirenal hematoma. Delineation of capsule is in favor of the first hypothesis. The second hematoma (*black arrowhead*) is separated from the renal lower pole by a fatty strip (*white arrow*). This indicates extracapsular location of the hematoma

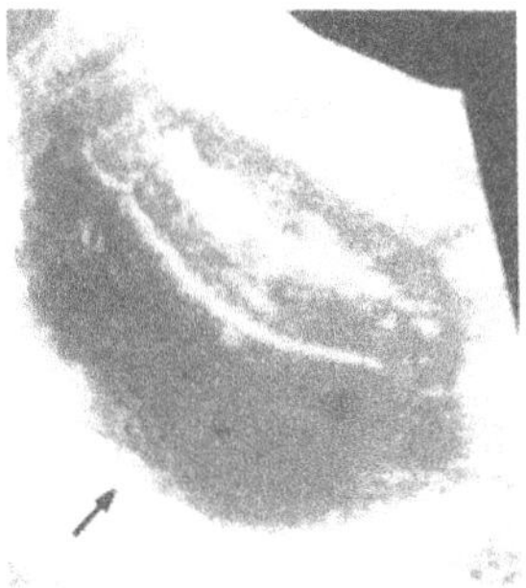

Fig. 10.9. Trauma. Typical fresh anterior perirenal hematoma (*arrow*)

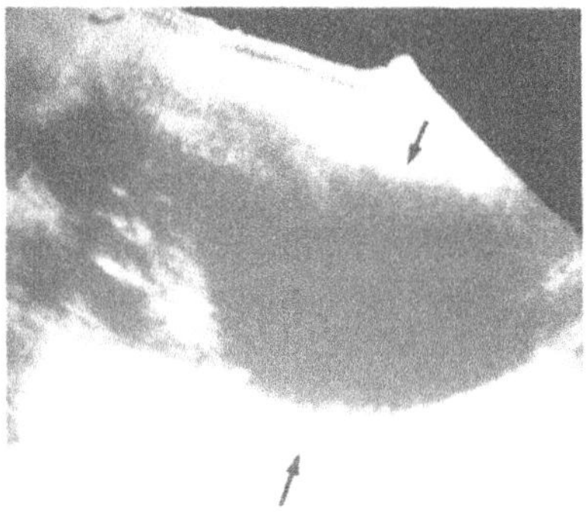

Fig. 10.10. Trauma. Typical fresh posterior pararenal hematoma (*arrows*). Note deformity of the kidney

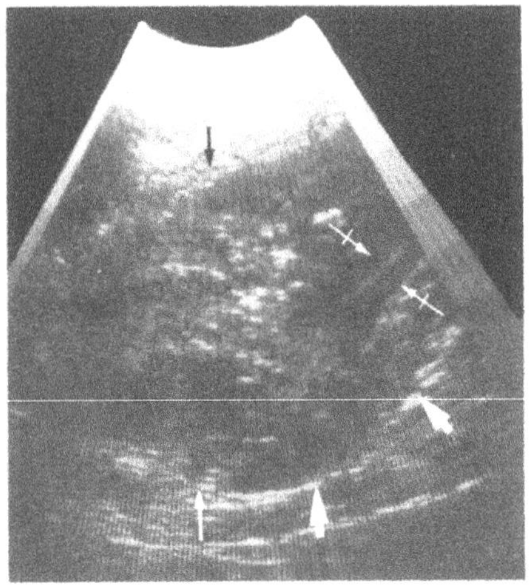

Fig. 10.11. Trauma: complex lesions. The kidney (*arrows*) is enlarged and heterogeneous. There is blood in the anterior perirenal (*crossed arrows*) and pararenal (*broad arrows*) compartments

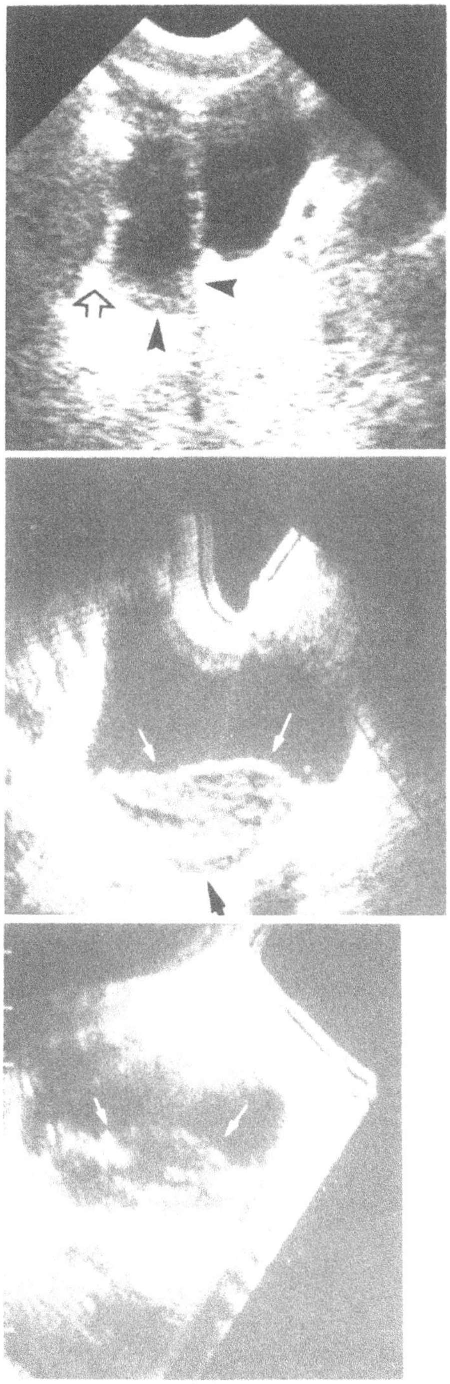

a b c

Fig. 10.12 a–c. Traumatic hematic effusions. **a** Pelvic hemoperitoneum: sagittal suprapubic section in patient of Fig. 10.2 b shows collection (*black arrowheads*) between urinary bladder and intestinal loop (*open arrow*). **b, c** Associated abnormality in the urinary bladder. **b** Transverse section of the pelvis in young male patient shows pseudouterine structure (*arrows*), seemingly behind the bladder. The structure is in fact intravesical and corresponds to blood clots, as demonstrated in **c**. **c** Patient is turned to the left oblique position. Blood clots move into new dependent situation, keeping identical shape. Note, in **b**, narrow retrovesical sonolucent strip (*black arrow*), indicating hemorrhage in Douglas' sac

10.4 Traumatic Urinomas (Uriniferous Cysts) and Nontraumatic Collections

Abundant juxtarenal collections are usually due to the presence of both blood and urine. Pure urinomas are, however, possible (Fig. 10.13). Urinomas can extend within the retroperitoneal compartments and even surround the aorta and vena cava (HEALY 1984). Such collections are sometimes disclosed weeks or months after the initial trauma (uriniferous cysts). Similar images of fluid collections, proximal to the kidney, are encountered in spontaneous urinomas, after impaction of ureteral calculi or after ureteral surgery (Figs. 10.14, 10.15).

We shall not examine again purulent juxtarenal collections arising from renal abscesses (see Chap. 7). Juxtarenal collections can be due to the migration of collections of pancreatic origin, during the course of acute pancreatitis, from the anterior pararenal space to the perirenal space (Fig. 10.16), or even to the subcapsular compart-

Table 10.1. Juxtarenal collections

Nontraumatic	Perinephric abscesses Tuberculous abscesses Nontraumatic hematomas (hemopathies, anticoagulant therapy) Spontaneous urinomas (stone impaction) Fluid of pancreatic origin (acute pancreatitis)
Traumatic	Traumatic hematomas Traumatic urinomas Lymphoceles (after transplantation)
Postoperative	Hematomas Urinomas Lymphoceles Abscesses

Table 10.2. Etiology of subcapsular collections

Abscesses
Acquired hematomas
anticoagulants
trauma
surgery
biopsy
interventional procedures
Spontaneous hematomas
hemopathies
coagulation disturbances
hemorrhagic tumors (malignant or benign)
Collections of pancreatic origin

ment. As hepatic tumoral processes, renal tumors, whether benign or malignant, can bleed, inducing subcapsular or extracapsular hematomas. Such hematomas can constitute the first symptom of the tumor. The various kinds of juxtarenal collection are set out in Table 10.1.

In Table 10.2 the different kinds of subcapsular collections are given.

Trauma and Preexisting Lesions

Any preexisting renal pathological process can be disclosed by a post-traumatic examination. A cyst or a hydronephrosis must not be misinterpreted as a hematoma, nor a renal enlargement of tumoral origin as a contusion with a subcapsular hematoma.

This possibility represents the only occasion for differential diagnosis in the context of renal trauma.

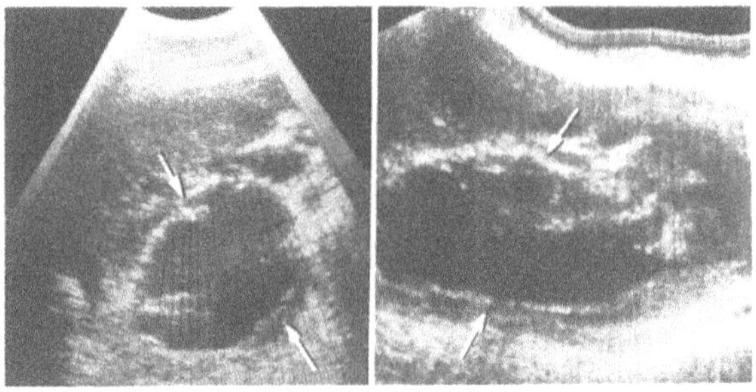

a, b

Fig. 10.13 a, b. Right post-traumatic urinoma. **a** Intercostal scan. **b** Sagittal scan; abundant collection (*arrows*)

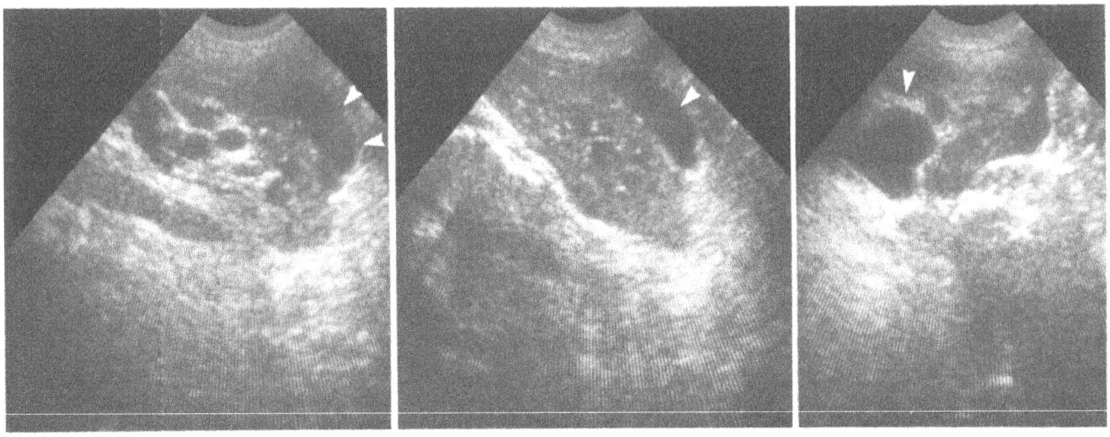

a–c

Fig. 10.14 a–c. Urinoma due to impaction of a stone in the left ureter. **a** Left coronal scan shows slight dilatation of the collecting system and discloses fluid collection (*arrowheads*). **b** Parallel scan. **c** Intercostal scan. The pattern of collection in **a** and **b** is in favor of perirenal location. In **c**, the concave shape of the parenchyma can lead to consideration of subcapsular collection – which in this case was finally perirenal

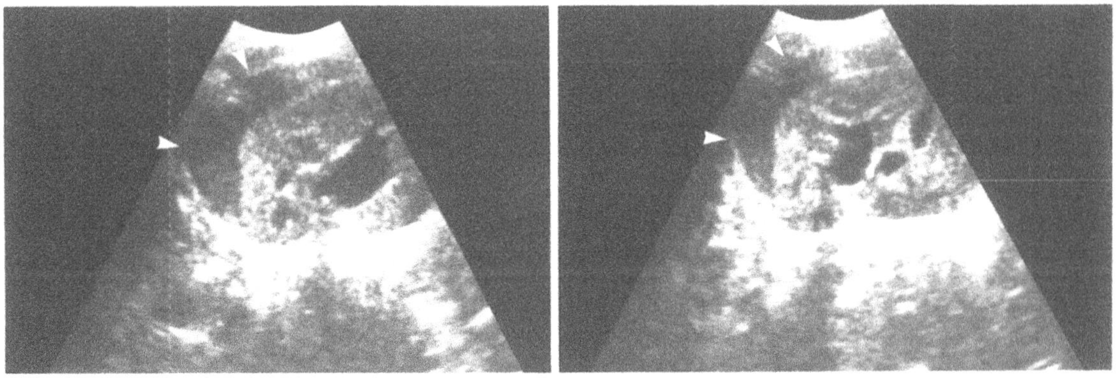

a b

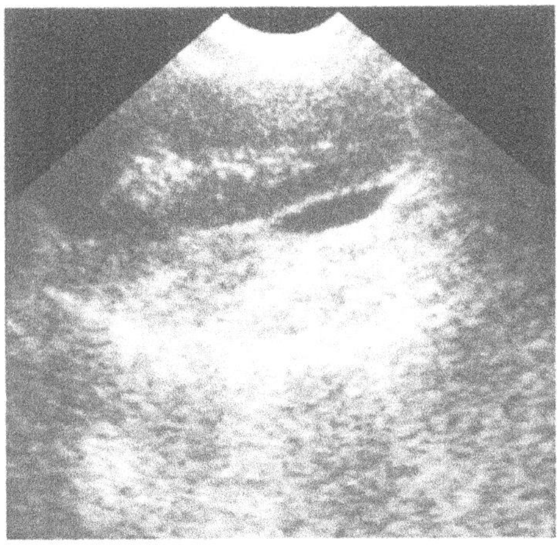

Fig. 10.16. Left perirenal collection discloses posterior to acute pancreatitis

10.5 Associated Lesions

High-resolution real time makes possible an excellent evaluation of the spleen through the left intercostal spaces. Since 1 October 1978, we have completely given up splenic angiography in post-traumatic evaluation without turning to CT in that particular field.

Hepatic and splenic evaluation must be associated with renal evaluation, looking for heterogeneities and/or subcapsular hematomas (Figs. 10.1 b and 10.17).

On the other hand, it is very easy, while examining the right kidney, to assess the condition of the liver. As mentioned above, a complete evaluation of the upper abdomen can also demonstrate suffusion of blood into Morison's pouch (WEILL 1978; WEILL et al. 1979), the juxtasplenic recesses, the cul-de-sac of Douglas (Fig. 10.12), the paracolic gutters, or the lesser omental sac ("butterfly sign," WEILL et al. 1983). The main ultrasonic patterns of renal trauma are summarized in Fig. 10.18.

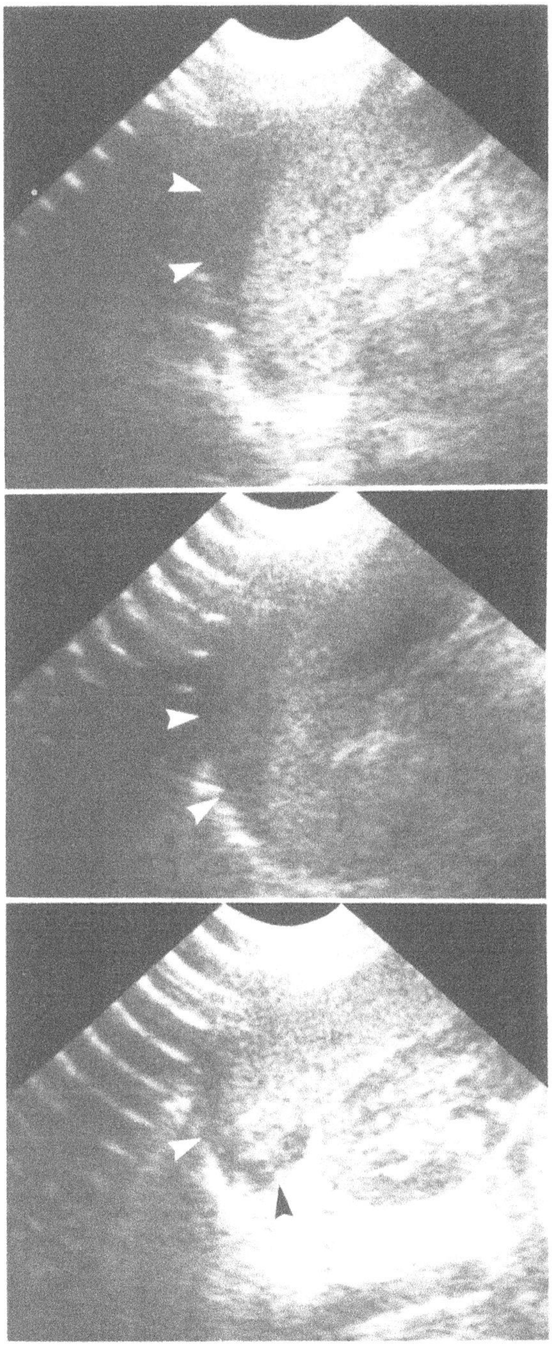

a

b

c

Fig. 10.17 a–c. Splenic subcapsular hematoma (*arrowheads*): three intercostal scans

◄ **Fig. 10.15 a, b.** Urinoma: perirenal collection (*arrowheads*), causing pain, is discovered in a 12-year-old child 1 week after surgery for ureteral reflux. **a, b** Two left intercostal scans

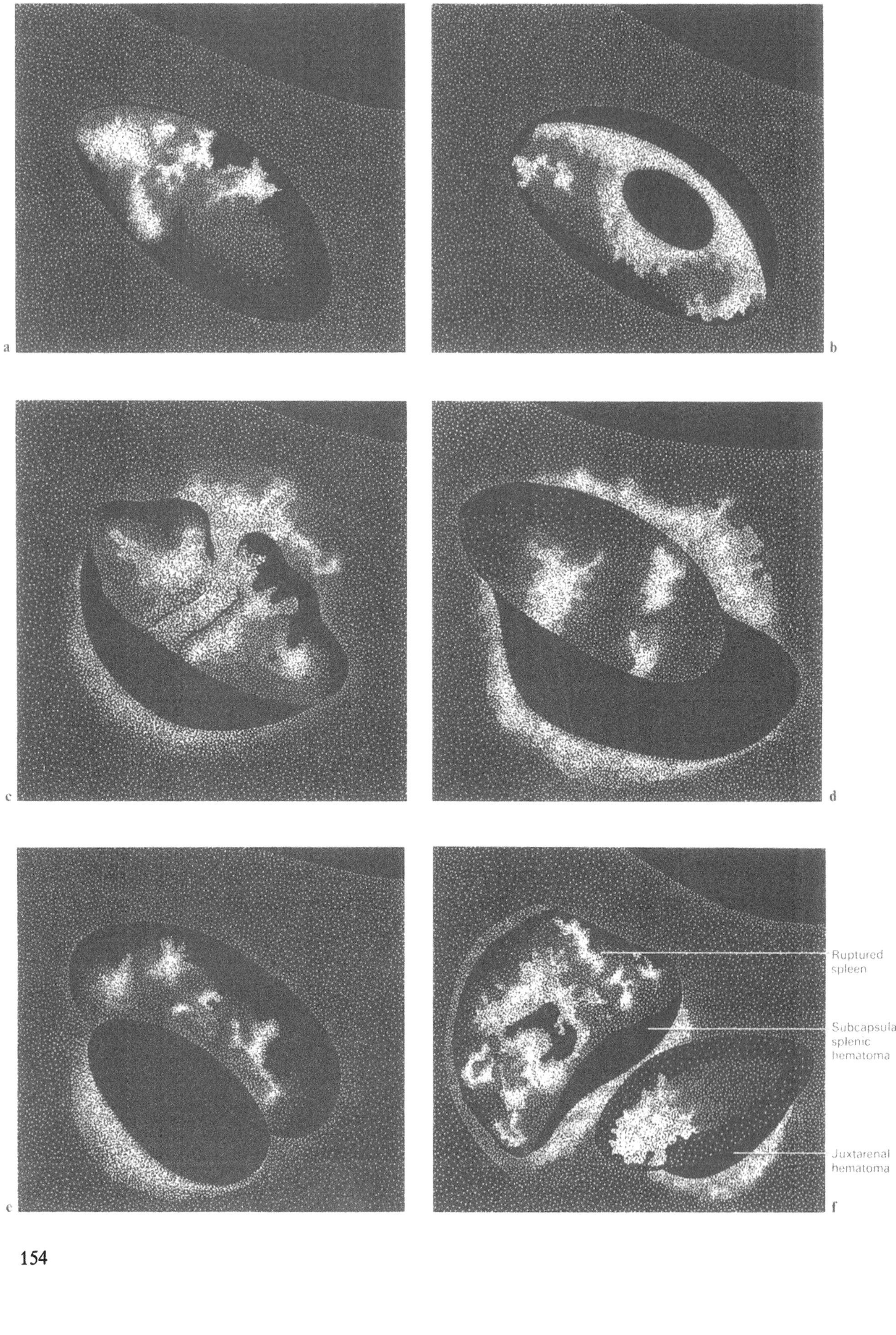
a
b
c
d
e
f
Ruptured spleen
Subcapsular splenic hematoma
Juxtarenal hematoma

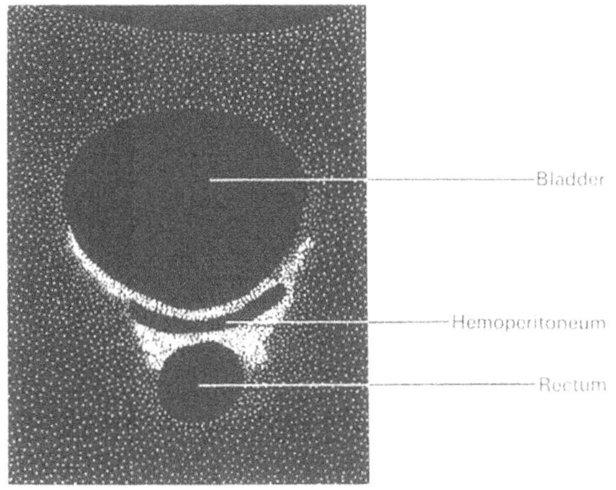

g

Fig. 10.18 a–g. Pattern of renal traumatic lesions and of juxtarenal hematomas (schemes). **a** Renal contusion; **b** tear with intrarenal hematoma; small juxtarenal hematoma; **c, d** renal fracture; large juxtarenal hematoma; **e** hematoma in anterior pararenal compartment; hematoma in posterior perirenal fat; **f** urinoma; **g** associated sign: hemoperitoneum

10.6 Radiological Policy

In light trauma, or after renal biopsy, sonography alone is sufficient for reliable confirmation that the kidney is normal. If a small hematoma is found, follow-up examinations will permit one to monitor its evolution. A large hematoma, a hematoma that does not subside, demands a CT scanning, or at least an IVU if not angiography. CT does not produce much more morphological information than ultrasound, but permits one to check the functional value of the kidney, and to rule out an asymptomatic arterial rupture, which remains a permanent worry, since such a rupture can exist without associated hematoma and without frank renal lesions (Fig. 10.19). Therefore severe trauma requires a CT or an IVU, even if the sonography is normal. IVU can be restricted to a few exposures, since its aim is functional rather than morphological. Where appropriate, we use the algorithm set out in Table 10.3. It will perhaps change in the best future, due to use of duplex Doppler.

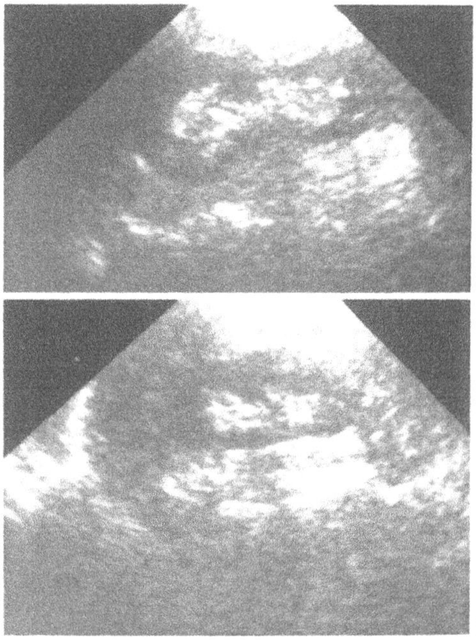

a

b

Fig. 10.19 a, b. Renal trauma. **a** Kidney is apparently normal. **b** Scan 3 weeks later shows renal atrophia due to ischemia. Normal ultrasonic pattern does not permit one to rule out asymptomatic rupture of the renal artery. IVU or CT must be carried out as complement to ultrasound

Table 10.3. Algorithm for severe lumbar trauma

Normal sonography or slight renal or juxtarenal abnormalities
↓
IVU
- → Normal STOP
- → Slight changes ↓ Ultrasonic follow-up STOP
- → Poor secretion No secretion ↓ Angiography

Abnormal sonography
↓
CT
- → Normal secretion Patent renal artery
  - No or slight extravasation ↓ Ultrasonic follow-up
    - ↓ Improvement STOP
    - → Deterioration ↓ Angiography
- → Poor secretion Renal artery damaged ↓ Angiography
- → Extravasation Calciceal amputation → Angiography

11 Adrenals

Despite many successes, adrenal sonography is not, in our experience, as reliable as renal sonography.

11.1 The Normal Adrenal

The late FRED SAMPLE (1977) described a very precise technique of displaying the adrenal, using contact scanning. We have not been able to achieve the same results – but this is not too surprising, considering how thin the glandular tissue appears when displayed on CT scans (Fig. 11.1). YEH (1980) has shown that the right adrenal can be visualized as a sonolucent retrocaval element. In exceptional cases, we have obtained the display of the thin pattern of the right adrenal on transverse ultrasonic sections (Fig. 11.2). The retrocaval image of the gland is then quite similar to that obtained by CT. It is more common to identify the adrenal posterior to the vena cava on sagittal or coronal scans (Fig. 11.3). However, such linear images lack specificity; often several similar images are displayed on the same scan, due to the vicinity of the right crux of the diaphragm.

In other subjects the adrenal has the appearance of a small juxtarenal element, surrounded by echogenic fat (Fig. 11.4). The right adrenal is internal to the kidney since it is retrocaval. On the left side the gland is prerenal. In most patients ultrasonic scans display the triangle-shaped fatty surrounding of the adrenal rather than the gland itself (Figs. 11.5, 11.6). Demonstration of the normal adrenal is quite easy in the neonate and premature infant: the size ratio adrenal:kidney is much greater.

Examination Procedure

It is possible to infer from the anatomical features depicted above that, on the right side, the examination technique of the adrenal is precisely that of the vena cava, that is sagittal and transverse scans. Sagittal and coronal scans also show the suprarenal fatty triangle. On the left side, since the adrenal is prerenal, the adrenal and surrounding fatty triangle are shown by posterior sagittal scans, and by coronal, intercostal, and transverse scans. Finally, even in adult, transverse intercostal scans through the liver can show the normal right adrenal in most subjects. A trans-splenic approach can be used on the left side (ZAPPASODI, 1986).

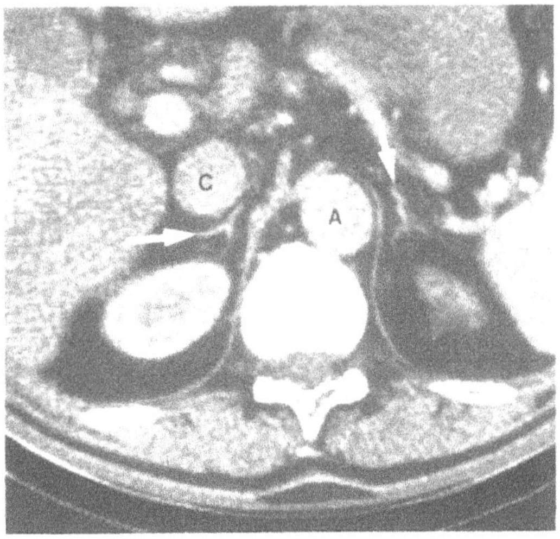

Fig. 11.1. Pattern of adrenals (*arrows*) on CT scan. The thin right gland is retrocaval. The left adrenal, triangle shaped, is frankly prerenal. *A*, aorta; *C*, cava

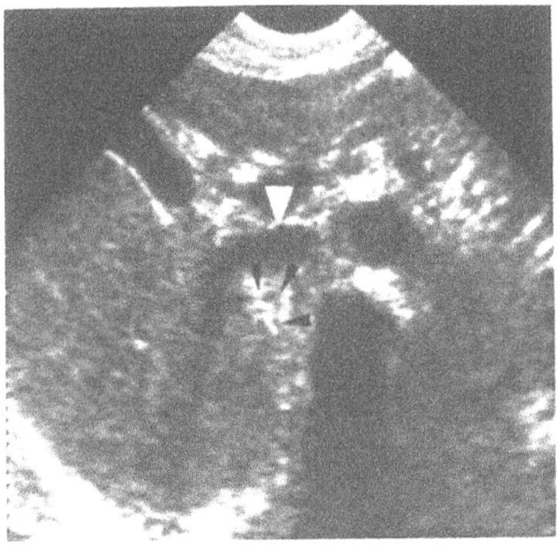

Fig. 11.2. Transverse section of the normal right adrenal: the "V"-shaped pattern of the gland (*black arrowheads*) is shown behind the cava (*white arrowhead*)

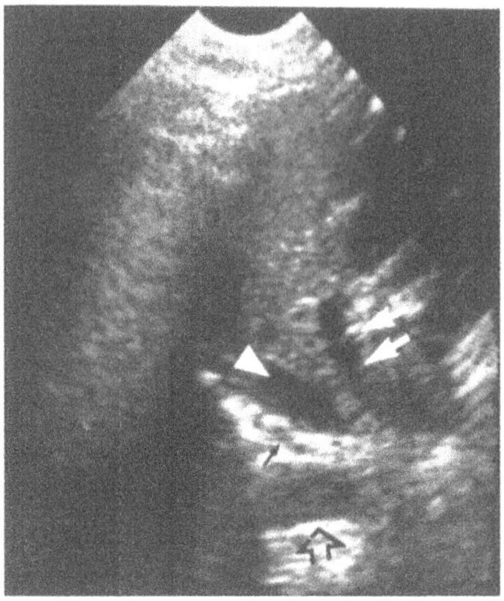

Fig. 11.3. Intercostal scan of the right adrenal (*small black arrow*). *Double arrow*, portal vein; *white arrowhead*, cava; *open arrow*, aorta

a

b

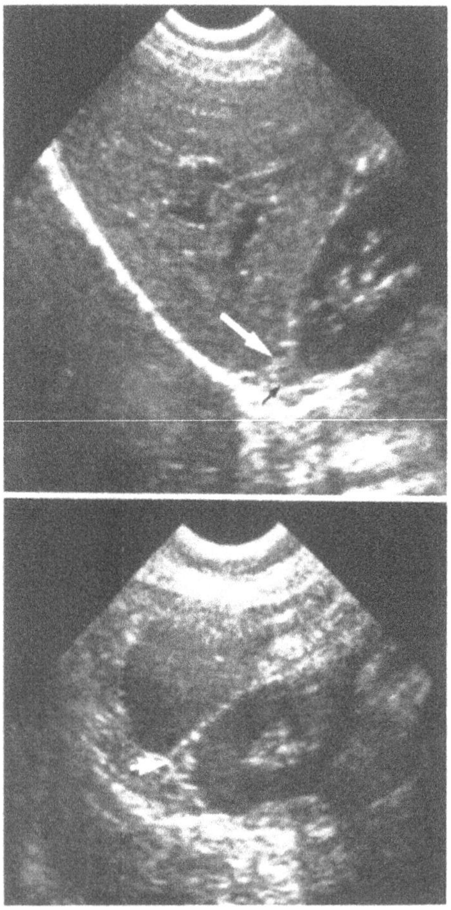

Fig. 11.4 a, b. Normal suprarenal fatty triangles (*arrows*). **a** Sagittal scan of the right suprarenal area; **b** coronal scan of the left suprarenal area

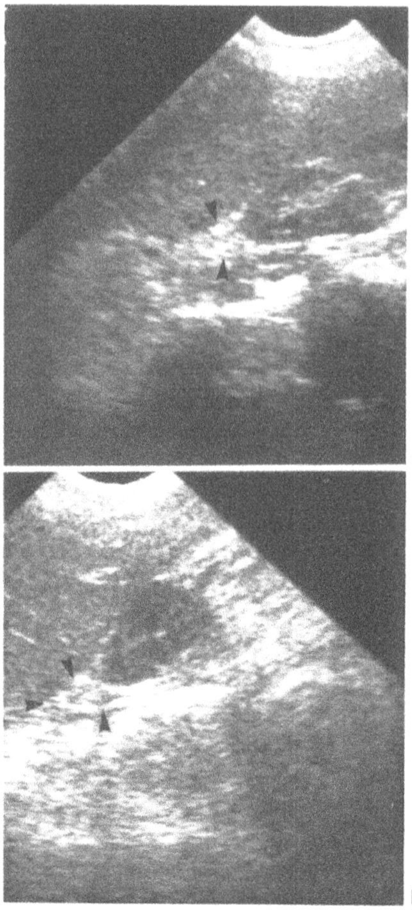

a

b

Fig. 11.5 a, b. Right suprarenal fatty triangle (*arrowheads*) and adrenal

11.2 The Pathological Adrenal

Tumors

The different kinds of adrenal tumors are listed in Table 11.1. An adrenal lesion can only be displayed, in our experience, providing one of two conditions is met:

1. The pathological process must be larger than the triangle (Fig. 11.7)
2. If it is smaller, its level of echogenicity must be markedly different from that of the fatty triangle (Fig. 11.8)
3. A small tumor of the right adrenal, in the retrocaval position, can push forward the posterior venous wall and become outlined by the echo-free venous lumen (see Figs. 11.9, 11.10).

Very small tumors, such as Conn's adenomas, (Fig. 11.11) are, in most cases not visualized. Hyperplasia is usually also not visualized with ultrasound, at least on the left side. Nodular hyperplasia has the same pattern as adenomas.

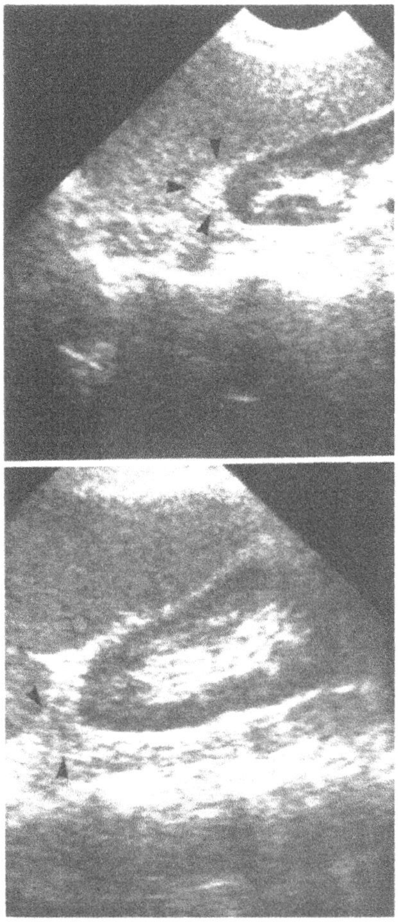

a

b

Fig. 11.6 a, b. Left suprarenal fatty triangle (*arrowheads*)

Table 11.1. Tumors of the adrenal

Tissue	Tumor	
Stroma	lipoma, angio-myo-lipomas, fibroma etc. cysts (see also Table 11.2)	usually benign; usually nonfunctional
Cortex	adenoma; carcinom hyperplaxia, nodular hyperplaxia	
Medulla	Pheochromocytoma neurogenic tumors	Pheochromocytoma 10% malignant; 10% multiple 10% extra-adrenal in location
Other	Metastases	lung; breast; ovary; any other carcinoma

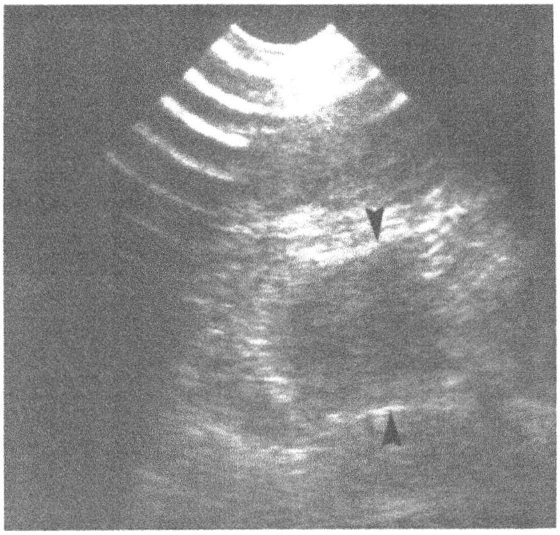

Fig. 11.7. Left adrenal mass (*arrowheads*) (intercostal scan). The mass, which corresponds to a deposit of lung carcinoma, is broader than the suprarenal fatty triangle. This kind of image requires a follow-up examination in the standing position in order to rule out a false image due to the colon

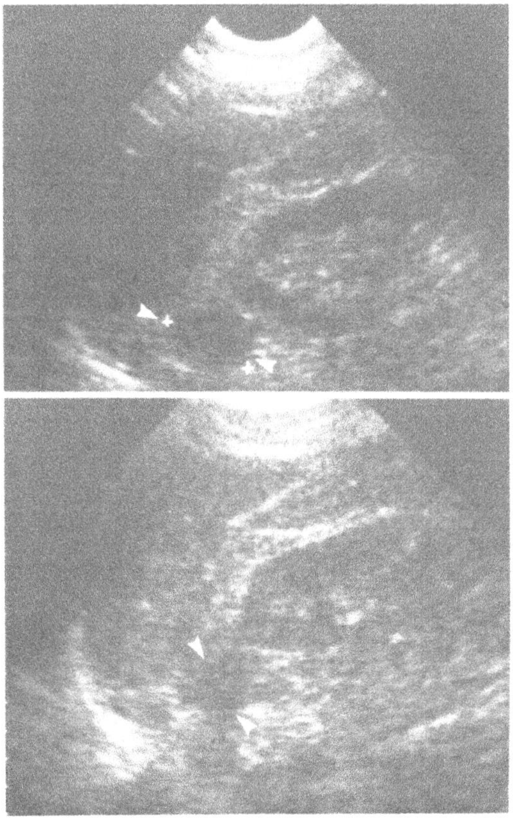

a

b

Fig. 11.8 a, b. Small left adrenal mass (*arrowheads*): two intercostal scans. Section of the mass is smaller than suprarenal fatty triangle. It is well visualized thanks to its sonotransparency. Mass corresponds to a deposit

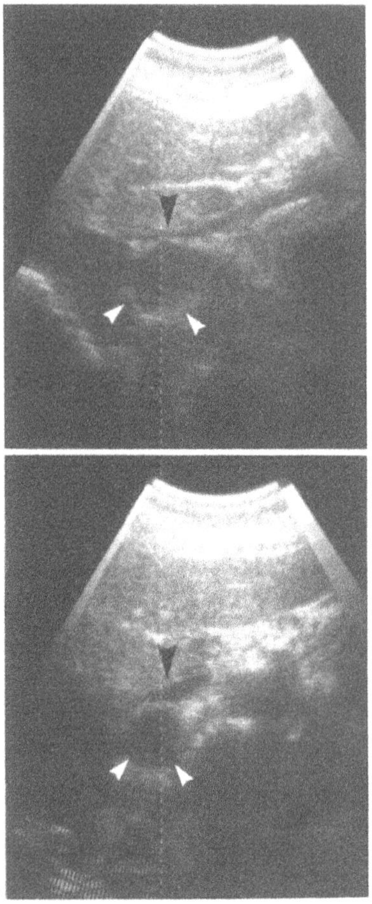

Fig. 11.9 a, b. Small right adrenal mass. **a** Sagittal scan shows mass (*white arrowheads*) posterior to the cava (*black arrowhead*). **b** Transverse scan. Note impression of mass on cava. Mass corresponds to deposit of lung carcinoma

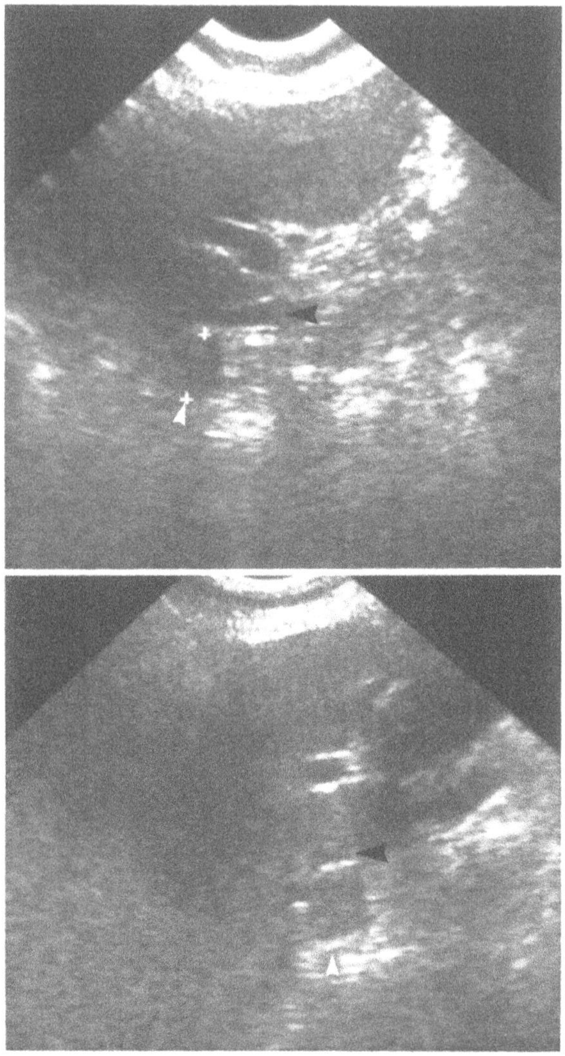

Fig. 11.10 a, b. Small right pheochromocytoma. **a** Sagittal scan shows a mass (*white arrowhead*) posterior to cava (*black arrowhead*). **b** Transverse scan: cava is pushed forward by mass and has lost its direct relationship with spine

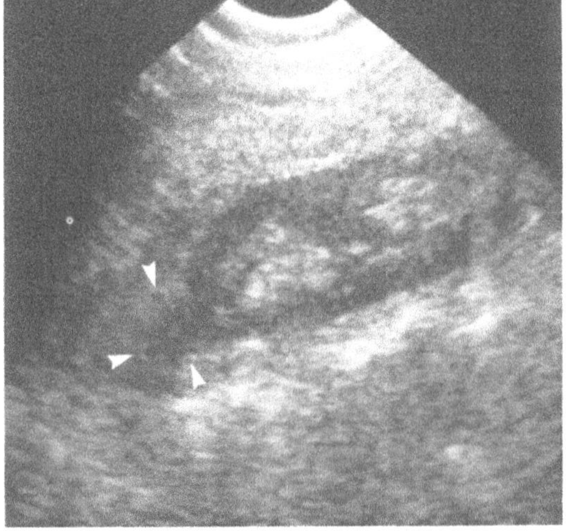

Fig. 11.11. Left Conn's adenoma (*arrowheads*) ▸

Phéochromocytomas

Pheochromocytomas can be small (Figs. 10.10, 10.12) or quite large. Their echopattern is usually frankly solid and more or less heterogeneous (Fig. 11.12). Sonotransparence can arise from necrosis or intratumoral bleeding (Fig. 11.13) (BOWERMAN et al. 1981). The development of large adrenal tumors is sometimes paradoxical: some masses arising from the right gland extend anteriorly to the kidney (Figs. 11.12) instead of being retrocaval.

Pheochromocytomas (10%) can be multiple and have atypical locations.

Multiple and atypical pheochromocytomas are much more readily disclosed by CT. But when considering CT, the occurrence of grave hypertensive crises induced by injection of contrast medium should be kept in mind.

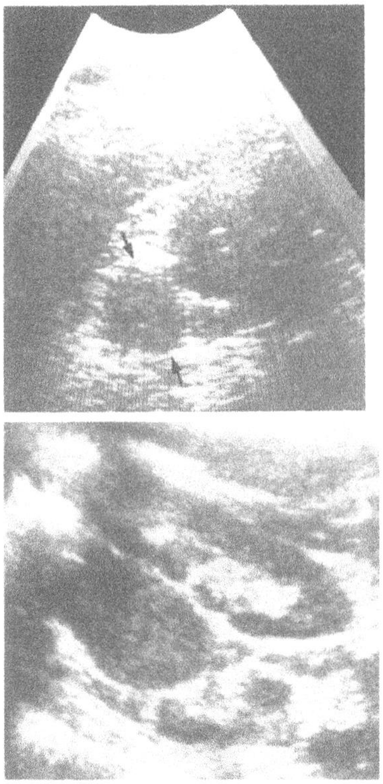

Fig. 11.12 a, b. Pheochromocytomas. **a** A small sonotransparent mass (*arrows*) is surrounded by suprarenal fat. **b** Left pheochromocytoma: a sagittal scan of the left kidney in the prone position shows a large mass in front of the kidney. (by courtesy of Prof. Tran-Minh, Lyon)

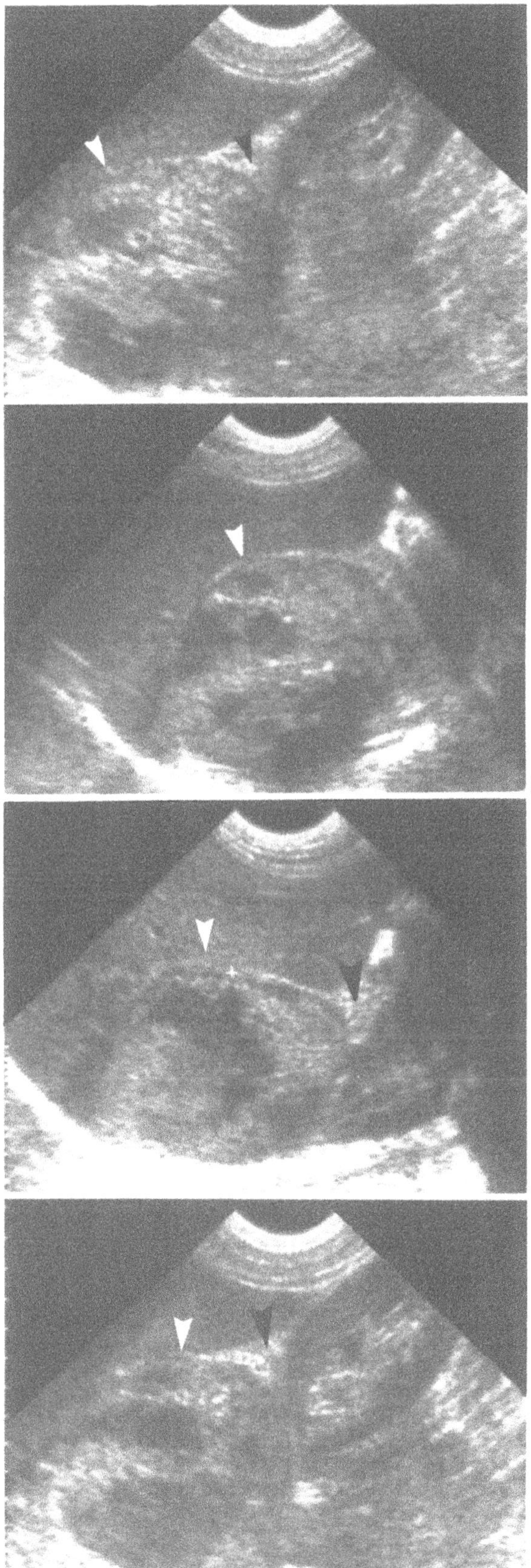

Fig. 11.13 a–d. Pheochromocytoma. **a** Sagittal scan of right ▸ upper quadrant shows large suprarenal mass (*white arrowhead*), separated from the renal upper pole by fatty cleavage plane (*black arrowhead*). Echotexture is heterogeneous. **b** Intercostal scan shows sonotransparent areas of liquid appearance. **c** Parallel intercostal scan. **d** Coronal scan

Other Tumors

Adrenocortical Carcinomas (see Table 11.1). The pattern of adrenocortical carcinomas is solid and heterogeneous (Figs. 11.14, 11.15). Nonsecreting or poorly secreting tumors can reach a large volume before they induce clinical symptoms and trigger imaging.

Angiomyolipomas possess the same reflective pattern in the adrenals as they do in the kidneys (GEE et al. 1975).

Cystic processes possess a particularly clear pattern (see Table 11.2), (Fig. 11.16, 11.17).

Table 11.2. Cystic processes of adrenal

0.06 of autopsies; twice more frequent in female patient
Nature
Lymphangioma (endothelial)
Epithelial cysts (9%) = embryonic cystic adenomas
Pseudocysts (40%) = liquefacted hematomas in normal and pathologic adrenal; neonate but also adults

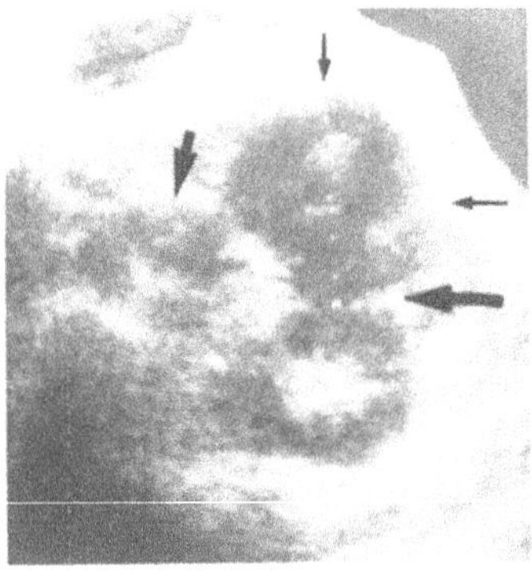

Fig. 11.14. Large tumor: carcinoma of the adrenal cortex. Transverse scan shows a large mass (*small arrows*) with echogenic nodules, in front of the left kidney. Note the frank cleavage plane and precaval lymph nodes (*broad arrows*). (Courtesy of Prof. Tran-Minh, Lyon)

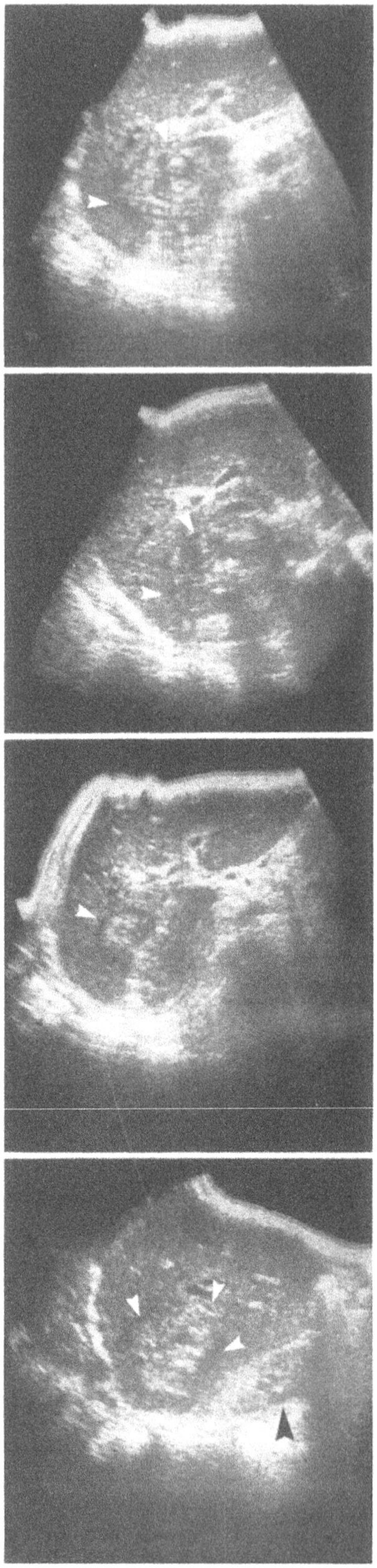

Fig. 11.15 a–d. Adrenocortical carcinoma (*arrowheads*). **a–c** ▶ Coronal scans. **d** Sagittal scan. Delineation of the mass with liver is unsharp. On sagittal scan, hepatoma could be considered, the more so since mass seems to be at a distance from kidney (*black arrowhead*)

Many of these cystic lesions are discovered on ultrasonic abdominal screening. Cystic lymphangiomas have a cystic or multilocular pattern (Fig. 11.17). Most cystic masses are in fact pseudocysts, following hemorrhage within the normal or tumoral adrenal (GEORGI et al. 1982). Plain X-ray, and still better, CT, can show a calcified pericystic rim.

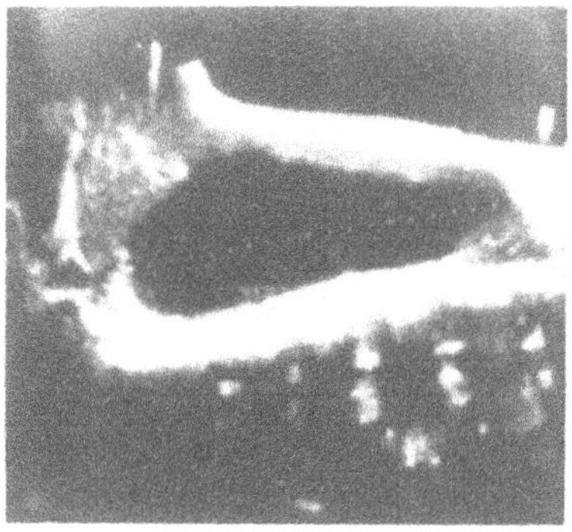

Fig. 11.16. Giant adrenal cyst. Right kidney is displaced and flattened (sagittal scan in the supine position); axial length of the cyst is 18 cm. (Courtesy of Prof. Tran-Minh, Lyon)

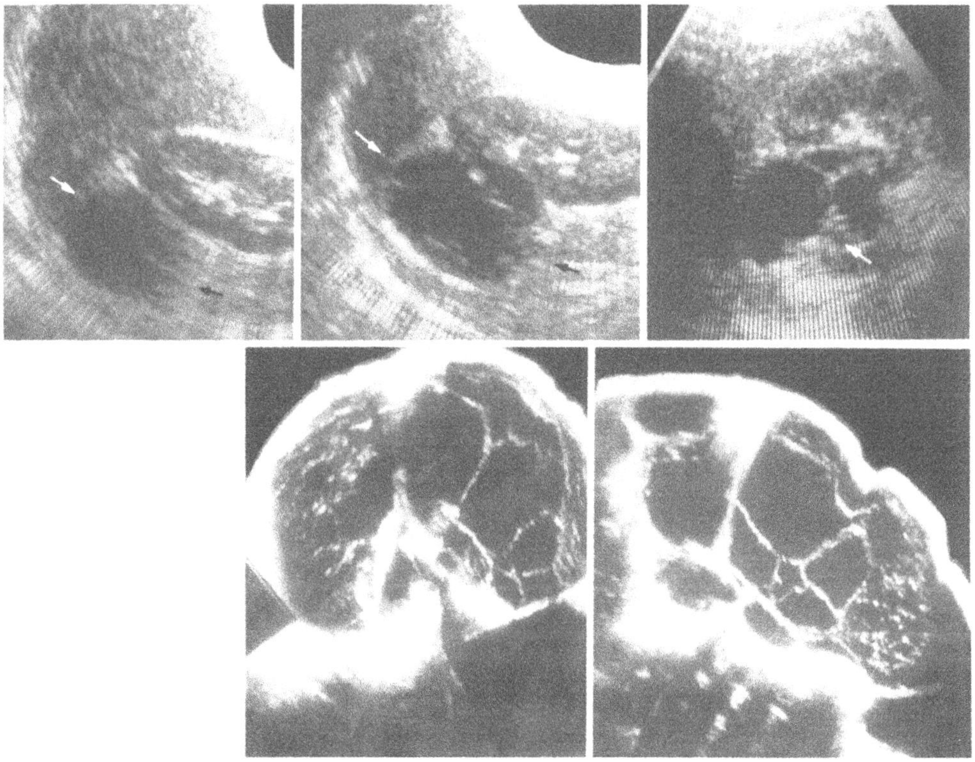

a–c

d, e

Fig. 11.17 a–e. Cystic adrenal masses. **a–c** First case. **a** Sagittal scan of right upper quadrant shows rounded cystic mass (*arrows*) posterior to renal upper pole. **b** Parallel scan shows multilocular pattern of the mass. **c** Same pattern is displayed on transverse scan. Note posterior, retrorenal situation of the adrenal mass. Multilocular pattern is typical of cystic lymphangioma. **d, e** Another case. Giant left cystic lymphangioma occupies whole-hemiabdomen in neonate. **d** Transverse scan. **e** Sagittal scan. (**d, e** Courtesy of A. Le Mouel, Besançon)

Metastases

Metastases, when discovered by screening, can be of any size (Figs. 11.18, 11.19). Their echotexture is either sonotransparent or echogenic, either homogeneous or heterogeneous (MORLEY 1976; FORSYTHE 1976). They can necrotize (Fig. 11.20) (FORSYTHE 1976).

Bilateral Tumors

Bilateral tumors are due either to pheochromocytoma or to metastases (mainly breast and lung carcinoma) (Figs. 11.21, 11.22). Systematic screening of the suprarenal areas, after evaluation of the liver, in patients having lung or breast carcinoma confirms the frequency of these bilateral deposits, a classical feature for pathologists. Some latent bilateral deposits can reach a large volume (Fig. 11.22).

Tumoral Spread

Malignant adrenal tumors are liable to spread into the caval lumen, as do renal carcinomas (see Fig. 6.18). The frequent extension of adrenal tumors behind the vena cava (Fig. 11.13) must not be confused with true caval involvement. Malignant tumors can also give rise to metastatic lymph nodes.

Hematomas

Hematomas, sometimes bilateral, produce a frank glandular swelling. Classical in the neonate (POND and HABER 1976), they can also be encountered in the adult. Most hematomas rapidly lose their sonotransparent pattern. Their echotexture, due to the presence of blood clots, becomes strongly echogenic: this pattern must be kept in mind to avoid false-negative diagnoses. On the other hand, as stated above, hematomas can transform into pseudo-cysts.

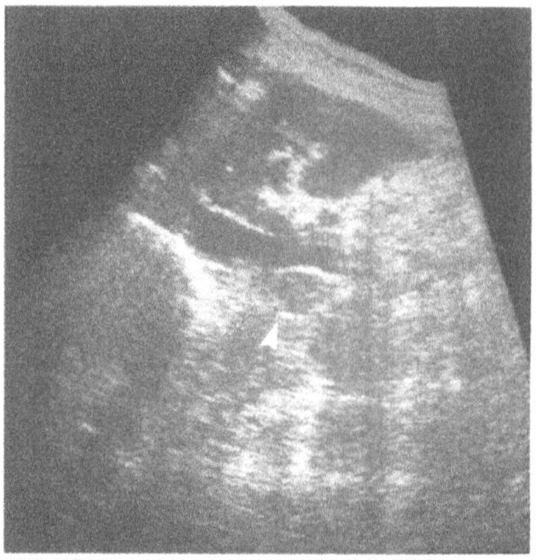
a

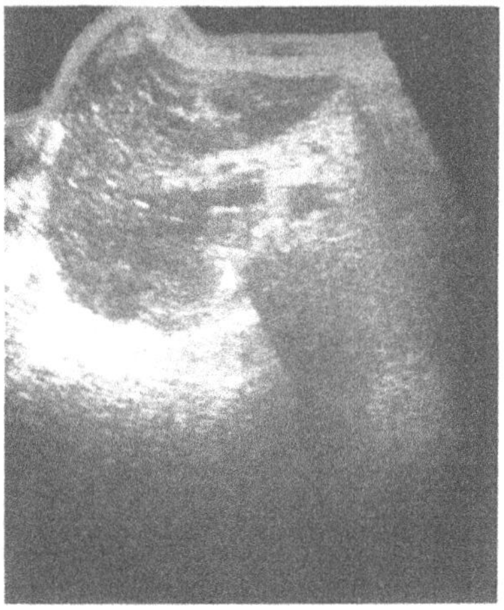
b

Fig. 11.18 a, b. Small right adrenal metastasis (*arrowheads*) of lung carcinoma. **a** Sagittal scan; **b** transverse scan

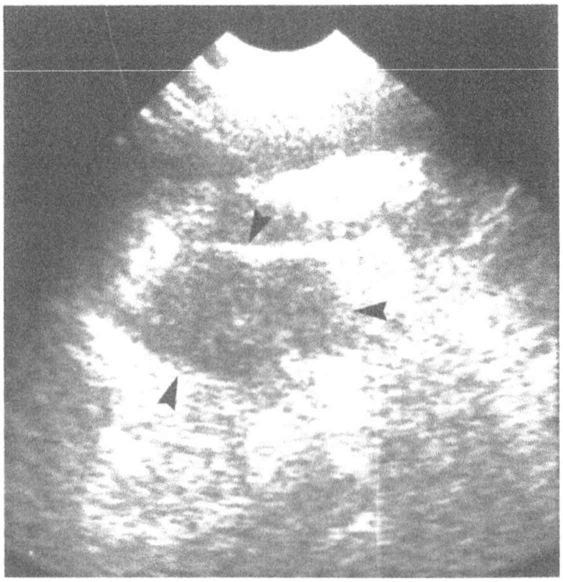

Fig. 11.19. Coronal scan of left renal deposit (*arrowheads*) from lung carcinoma

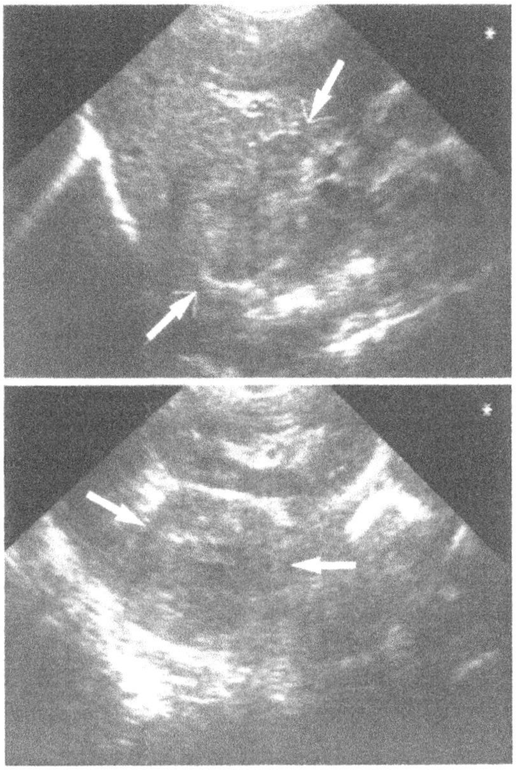

Fig. 11.20 a, b. Bilateral adrenal metastases consecutive to bronchial carcinoma. **a** Intercostal scan shows mass (*arrows*) between liver and kidney. **b** Posterolateral scan of left kidney discloses prerenal mass (*arrows*)

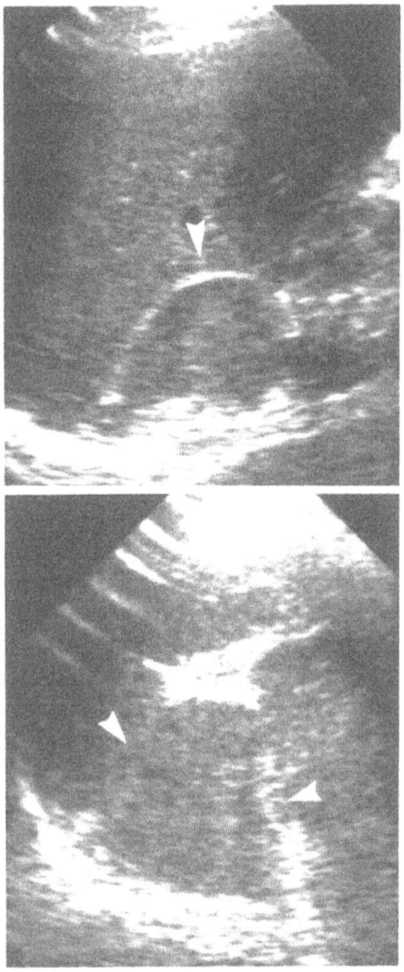

Fig. 11.21 a, b. Large bilateral adrenal metastases (*arrowheads*). **a** Right intercostal scan; **b** left intercostal scan

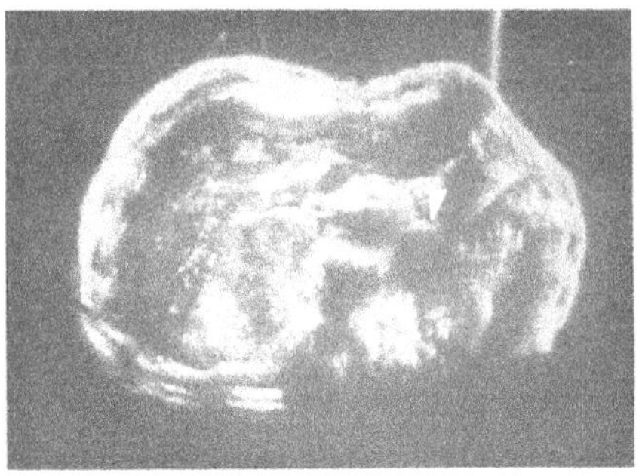

Fig. 11.22. Large bilateral adrenal metastases (*arrowheads*) (global transverse scan)

11.3 Diagnosis

Differentiation between an adrenal mass and a mass arising from the renal upper pole relies on the display of a fatty cleavage plane (Fig. 11.13 a). On the right side, a retrocaval mass raises the question of adenopathy. A solitary mass, proximal to the kidney, is likely to be suprarenal. A definite diagnosis relies on CT scans, which will show that the normal image of the adrenal has disappeared. On the left side, the colonic flexure can mimic an adrenal mass. Before formulating the diagnosis of tumor, the permanence of the image must be checked by a positional study: a colonic image will disappear in the standing position, whereas the pattern of a suprarenal mass will not be modified. Spontaneous splenorenal shunts due to portal hypertension can mimick small left adrenal masses. Multiple collaterals or varices make a correct diagnosis possible. In other cases, contrast-enhanced CT will show the vascular nature of the pseudo-mass.

Difficult diagnostic problems can arise with large tumors, as regards their suprarenal origin. To be able to confirm that origin, the normal right and left kidneys, the spleen or the liver must be clearly delineated in the vicinity of the tumor. Some adrenal tumors develop in front of the kidney, while their plane of cleavage with the liver tissue is not sharply delineated (Figs. 11.15, 11.23, 11.24). Thus without other procedures it is quite impossible to differentiate between an adrenal tumor spreading into the liver and the caudal development of a tumor arising from the liver.

CT will be employed first, and if it is not conclusive, arteriography. Arteriography itself can lead to false conclusions since adrenal tumors can draw their vascularization from the inferior diaphragmatic artery. When the latter arises from the celiac trunk or its branches, the tumoral blood supply seems to be digestive. In some confusing patterns, guided puncture is finally the best procedure.

11.4 Reliability and Diagnostic Policy

Sample (1978) reported a correct diagnosis in 20 out of 22 cases of adrenal masses and a correct diagnosis of normality in 36 out of 38 cases (93% accuracy). Abrams et al. reported comparative results of CT and ultrasound in a series of 56 adrenal masses (1982). Their results are as follows:

	Sensitivity	Specificity
CT	84%	98%
Ultrasound	79%	61%

Thus, this study is clearly in favor of primary utilization of CT when a suprarenal mass is considered.

However, adrenal sonography is invaluable as a complement to liver screening in the search for metastases. Ultrasound is also invaluable for the positive diagnosis of pheochromocytoma in very fragile patients. Lastly (and paradoxically) ultrasound, which makes it possible to perform sagittal and coronal scans, can show more readily the adrenal nature of some large right masses. Lastly, the false negative diagnoses of CT and ultrasound do not superimpose: rarely tumors are better displayed by ultrasound, since their impedance gradient is greater than their density gradient.

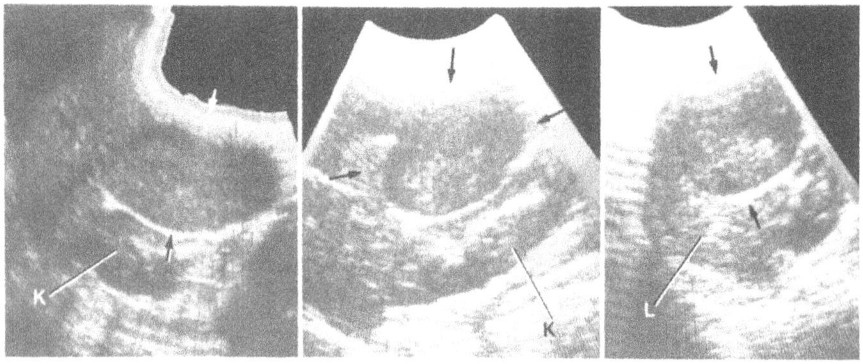

Fig. 11.23 a–c. Pseudohepatic tumor of suprarenal origin. A large mass is palpated in the upper quadrant of a 7-year-old child. **a** Sagittal right upper quadrant scan shows mass (*arrows*) in front of right kidney (*K*). No cleavage plane is outlined between liver tissue and mass. Echogenicities of the liver and of the mass are similar. Liver scintigram is normal. **b** More external scan, parallel to scan in **a**, shows cleavage plane. **c** Cleavage plane is also outlined on the transverse scan (*L*, liver). Ultrasonic diagnosis is liver adenoma, arising from an inferior liver surface. The surgeon found huge adrenal tumor

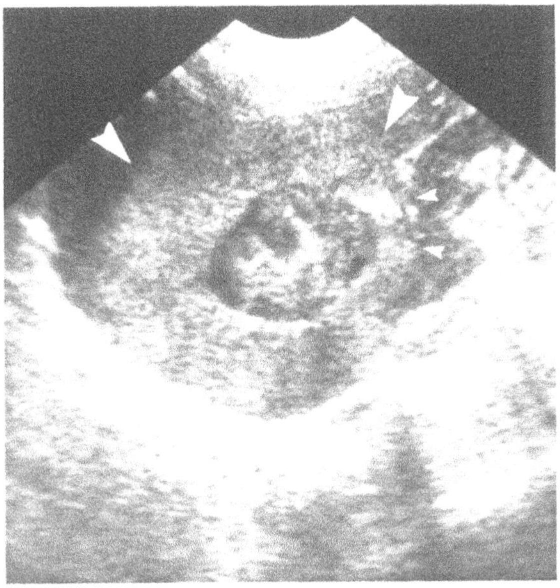

Fig. 11.24. Right sagittal scan shows large mass of right upper quadrant (*broad arrowheads*) depressing upper pole of right kidney (*small arrowheads*). Cleavage plane of mass with liver is ill defined. Image is consistent with hepatoma, but corresponds to malignant cortical tumor

12 Lower Urinary Tract

We shall deal with the lower urinary tract only briefly, considering its ultrasonic study merely as a complement to renal examinations, as for instance after discovery of hydronephrosis.

For us, pelvic evaluations is mandatory and systematic while examining the abdomen. This of course requires repletion of the urinary bladder, and means therefore that the patient *must not* be *prepared by complete fasting:* normal fluid absorption is required before sonography.

We shall not detail the important research work published by Japanese authors, such as WATANABE (1971, 1974, 1979), especially regarding the possibility of differentiating between malignant and benign prostatic lesions. Nor shall we detail the patterns of mucosal and transmucosal spread of bladder tumors (MORLEY 1978, 1979). Many such studies were carried out with the help of special intrarectal (WATANABE) or intravesical transducers (HOLM and NORTHERED 1974; FORNAGE 1979; FRENTZEL-BEYME 1982).

The expectation of a definite histological diagnosis based on improved imaging has not been met. Precise diagnosis requires, in the prostate as in other parenchymas, guided biopsy, which of course is rather easy now with intrarectal probes. Such probes are now currently available, as extensions to standard realtime machines. Thus intrarectal prostatic sonography has become a routine procedure (FORNAGE 1985; DAHNERT 1986; LEE 1986; RIFKIN 1986). Intraversical sonography, on the contrary, remains a specialized, interventional technique.

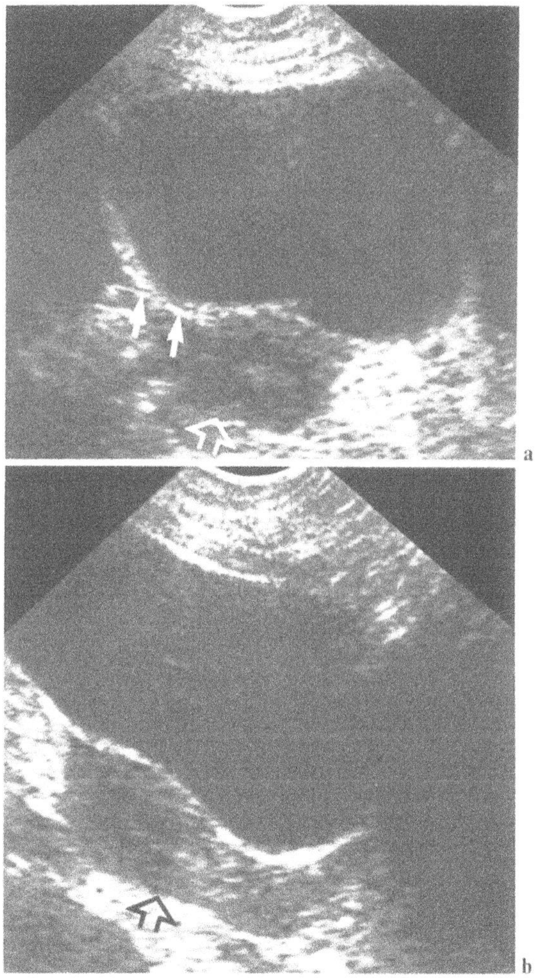

Fig. 12.1 a, b. The normal urinary bladder. **a** Transverse scan in female patient. The vesical wall (*arrows*) is displayed between the uterus (*open arrow*) and the vesical contents. **b** Sagittal scan

12.1 Bladder

The bladder is an ideal organ for sonography, thanks to the high contrast between contents and container (Fig. 12.1). The wall of the urinary bladder is smooth. Proper scans can display several parietal layers (mucosa, muscle, etc.). Mirror artifacts can intervene, however, and must be kept in mind while analyzing these patterns (Fig. 12.2). Interfaces do not necessarily correspond to anatomic structures.

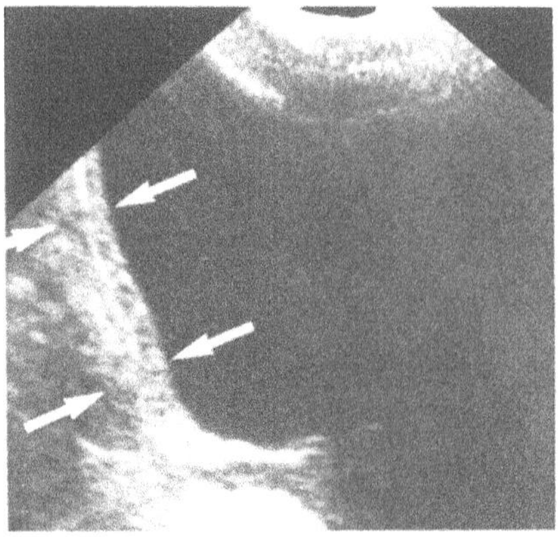

◂ **Fig. 12.2.** Transverse scan of vesical wall. External layer image is due to artifact

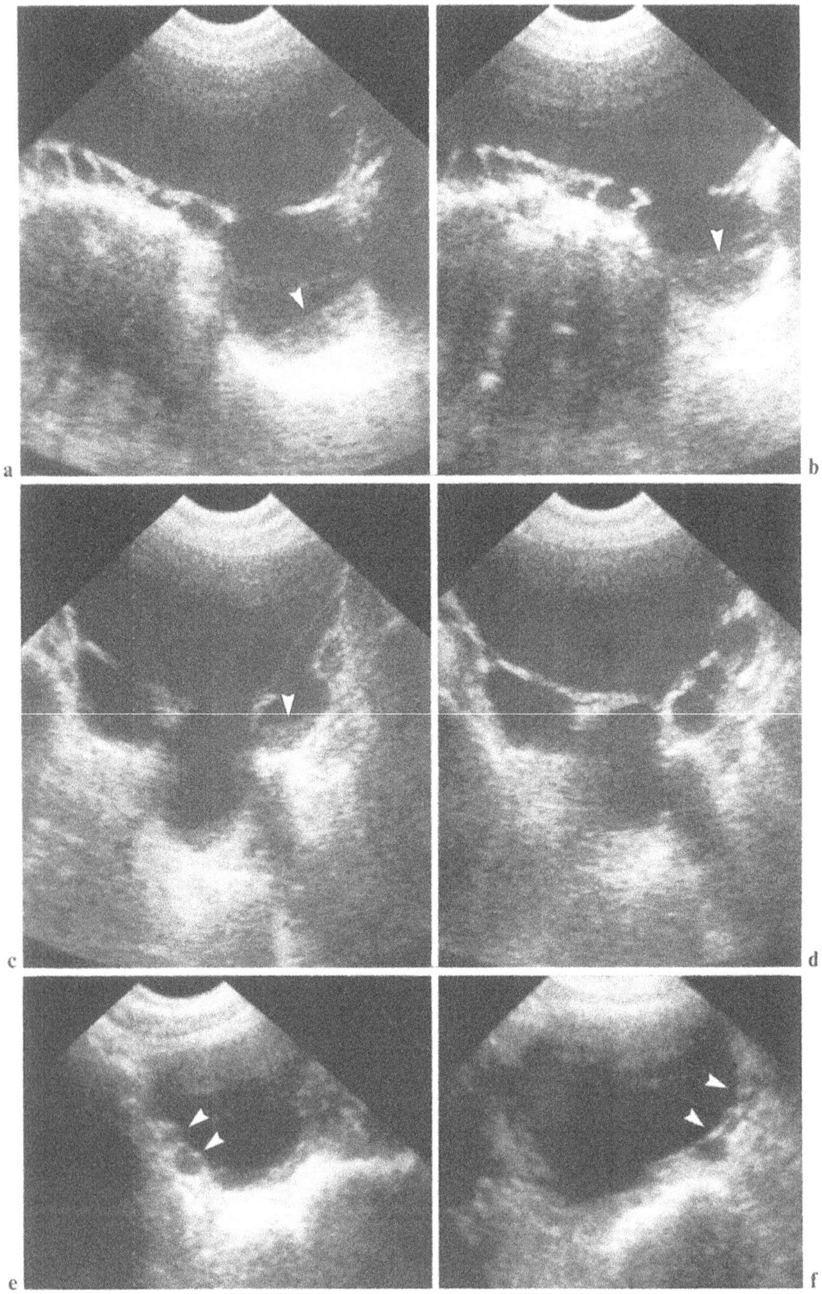

Fig. 12.3 a–f. Dysectasia. **a–d** First case: multiple pseudodiverticula due to muscular hypertrophy. Note in **a–c** pseudodependent accumulations corresponding to margin artifacts. **e, f** Another case: pseudodiverticula are smaller

True and False Diverticula-Stones

Parietal irregularities, due to the muscular hypertrophy and trabeculation arising from chronic interference with bladder emptying, are readily displayed (Fig. 12.3). Bladder scanning before and after micturition will show the presence of a residual volume.

The contents of the urinary bladder are perfectly sonotransparent. Accumulation of pus or of blood (see Fig. 10.12b, c) can give rise to an image of dependent echogenic layers: such images can, however, be mimicked by margin artifacts (Fig. 12.3a, b), which are more frequent.

Acquired or primary diverticula give rise to saccular, juxtavesical features (Figs. 12.4, 12.5). In the female pelvis, such images can mimic ovarian cysts (Fig. 12.4). Demonstration of an open communication between the bladder and diverticulum and examination after micturition will prevent such an error. *Stones,* whether intravesical or intradiverticular, usually cast clear acoustic shadows (Fig. 12.5). An ectopic ureteric implantation can be demonstrated on proper scans (Fig. 12.6). A dilated pelvic ureter will show, on transverse scans, the pattern of a retrovesical pseudodiverticulum (Fig. 12.7).

From time to time one encounters huge abdominal cystic masses – due to slowly constituted giant bladder dilatation (Fig. 12.8) which escaped the clinician's attention (neurogenic bladder, urethral stenosis, congenital or acquired) and which the patient tolerated for many years.

Ureteroceles

An intravesical diverticular image, in contact with the posterior wall, indicates a ureterocele. Ureteroceles (Fig. 12.4d, e, see also Fig. 3.11) cannot be confused with common diverticula, the more so since the relationship of the intraparietal segment of the ureter with the uterocele is readily demonstrated.

Intramural Ureter

The location of the ureteral confluence is marked by the transitory echogenic turbulences of the ureteral jet (Fig. 12.9). Proper scans can display the intramural segment of the ureter (Fig. 12.10). The narrow angle which the latter outlines with the vesical wall is readily evaluated (Marchal 1982). Abnormal implantations, responsible for reflux, can be demonstrated (Fig. 12.11), and also oral dilatations in some neurogenic bladders.

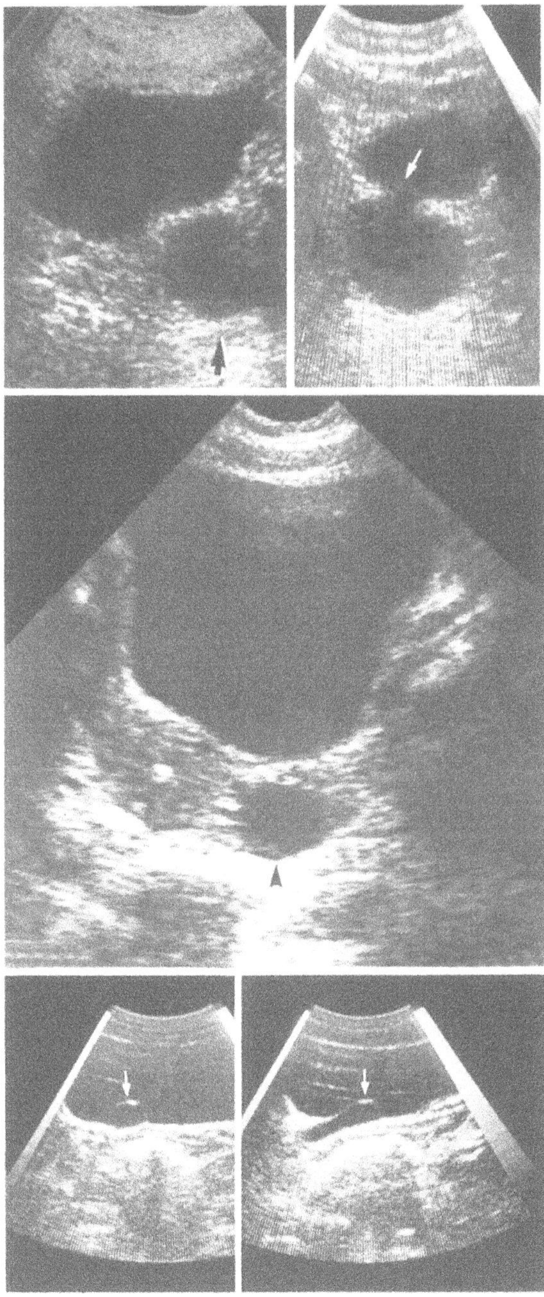
a, b
c
d, e

Fig. 12.4a–e. True and false diverticula. **a** Fluid collection (*arrow*) adjacent to bladder. **b** Parallel scan demonstrates confluence (*arrow*) with bladder: the collection represents diverticulum. **c** Other juxtavesical cystic image (*arrowhead*): this is true ovarian cyst. **d, e** Ureterocele (*arrow*): **d** transverse; **e** oblique scan. Note, in **e**, continuity with ureter

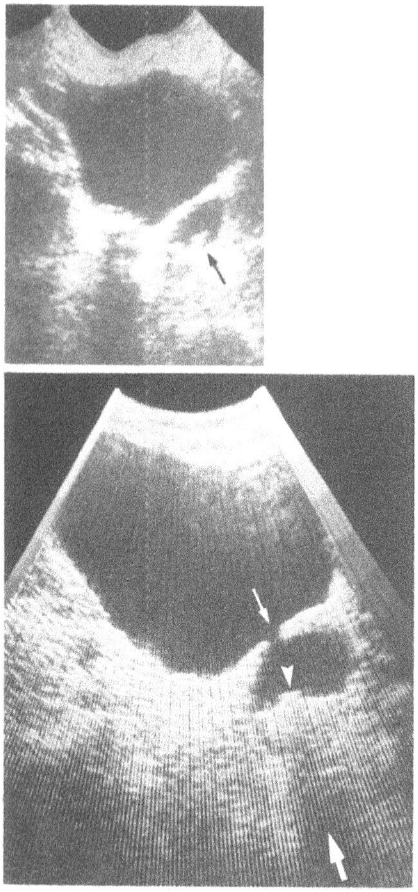

a

b

Fig. 12.5 a, b. Lithiasis within diverticulum: **a** First case: stone is indicated by an arrow. **b** Another case: note orifice of diverticulum (*small arrow*) and shadow (*broad arrow*) of stone (*arrowhead*)

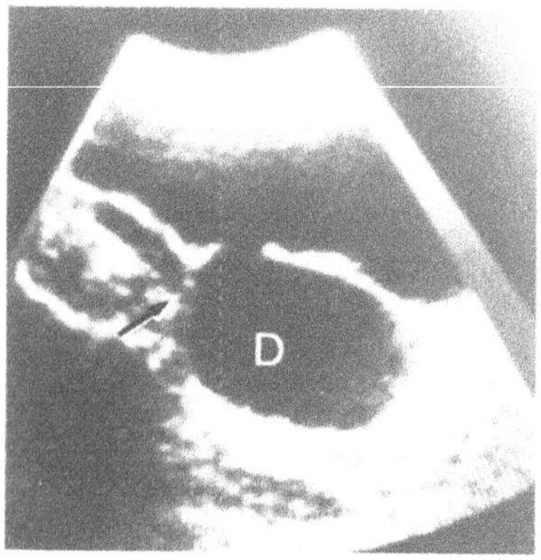

Fig. 12.6. Vesical congenital diverticulum (*D*). Note implantation of right ureter (*arrow*) into the diverticulum (*sagittal scan*). (Courtesy of Dr. Barc, Vannes France)

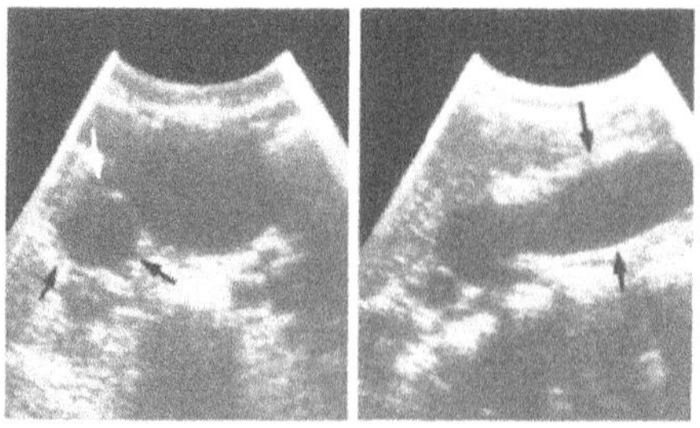

a, b

Fig. 12.7 a, b. Congenital diverticula; differential diagnosis. **a** Retrovesical septated fluid collection (*arrows*) does not correspond to a diverticulum, but to a dilated ureter. **b** The diagnosis is evident on a parasagittal scan

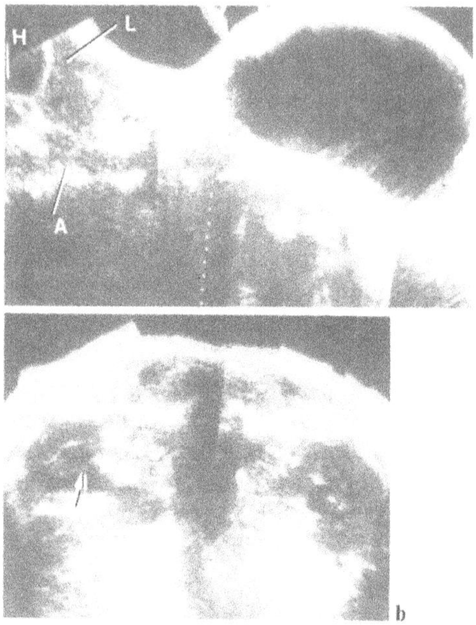

a

b

Fig. 12.8 a, b. Male patient, 25 years old, is referred for abdominal mass. **a** Sagittal scan from xyphoid process down to the pubis shows huge cystic mass extending higher than umbilicus. There is no distinct bladder image. *H*, heart; *L*, liver; *A*, aorta. **b** Transverse dorsal scan shows pelvic dilatation. Cystic mass corresponds to hugely dilated bladder above a clinically undiagnosed urethral valve

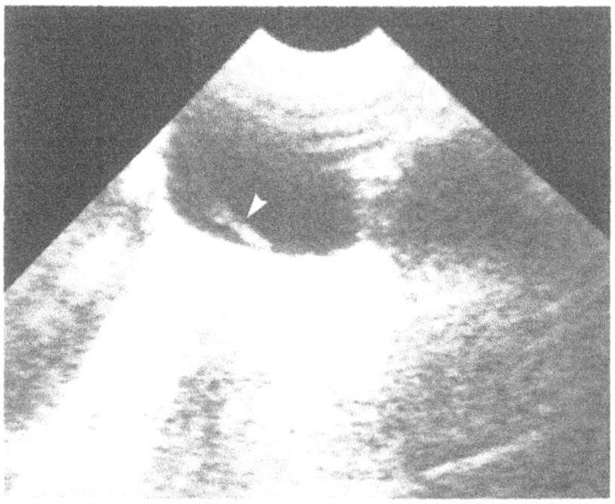

a

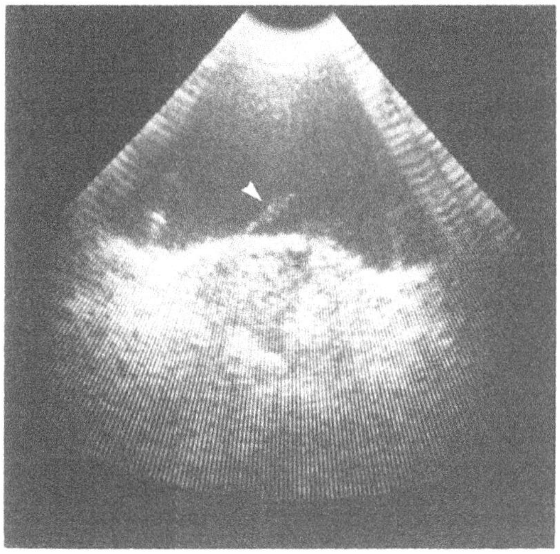

b

Fig. 12.9 a, b. Ureteral jets (*arrowheads*)

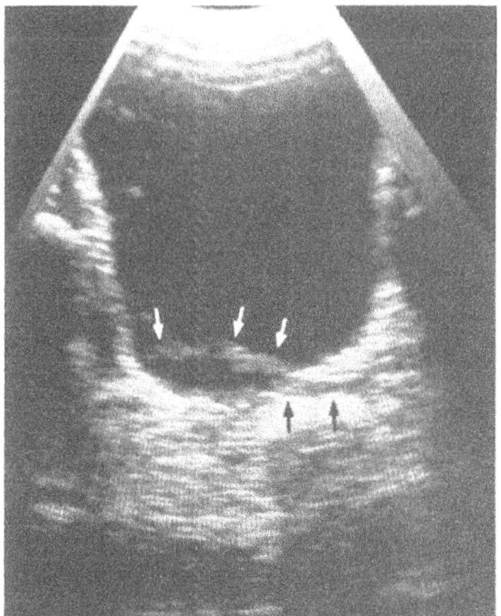

Fig. 12.10. Juxtavesical ureter (*black arrows*) and its intravesical jet (*white arrows*)

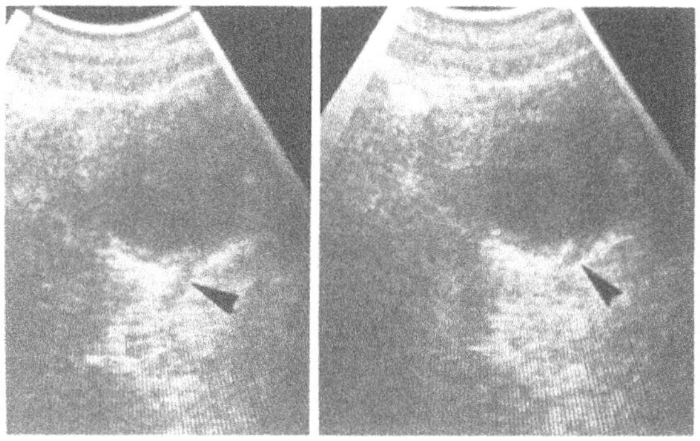

a, b

Fig. 12.11 a, b. Abnormal right ureteral implantation (*arrowheads*)

Tumors

Bladder tumors give rise to growths clearly delineated by the surrounding fluid.

Multidirectional scanning enables one to display the different elements of a case of papillomatosis, even when small (Figs. 12.12–12.14). The scalloped contours of some papillomas are well demonstrated (Figs. 12.12, 12.14). The size, shape, and pattern of implantation of vesical tumors are readily assessed (Fig. 12.15).

The tumoral infiltration can be followed along the vesical wall (Figs. 12.16, 12.17). However, insufficient repletion can increase the apparent thickness of the infiltrated wall. Such infiltrative patterns are frequent in sarcomas, particularly in children, and are also encountered in secondary processes (Fig. 12.17). Neurogenic processes, on the one hand (Fig. 12.18) and acute and chronic cystites on the other hand can also give rise to diffuse parietal thickenings.

Some pathological processes of the lower urinary tract are diagnosed following the display of hydronephrosis, during abdominal screening.

The ultrasonic analysis of the involvement of the muscular layer and perivesical compartments by malignant tumors still provokes discussion, despite already classical publications (Morley 1978–1979). It relies on the smooth character of the parietal muscular line (Fig. 12.15).

However, in our experience, when conventional techniques are used, the base of the tumor often appears as a continuous linear reflection despite direct transmucosal spread. The presence of a tumoral pattern beyond the bladder wall, with fields of heterogeneity (Fig. 12.16), contrasting with the normal homogeneous, intense juxtavesical reflectivity, is more relevant. Transurethral, intravesical devices are designed for this type of study with much more reliable results.

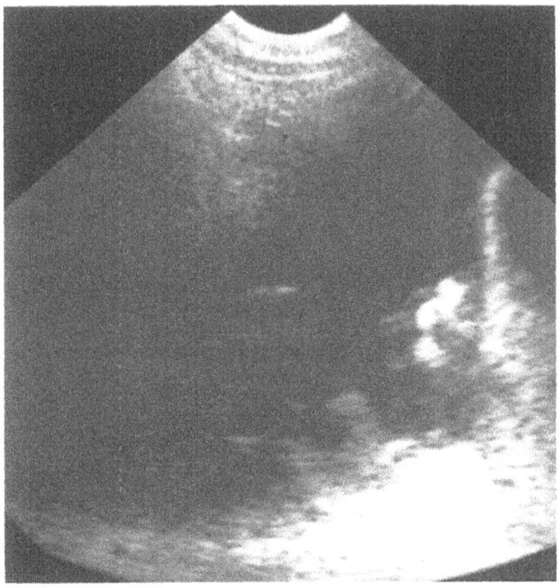

Fig. 12.12. Papilloma

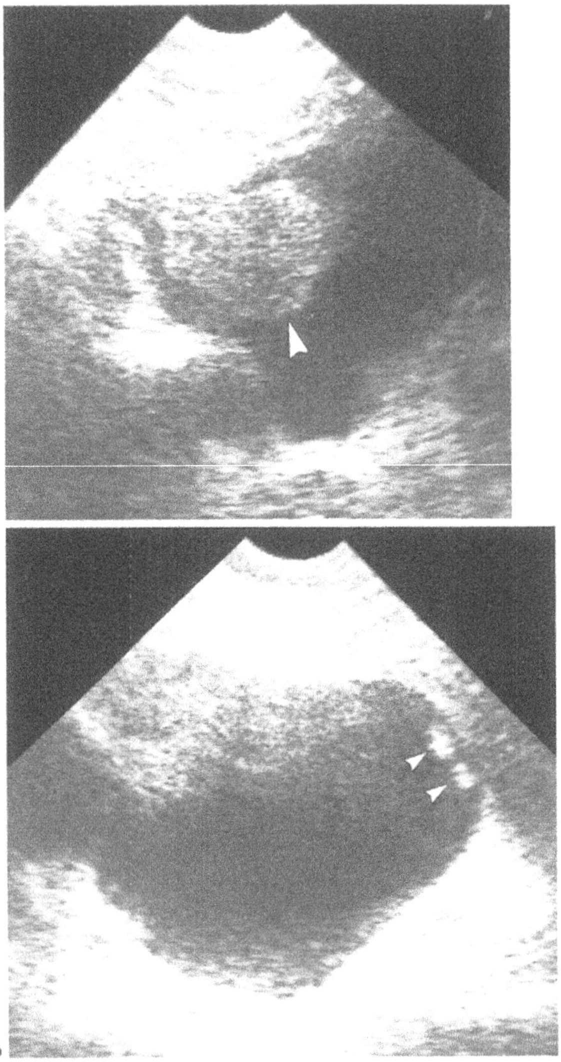

a b

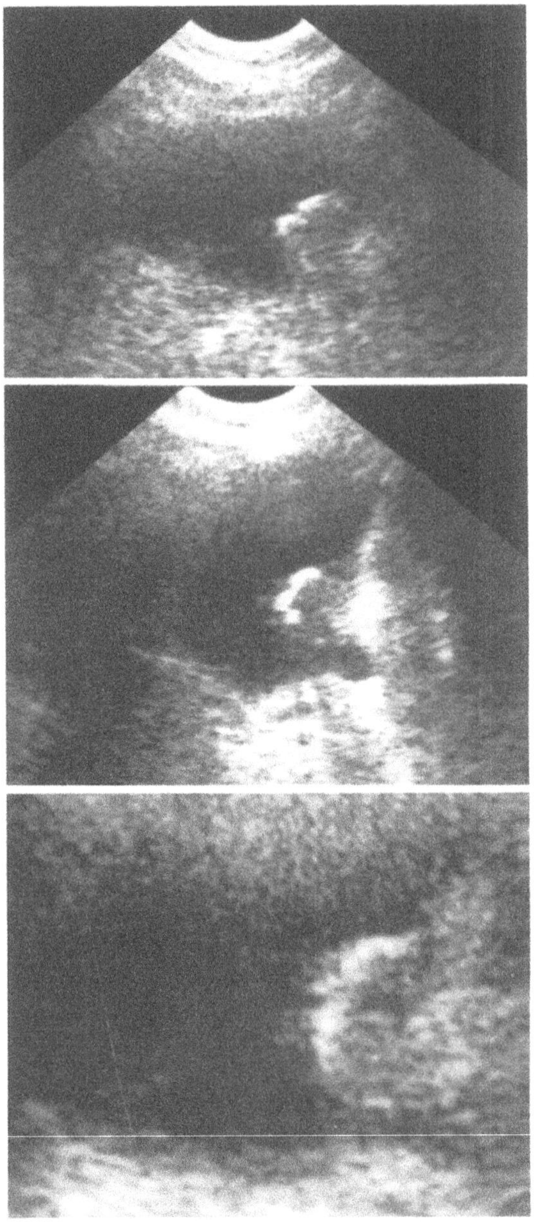

a b c

Fig. 12.14 a–c. Multiple papillomas

◀ **Fig. 12.13 a, b.** Recurrent multiple papillomas (*arrowheads*). **a** Large anterior papilloma; **b** small lateral papilloma

Fig. 12.15 a–g. Bladder carcinoma. **a** First case: tumoral implantation is heterogeneous; there is transmuscular extension (*arrowhead*). **b** Similar image in another case. **c** Third example: muscle (*arrowhead*) seems intact, but was invaded. **d–g** Another case. Four parallel sections carried out with an intrarectal probe. Tumor is readily demonstrated (*arrows*). The muscle seems not involved, except in **a** (*arrowhead*) ▶

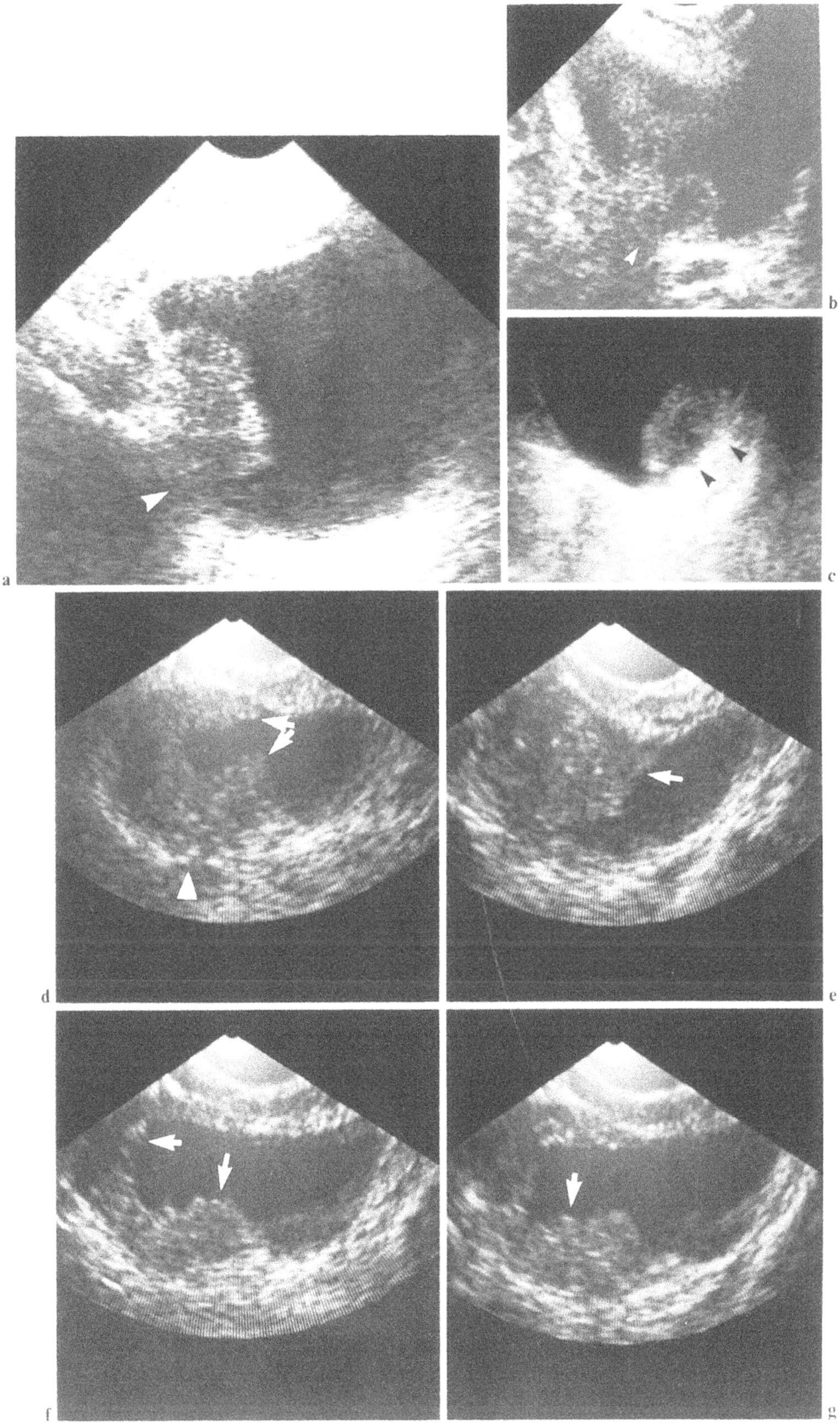

In this field of bladder tumors, only a few documented comparative studies with endoscopic ultrasound are available. CT also has limitations, particularly in the evaluation of tumors arising from the upper and lower walls of the bladder. The work of VON GREINER (1983) is promising for ultrasound.

Associated *blood clot* images can give rise to intravesical areas of reflection. These areas move with changes of position, while a tumor does not (see Fig. 10.12, p. 151).

The pattern of *malignant pelvic tumors* involving the bladder wall can be infiltrating, without specificity (Fig. 12.19). In other cases an impression on the vesical wall is indicative of an extrinsic process (Fig. 12.20).

Noninvading juxtavesical tumors depress the bladder wall. The most frequent, apart from gynecological tumors (Fig. 12.21), are lymph node tumors and lipomatoses. Lymph nodes are usually sonotransparent (Fig. 12.22), whereas lipomatoses are echogenic (RIZZATO 1982).

In gynecological masses, whether due to ovarian cysts or to fibromas, the bladder deformity constitutes an accessory symptom. We shall merely mention juxtavesical *pelvic abscesses*.

Urachus

Urachal cysts extend above the pubis, along the anterior abdominal wall. Exceptionally such cysts can contain malignant tumors, usually due to the extension of bladder carcinomas (Fig. 12.20).

Urethra

Micturition images of the urethra can be obtained with intrarectal linear arrays (SHAPEERO 1983). But in most cases, the urethra is examined because of a suprastenotic dilatation after the discovery of parietal bladder abnormalities consistent with dysectasia. The urethra is then examined by suprapubic approach.

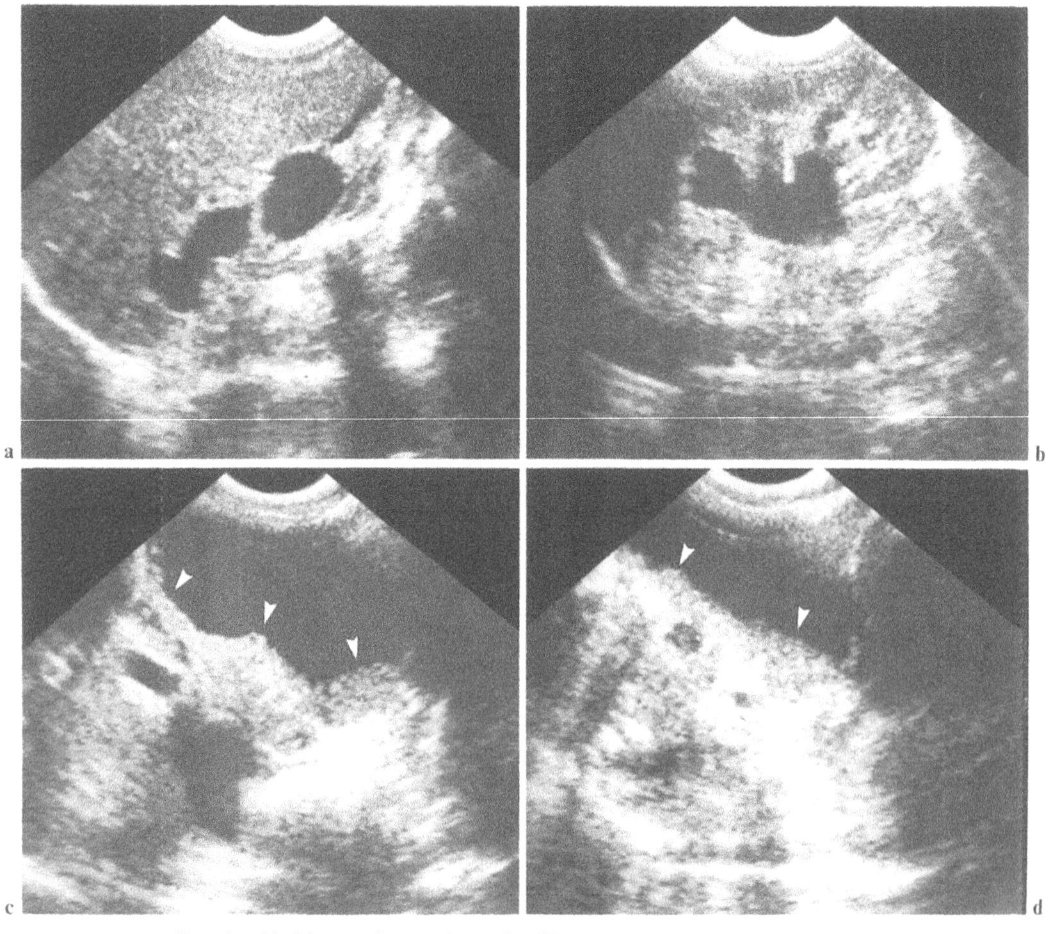

Fig. 12.16 a–d. Infiltrative bladder carcinoma (*arrowheads*), diagnosed after demonstration of hydronephrosis while screening abdomen. Note, in **b**, ill-defined posterior limit

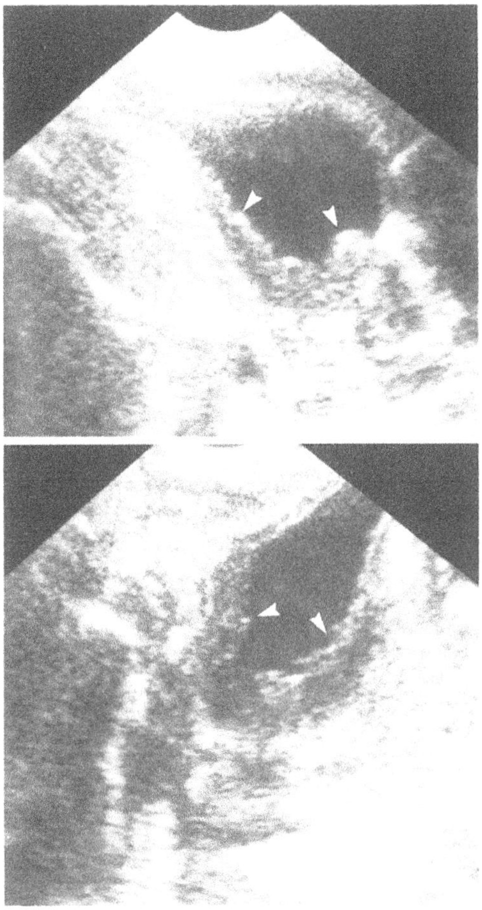

a

b

Fig. 12.17 a, b. Oblique scans show lymphomatous infiltration of bladder (*arrowheads*) (chronic lymphoid leukemia). Similar images are encountered in bladder sarcomas

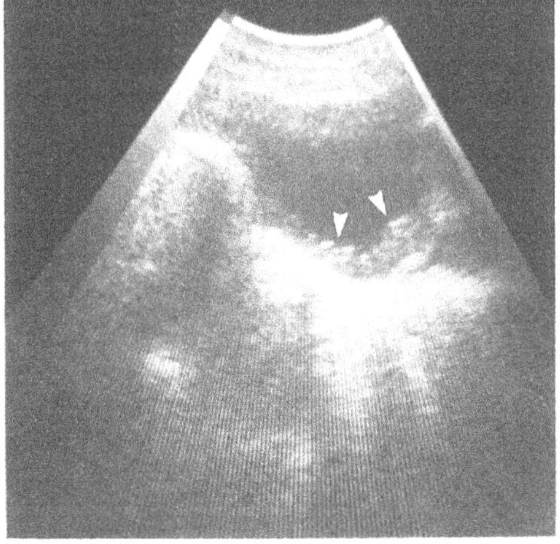

Fig. 12.18. Thickening of the bladder wall (*arrowheads*) due to subacute cystitis in patient with spinal cord injury

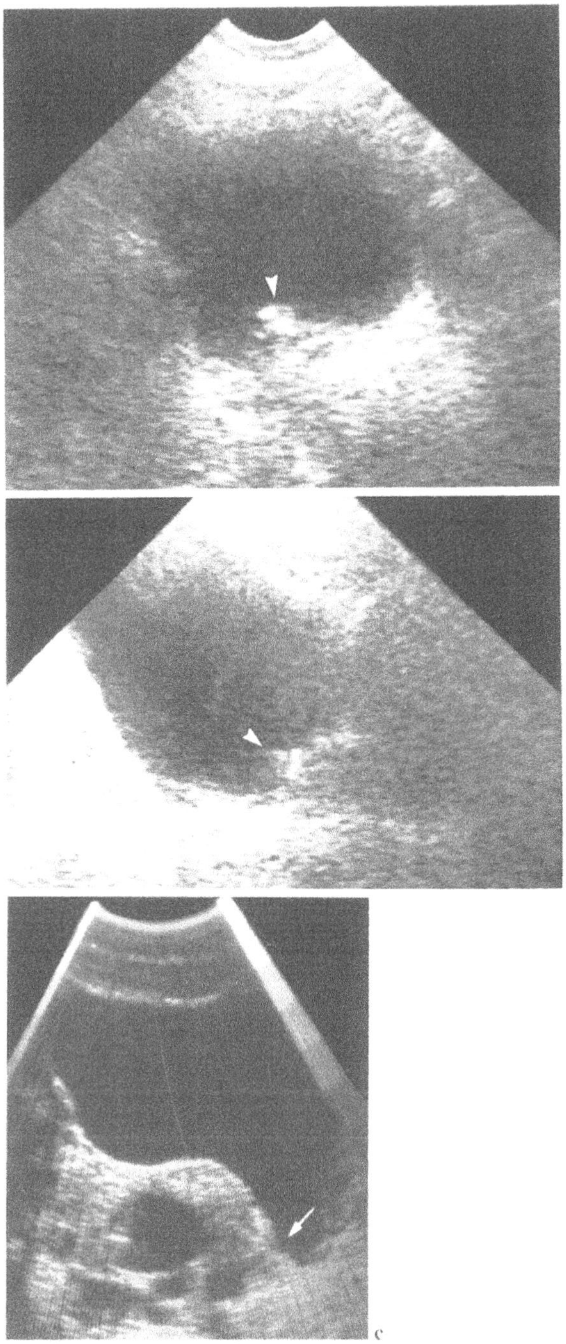

a

b

c

Fig. 12.19 a–c. Extrinsic lesion: **a, b** First case: intravesical growths (*arrowheads*) due to invading recurrent vaginal carcinoma. **c** Another case: invasive tumor. Multilocular ovarian carcinoma bulges toward vesical lumen. Small mucosal elevations (*arrow*) indicate direct spread through bladder wall

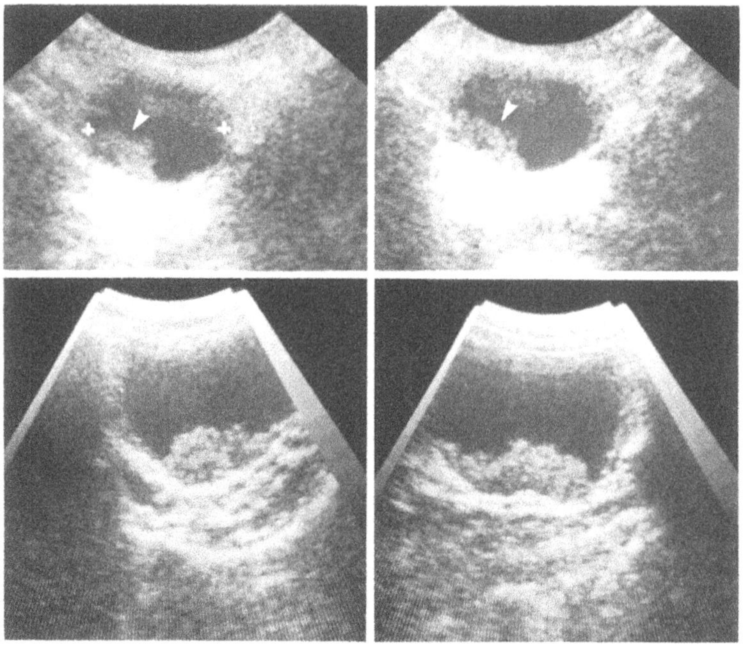

a b c d

Fig. 12.20 a–d. Deposit of bladder carcinoma in urachal cyst. **a, b** Two transverse scans show cyst posterior to the abdominal wall; it contains tumoral growth (*arrowheads*). **c, d** Follow-up examination 6 months later shows increase in tumoral size

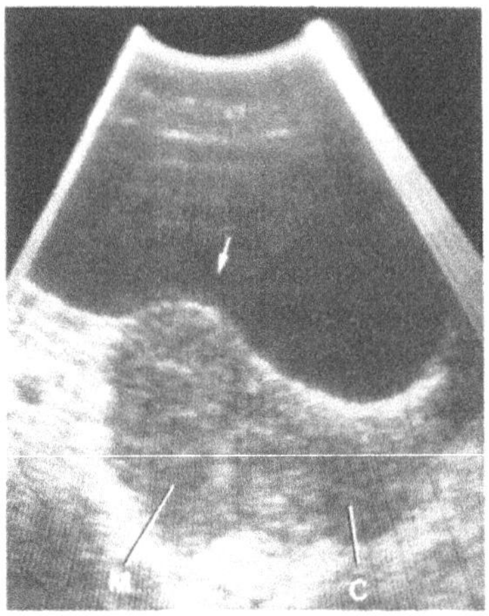

Fig. 12.21. Bladder wall deformity of extrinsic origin: corporeal myoma bulges toward bladder lumen (*arrow*). *C*, cervix; *M*, myoma

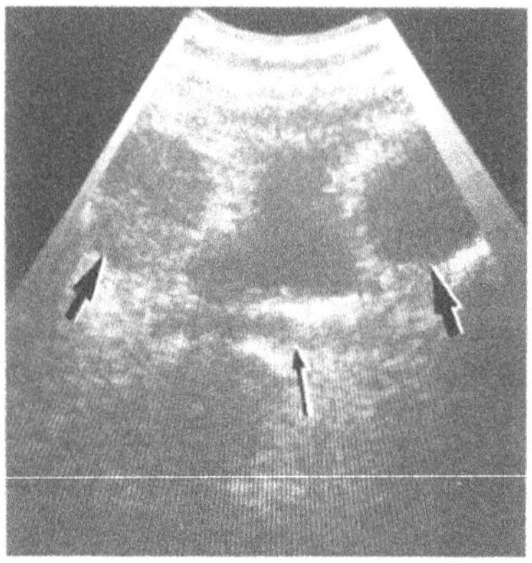

Fig. 12.22. Transverse scan of pelvis in adult male: bilateral sonolucent lymph nodes (*broad arrows*), depress wall of the urinary bladder. Sonolucent retrovesical strip corresponds to the seminal vesicles (*small arrow*). Similar pattern of bladder compression is also encountered in pelvic lipomatosis

12.2 Prostate

Scanning Technique

Transcutaneous prostate scanning is carried out transversally and sagittally. During transverse scans, proper angulation makes it possible to scan the retropelvic area; retropubic sagittal scanning is easy with the help of a small real time head as well as the conventional transducer. Perineal scanning can prove helpful, not foregetting intrarectal transducers.

There are two kinds of *intrarectal methods*: the first relies on a transducer revolving in a plane perpendicular to the axis of the rectum, and the second relies on a linear array; the scanning plane then contains the axis of the rectum. The successive use of both kinds of transducers is commendable. Guided biopsy is easier with linear arrays.

Normal Prostate

The normal prostate is difficult to display with conventional techniques, because of its small volume if the suprapubic approach is utilized (Figs. 12.23–12.24). The small prostate is more readily explored by perineal scanning (Fig. 12.25 a), which does not require bladder repletion, and of course by transrectal scanning (Fig. 12.25 b) which permits screeing of small carcinomas in nonenlarged glands. The normal echotexture is homogeneous. The anterior lobe is sonotransparent. On transverse scans, a central reflection corresponds to the section of the urethral canal. On sagittal scans the canal gives a linear reflection (Fig. 12.24).

The orifices of the ejaculatory ducts induce on transverse scans small symmetrical intraglandular areas of reflection (Figs. 12.22, 12.23).

The lateral limits of the gland are well delineated. Its upper pole does not bulge into the bladder. Retroprostatic acoustic shadows, due to intrarectal gas, can appear behind the gland. On transverse scans the seminal vesicles have a supraprostatic moustache-like pattern (Figs. 12.26, 12.27).

The thin seminal vesicles are displayed symmetrically on transverse sections (Fig. 12.22); each seminal vesicle can also be visualized unilaterally, by oblique scans (Fig. 12.23) and by sagittal scans (Fig. 12.27). Sagittal intrarectal scans show them posteriorly, immediately anterior to the linear array.

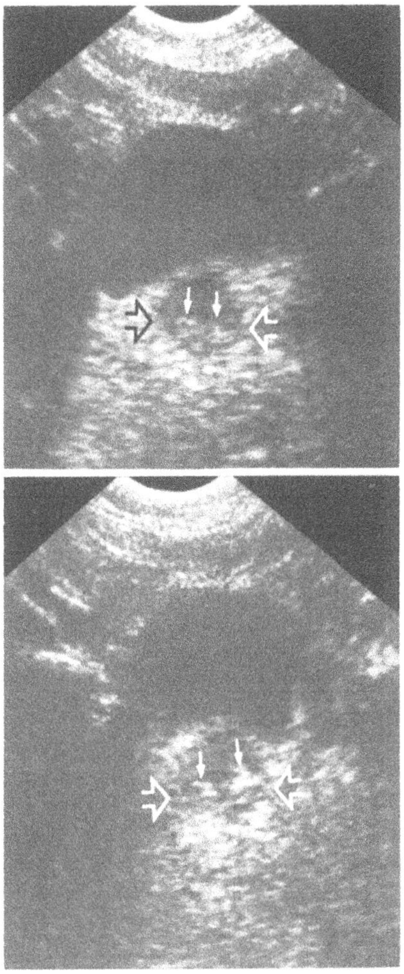

a

b

Fig. 12.23 a, b. Normal prostates (transverse scans). Note (*open arrows*) the well delineated lateral limit. *Small arrows* indicate orifices of seminal ducts. Anterior lobe, anterior to them, is sonotransparent

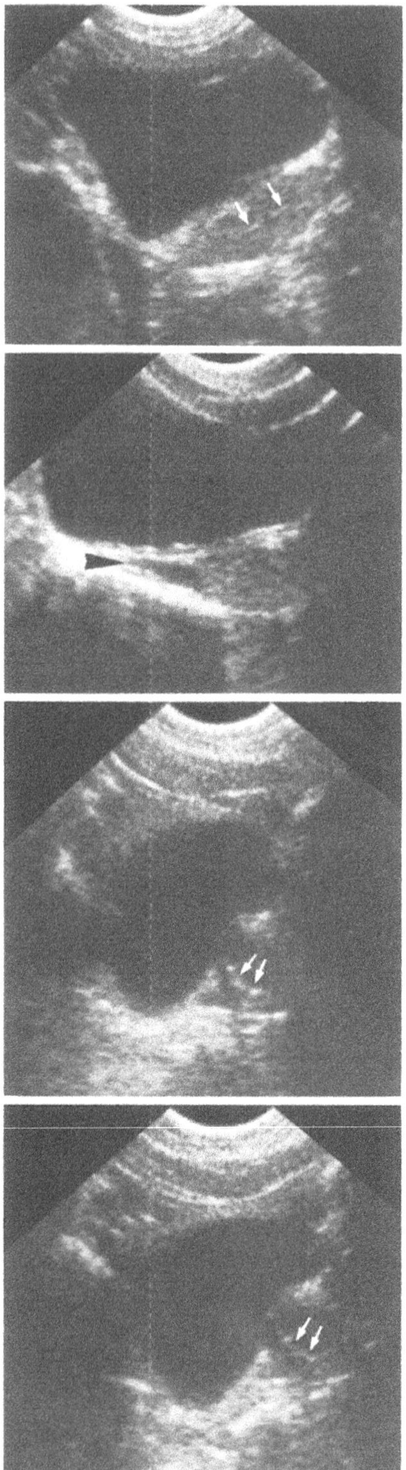

a

b

c

d

Fig. 12.24 a–d. Normal prostates: Suprapubic sagittal scans. *Arrows*: posterior urethra; *black arrowhead*: one of the seminal vesicles

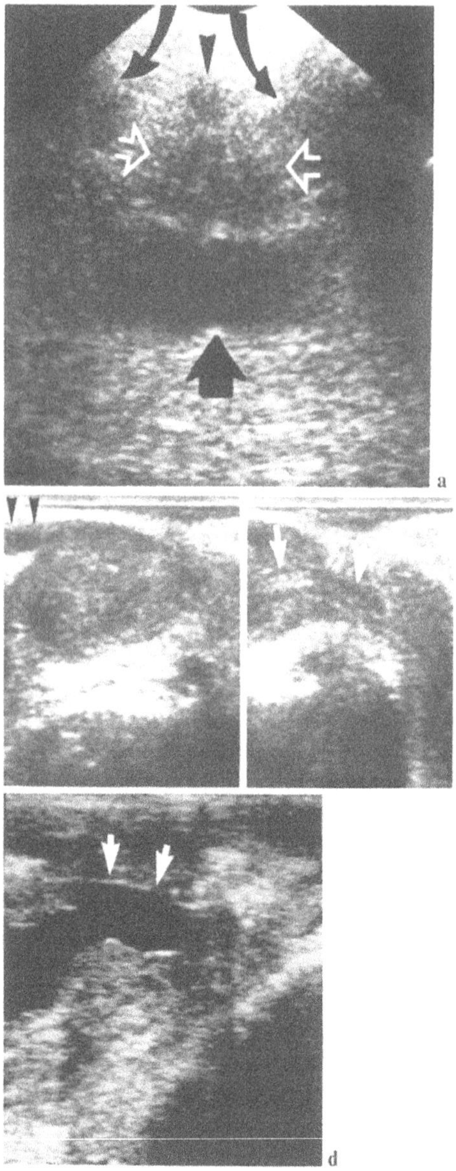

a

b, c

d

Fig. 12.25. a Coronal scan of the prostate (*open arrows*) obtained by perineal scanning. Note the sections of levators ani (*curved black arrow*) and of bulbus of corpus spongiosum (*black arrow*). Broad arrows indicate the bladder. **b–d** Linear intrarectal scanning; **b** parasagittal scan with seminal vesicle (*arrowheads*); **c** medial scan of lower pole with urethra (*arrows*); **d** in another subject the urethra during micturition

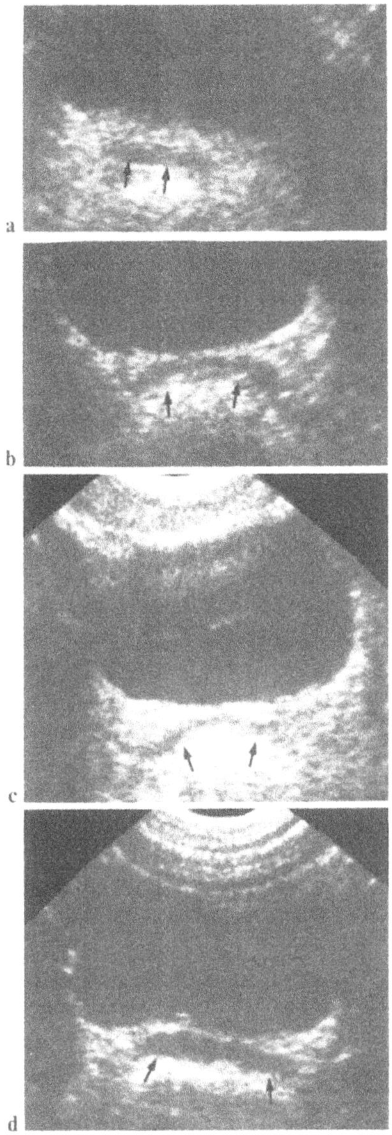

Fig. 12.26 a–d. Transverse scans of seminal vesicles (*arrows*)

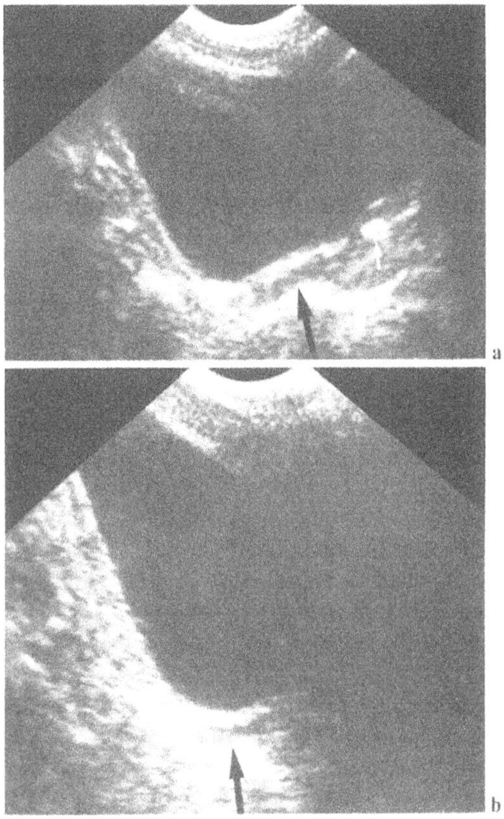

Fig. 12.27 a, b. Sagittal scans of seminal vesicles (*black arrows*). Note, in **a**, prostatic calcified focus (*white arrow*)

Tumors

In adenomas the gland is enlarged; there is a cephalad bulge.

The following formula enables one to evaluate roughly the volume of the prostate.

(Cranio-caudal diameter × transverse diameter × anteroposterior diameter): 3 = volume

Taking density into account, a reduction of 10% enables the passage from volume to weight to be made.

In adenomas the capsule boundaries remains well delineated. The basic texture is homogeneous (Figs. 12.28–12.31 a–f). However, calcifications, parenchymal and lithiasic, and also tissue alterations due to chronic infection, can give rise to heterogeneous reflective nodules (Fig. 12.32). This explains the utter unreliability of the simplistic binary rule: homogeneous echotexture = adenoma; heterogeneous echotexture = carcinoma. Superficial tumors and/or lateral spread blur the glandular limits.

Adenoma can feature multiple nodules with polycyclic contours (Fig. 12.33).

Most *malignant foci* are hypoechoic (Figs. 12.31 g–j). Suspicion of malignancy must lead to scrutiny of the capsule, in order to detect any effraction and spread to the neighboring tissues (Fig. 12.34). Recent publications (Denkhaus 1981; Frentzel-Beyme 1981) confirm that contour abnormalities are more specific of malignancy than mere hypoechoic nodules – not taking into account guided puncture. The presence of trigonal irregularities would also be consistent with a malignant process (Figs. 12.35, 12.36).

Upward bulging of the medial lobe (Fig. 12.37) must not be confused with malignant mucosal growths.

Sonography readily shows the involvement of the seminal vesicles (Fig. 12.38).

Our personal feeling is that CT evaluation of lateral extensions is more relevant than evaluation by transabdominal ultrasound thanks to the particular radiological transparency of pelvic fat. However, Denkhaus et al. (1983) draw opposite conclusions from a comparative study of 41 patients; real time suprapubic sonography gave a better appreciation of tumoral extension than CT.

Prostatitis

In acute prostatitis there is a sonolucent swelling. Collected abscesses give rise to echo-free areas (Figs. 12.39 a–b), as in other organs, and gas bubbles can give rise to echogenic elements. In chronic prostatitis, a reflective heterogeneous echotexture appears. Calcifications give rise to narrow acoustic shadows (Figs. 12.39 c, d).

Seminal Vesicles

Sonography can disclose agenesis of the seminal vesicles, spermatic cysts, tumoral involvement, and inflammatory processes. Vesiculites, acute, subacute, or chronic, is indeed the most frequent pathology. It gives rise to symmetrical swelling of the vesicles, with a sonotransparent echotexture (Fig. 12.40).

Diagnostic Policy in Prostatic Swellings

Posterior malignant nodules and large adenomas are readily diagnosed by ordinary digital rectal examination. Bulging adenomas and malignant spread to the bladder floor give rise to obvious abnormalities on films obtained during the cystographic phase of the IVU.

However, in our institution, we do not perform systematic IVU in prostate adenomas: ultrasound makes possible the morphological evaluation of the renal collecting system, and prostate and bladder; biological tests ensure the renal function is assessed.

What prostatic sonography will more specifically show is:

1. The presence of localized intraglandular abnormalities, whose display must lead to histological analysis by guided puncture.
2. The presence of any peripheral capsule effraction or tumoral spread, demonstration of which is relevant for diagnosis as well as for therapeutic management.
3. Confirmation of involvement of the seminal vesicles.

Finally, the indications for prostatic sonography are:

1. As just mentioned, the preoperative evaluation of the urinary tract.
2. The analysis of the echotexture of adenomas, after clinical sonographic, or urographic diagnosis: any heterogeneity is suspect, even if finally only of inflammatory origin.
3. The evaluation of the limits of the gland when clinical or imaging abnormalities are consistent with a malignant process.
4. In many cases, the shift of the transducer down to the pelvis will in fact follow the discovery,

in an upper abdomen ultrasonic examination, of hydronephrosis or chronic pyelonephritis.

5. Lastly, screening for small tumors, as advocated by WATANABE et al. (1979) either in the frame of general screening or after discovery of metastases. Screening is mandatorily associated to guided puncture.

Thus, we can expect to see the indications for prostatic ultrasound broadening in the years to come. Let us, however, keep in mind that as long as tissue characterization by ultrasound is not available, prostatic scanning implies guided biopsy.

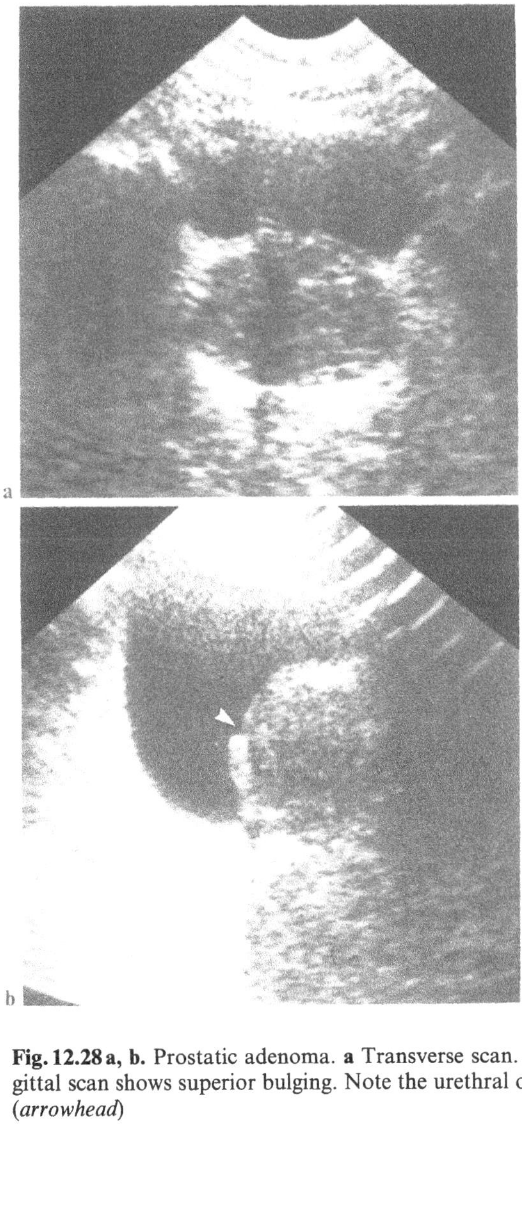

Fig. 12.28 a, b. Prostatic adenoma. **a** Transverse scan. **b** Sagittal scan shows superior bulging. Note the urethral orifice (*arrowhead*)

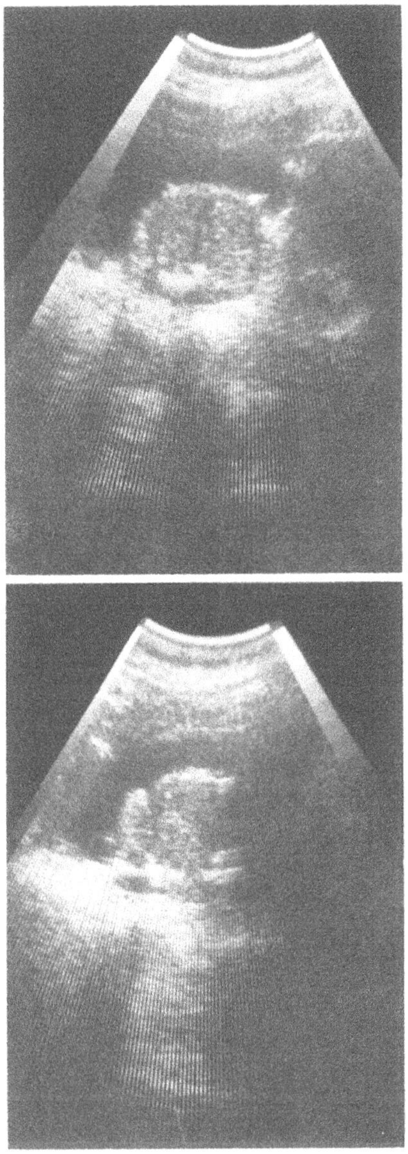

Fig. 12.29 a, b. Adenoma. **a** Transverse scan. **b** Sagittal scan: echogenic zones correspond to urethra on the one hand and to abnormal tissue on the other hand

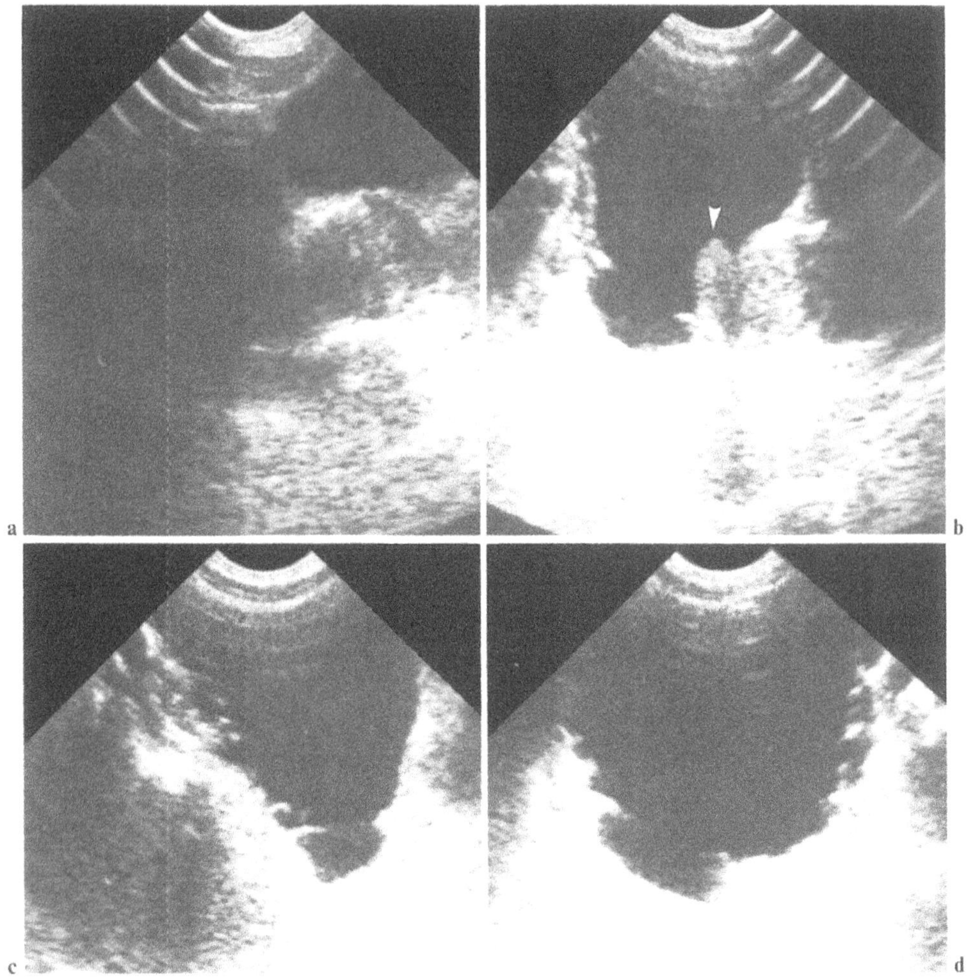

Fig. 12.30 a–d. Adenoma. Bladder pseudodiverticula. **a** Transverse scan of prostate. **b** Sagittal scan: note bulging of the medial lobe (*arrowhead*). **c–d** Scans of bladder show pseudodiverticula

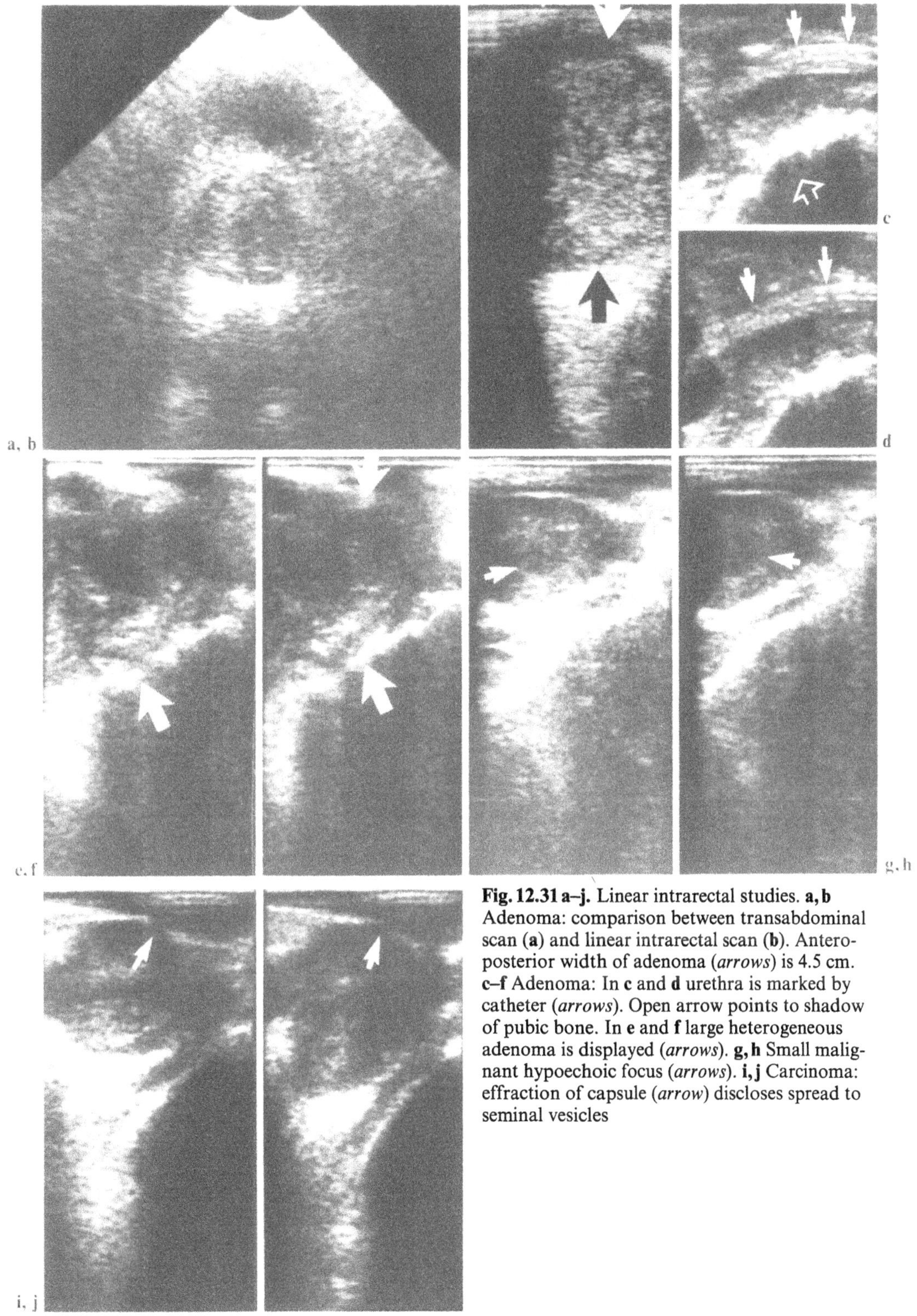

Fig. 12.31 a–j. Linear intrarectal studies. **a, b** Adenoma: comparison between transabdominal scan (**a**) and linear intrarectal scan (**b**). Antero-posterior width of adenoma (*arrows*) is 4.5 cm. **c–f** Adenoma: In **c** and **d** urethra is marked by catheter (*arrows*). Open arrow points to shadow of pubic bone. In **e** and **f** large heterogeneous adenoma is displayed (*arrows*). **g, h** Small malignant hypoechoic focus (*arrows*). **i, j** Carcinoma: effraction of capsule (*arrow*) discloses spread to seminal vesicles

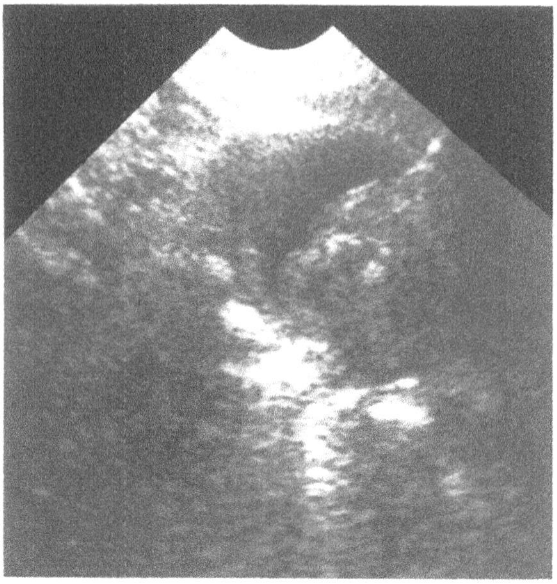

Fig. 12.32. Heterogeneous adenoma (sagittal scan)

▼ **Fig. 12.33 a–d.** Multinodular adenoma. Four transverse scans. Note smooth delineation of polycyclic contour

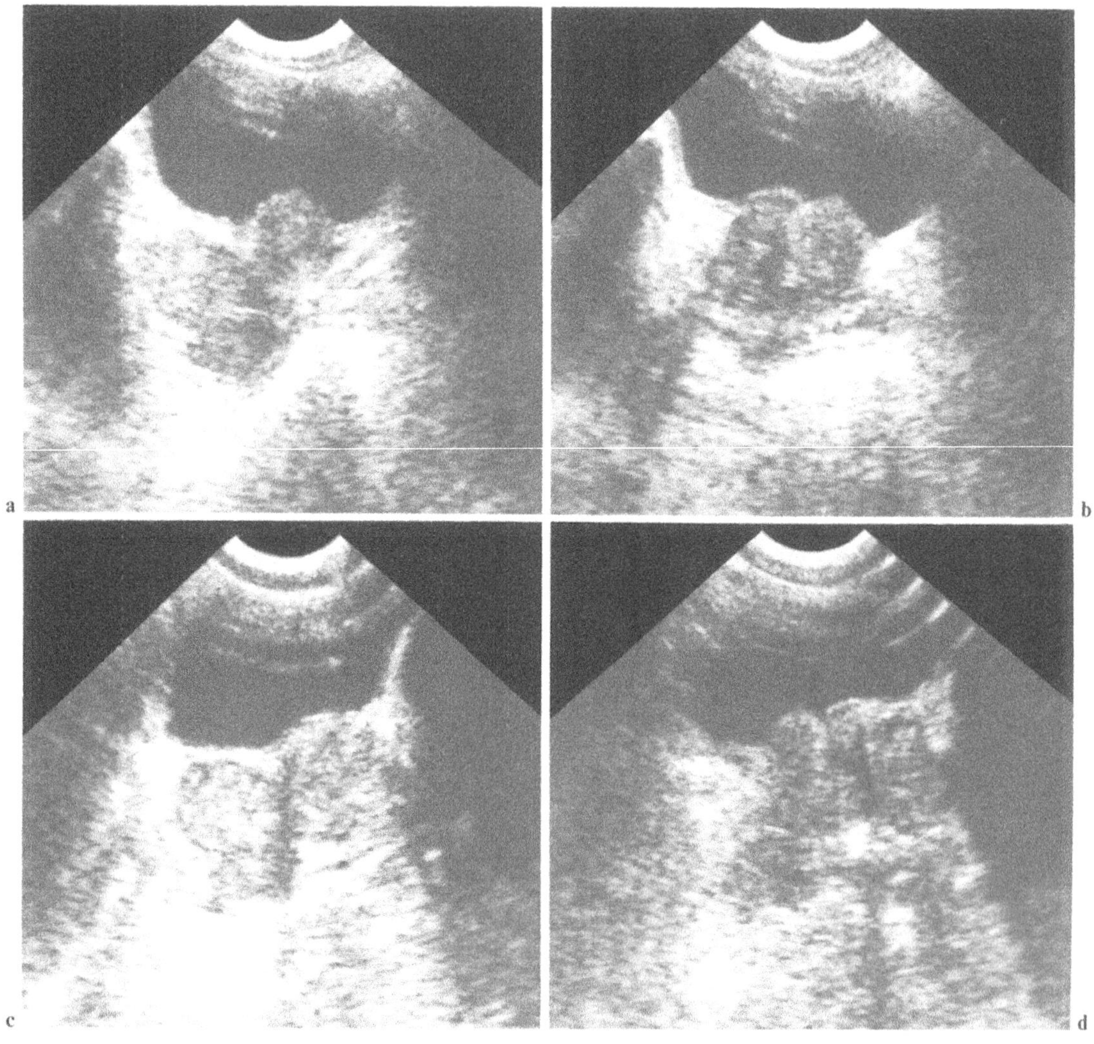

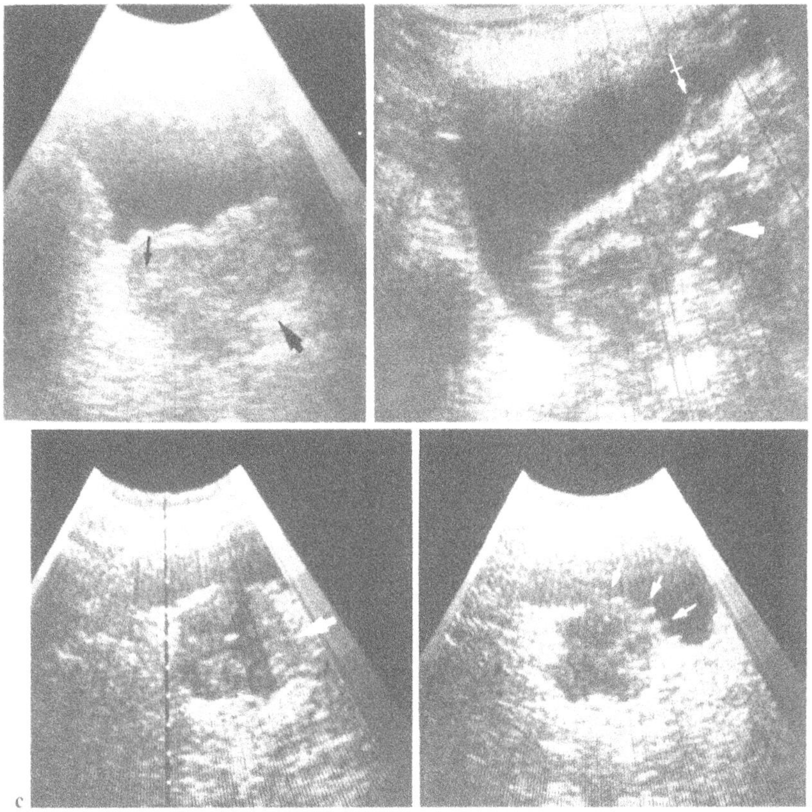

Fig. 12.34 a–d. Prostatic carcinoma. **a, b** First case: prostatic carcinoma developed on adenoma. **a** Transverse real time scan. There is a reflective nodule (*small arrow*) present. Posterolateral prostatic wall is irregular (*broad arrow*). Note the small mucosal irregularities. These patterns are indicative of malignancy. **b** Parallel transverse scan. Note again heterogeneous echotexture. Left lateral limit (*arrows*) is irregular. There is intravesical growth (*crossed arrow*). These last two elements count in favor of malignancy. **c, d** Prostatic carcinoma. Real time transverse scans show heterogeneous echotexture (*broad arrow*), irregular limits, and small intravesical growths (*small arrows*)

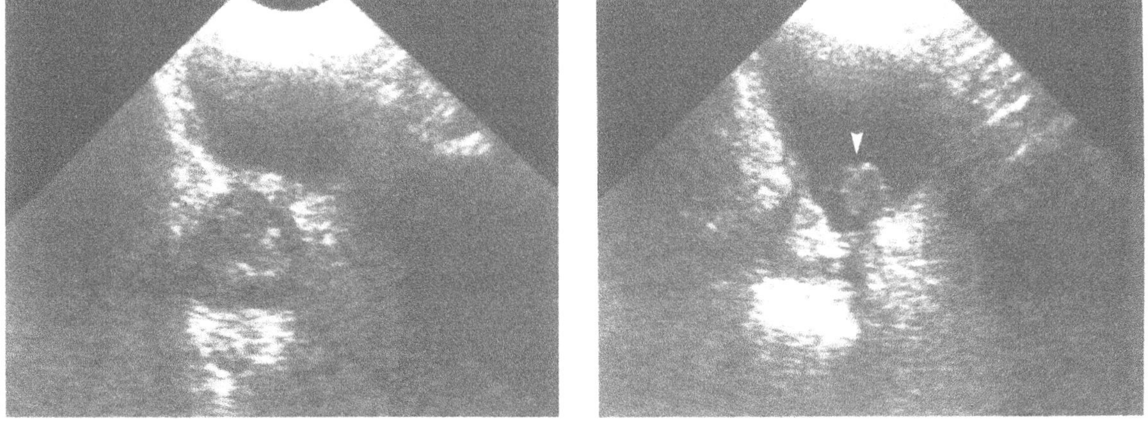

Fig. 12.35 a, b. Carcinoma. **a** Transverse scan shows common pattern of adenoma. **b** Sagittal scan discloses malignant mucosal growth (*arrowhead*)

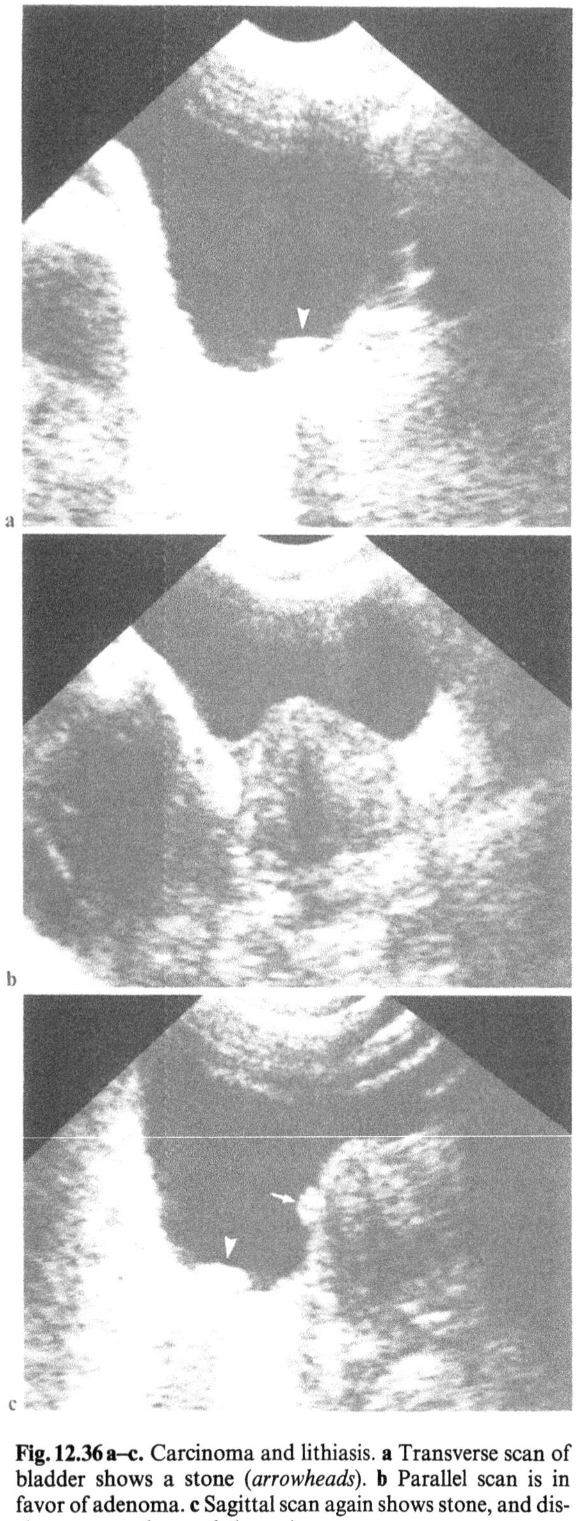

Fig. 12.36 a–c. Carcinoma and lithiasis. **a** Transverse scan of bladder shows a stone (*arrowheads*). **b** Parallel scan is in favor of adenoma. **c** Sagittal scan again shows stone, and discloses mucosal growth (*arrow*)

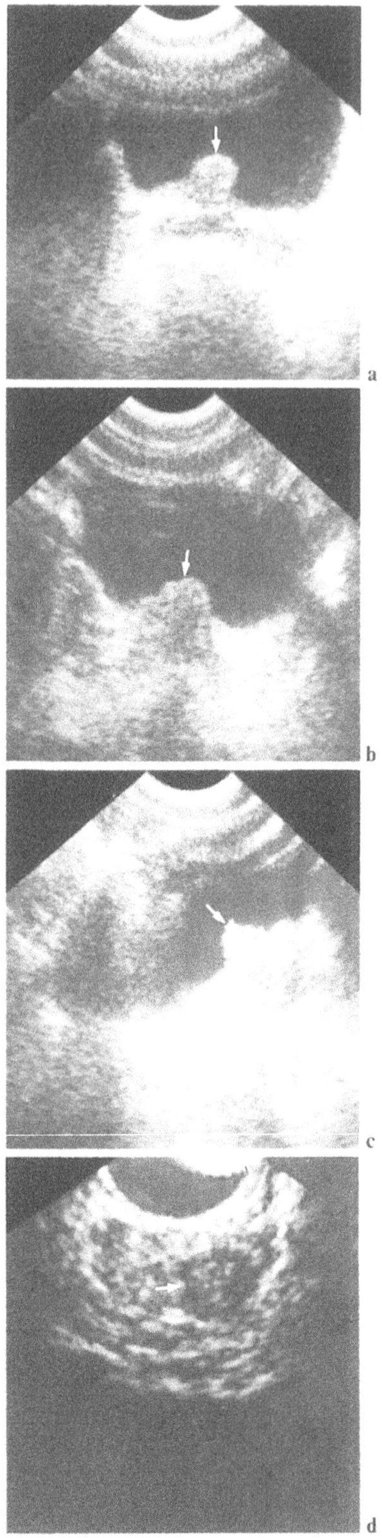

Fig. 12.37 a–d. Two benign prostatic abnormalities. **a–c** First case: hypertrophic medial lobe. **a, b** Transverse scans. **c** Sagittal scan. **d** Another case: intraglandular nodule displayed on a section obtained with an intrarectal probe with transverse scanning

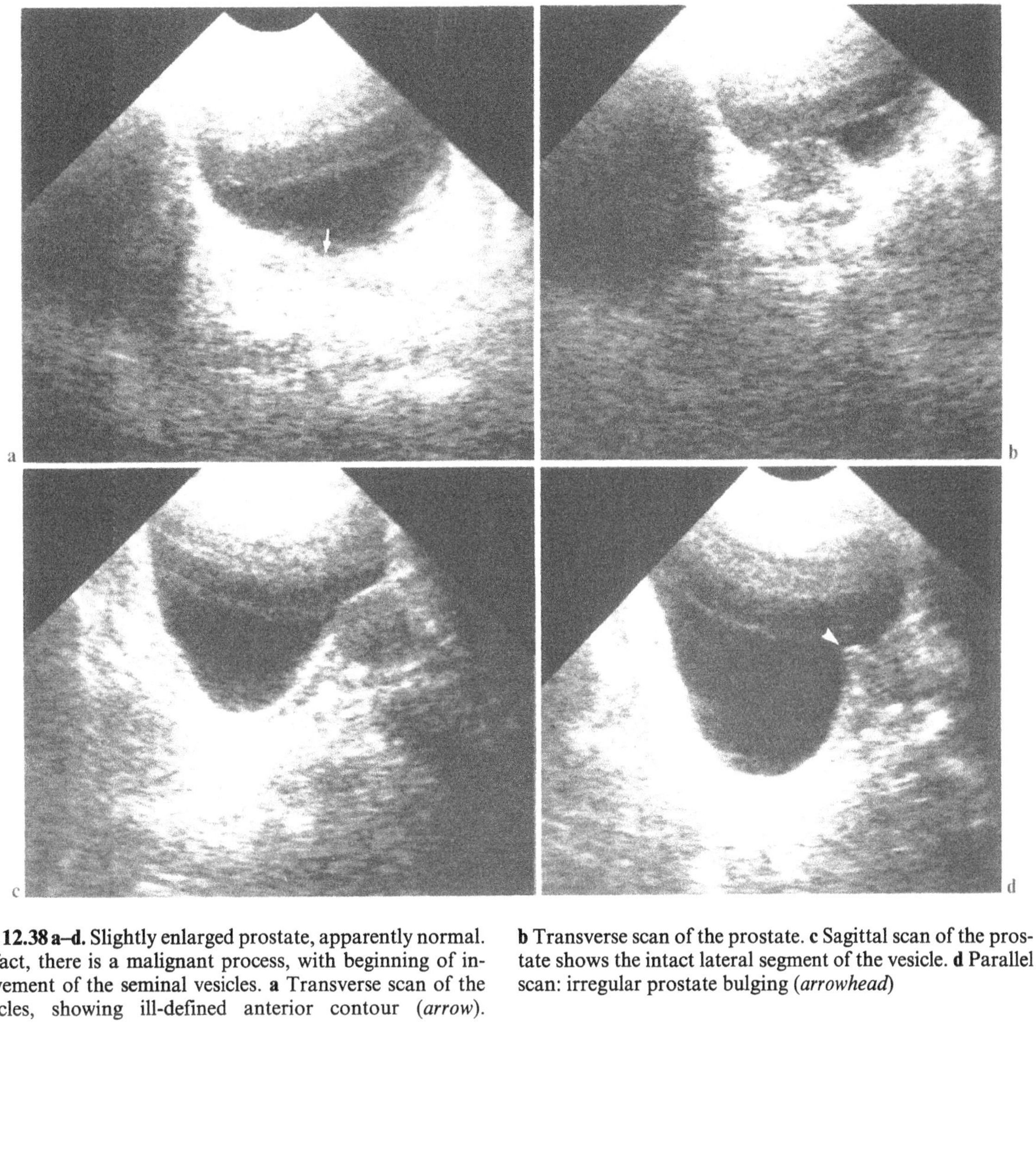

Fig. 12.38 a–d. Slightly enlarged prostate, apparently normal. In fact, there is a malignant process, with beginning of involvement of the seminal vesicles. **a** Transverse scan of the vesicles, showing ill-defined anterior contour (*arrow*). **b** Transverse scan of the prostate. **c** Sagittal scan of the prostate shows the intact lateral segment of the vesicle. **d** Parallel scan: irregular prostate bulging (*arrowhead*)

a, b

c–f

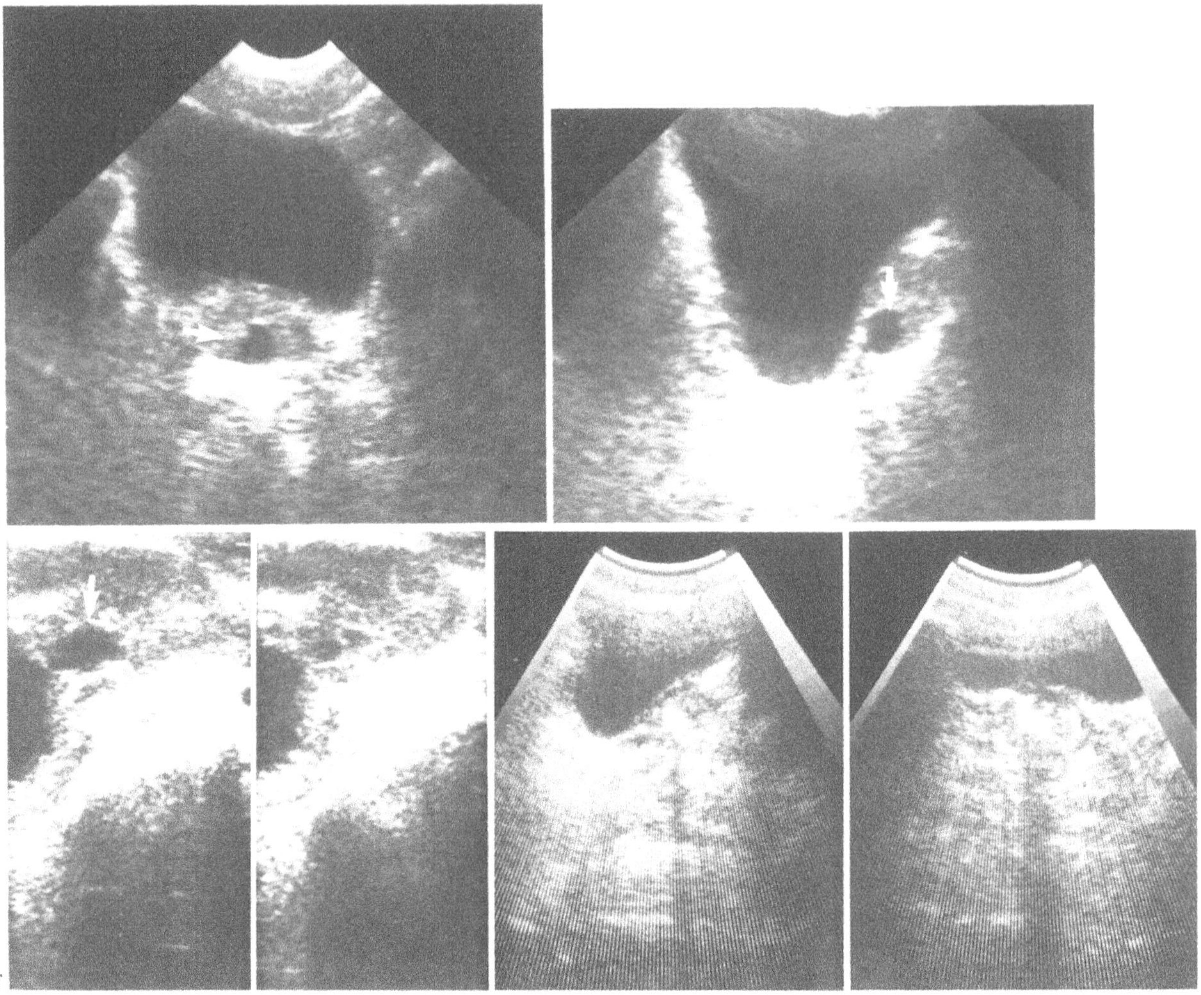

Fig. 12.39. a–d Abscess. **a** Transverse scan shows sonotransparent defect (*arrow*); **b** sagittal scan; **c, d** linear intrarectal scanning again shows defect (*arrow*); **e, f** chronic calcified prostatitis; **e** sagittal scan; **f** transverse scan

Fig. 12.40 a–c. Vesiculitis: swelling of vesicles. **a** First case: ▸ transverse scan; **b, c** another case; **b** right oblique scan; **c** transverse scan

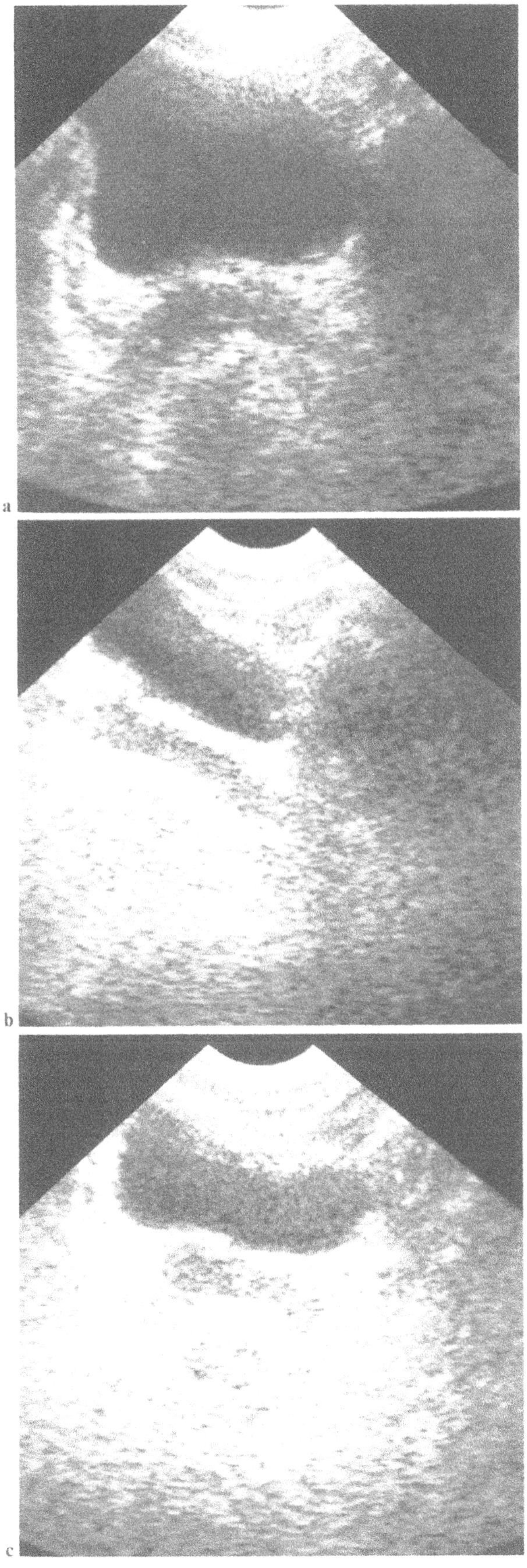

a

b

c

12.3 Testis and Its Covering

The availability of high-frequency real time heads of at least 7 MHz, with liquid delay, has made it possible routinely to obtain excellent testicular images (ARGER et al. 1981; VICK et al. 1982; BLEI et al. 1983; CARROLL et al. 1983).

Examination Procedure

Sagittal and transverse scans are carried out while the patient holds the penis upward. Since the testis is very mobile, the operator holds it with one hand while applying the transducer with the other hand.

Normal Testis

The contours of the normal testis are smooth and harmonious. Its echotexture is homogeneous, with a striking rich echo-amplitude (Fig. 12.41). Normally, size and echotexture are symmetrical. A small amount of fluid within the tunica vaginalis is displayed even in the normal subject.

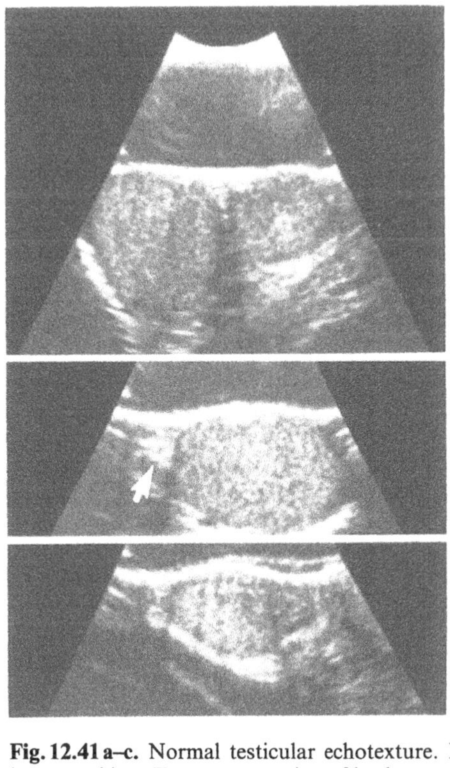

a

b

c

Fig. 12.41 a–c. Normal testicular echotexture. Left testis is hypotrophic. **a** Transverse section of both testes. **b** Right sagittal scan. *Arrow*, epididymis. **c** Left sagittal scan

The reflection of the tunica albuginea is marked by a small echogenic strip (Fig. 12.42). The epididymis is even more echogenic than the testis itself (Figs. 12.41 b and 12.44 b).

Miscellaneous Abnormalities

High-frequency real time examination enables one to localize the *undescended testis* (Fig. 12.43) (WOLVERSON 1983 a). Such localization is an important preoperative step, since undescended testis are liable to develope seminomas.

Hydroceles of the tunica vaginalis are readily demonstrated thanks to their typical liquid pattern (Figs. 12.44, 12.45).

Epididymal cysts are characterized by their supratesticular location (Fig. 12.46).

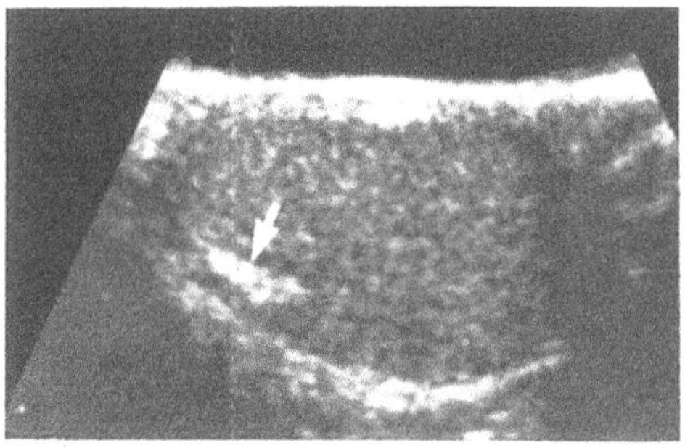

Fig. 12.42. Normal testis. Note zone of reflection of albuginea (*arrow*)

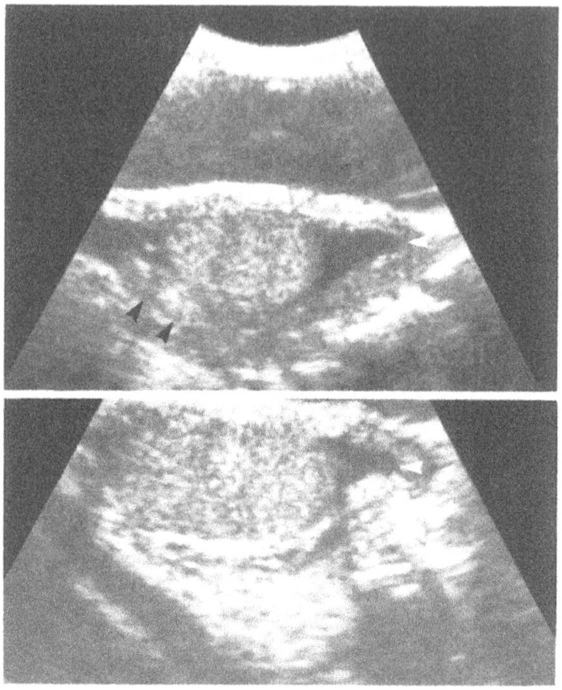

Fig. 12.44 a, b. Hydrocele with small amount of fluid (*white arrowheads*). Note in **a** pattern of epididymis (*black arrowhead*). (Two right sagittal scans)

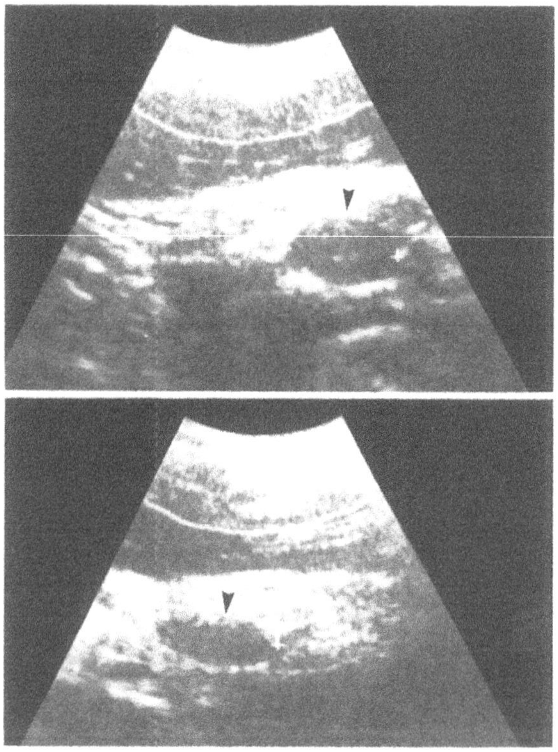

Fig. 12.43 a, b. Nondescended testes. Transverse scans above the groin show the oval pattern of both glands (*arrowheads*)

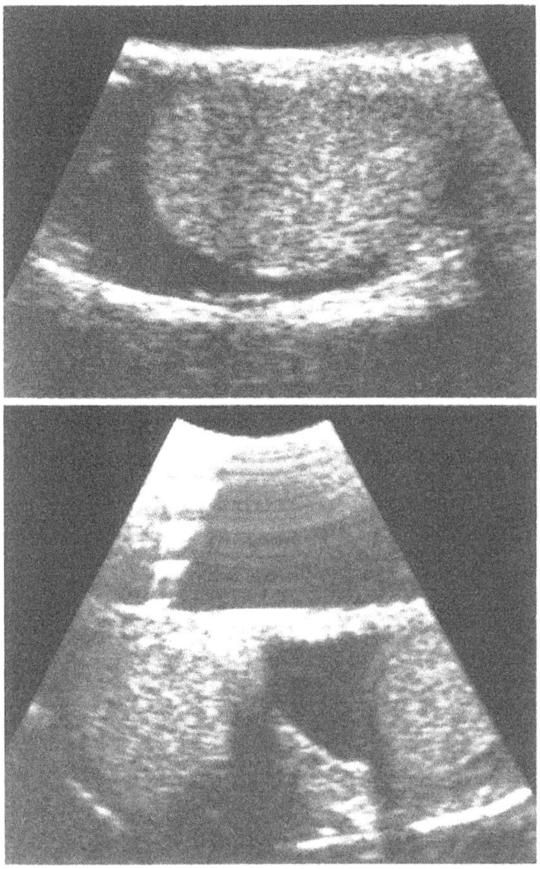

Fig. 12.45 a, b. Abundant hydrocele. **a** Sagittal scan; **b** transverse scan

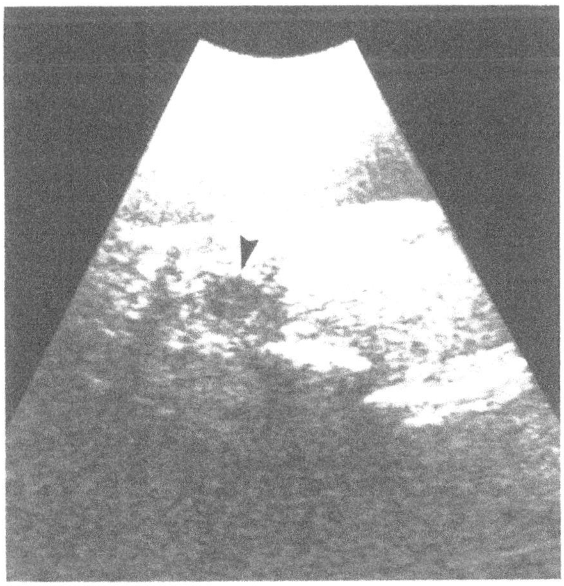

Fig. 12.46. Epididymal cyst (*arrowhead*). Sagittal scan

Varicoceles

Venous ectasia gives rise to multiple and adjacent cystic images (Fig. 12.47) (Wolverson 1983b). Doppler studies can demonstrate a blood flow.

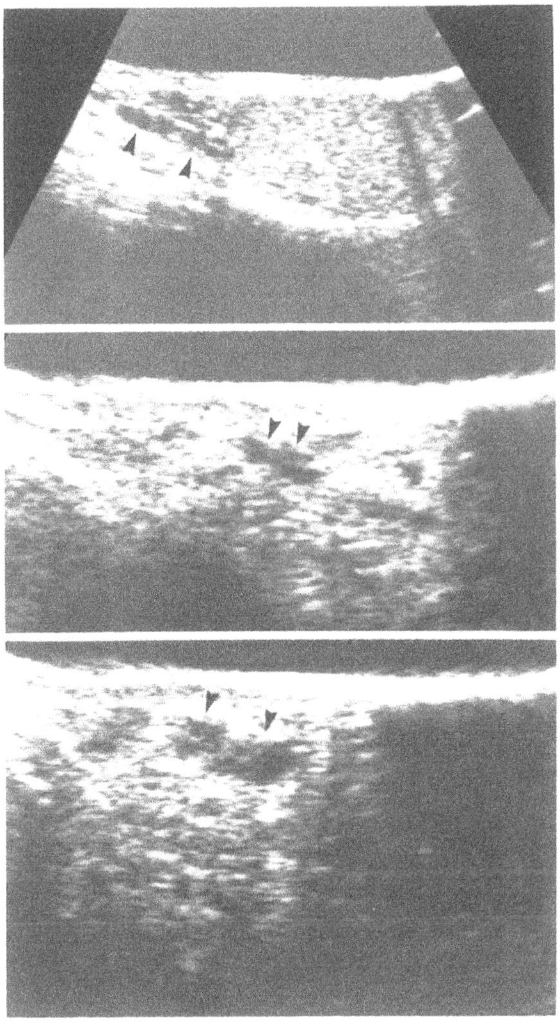

Fig. 12.47 a–c. Varicocele (*arrowheads*). Sagittal scans

Trauma

Examination of a traumatized scrotum enables one to differentiate swelling of the covering by hematoma or edema, from true testicular swelling by contusion or hematoma (Fig. 12.48), the latter requiring surgery (Cunningham 1983; Jeffrey 1983).

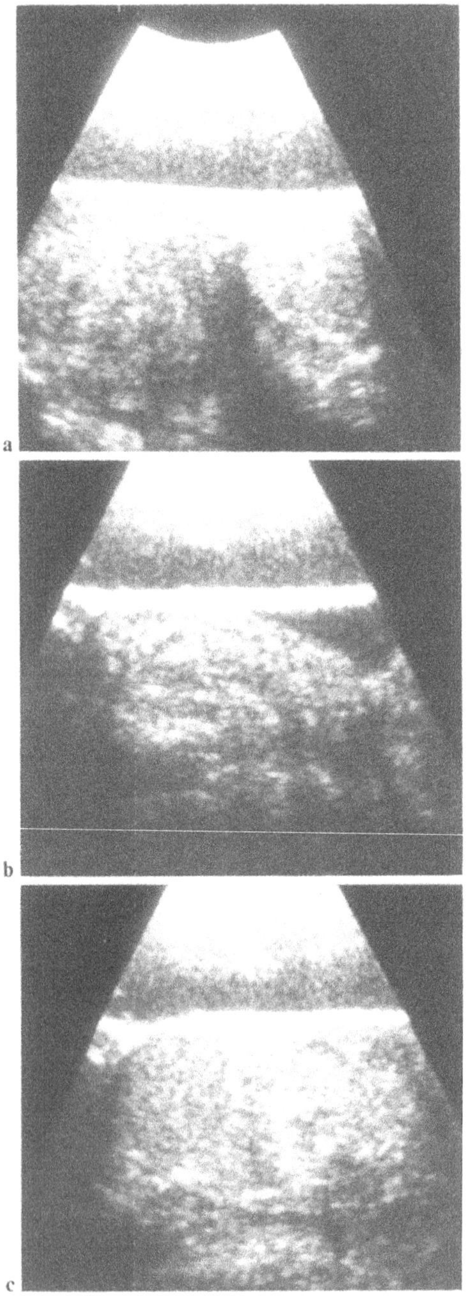

Fig. 12.48 a–c. Traumatic hematoma of right testis. **a** Transverse scan of both glands. Right testis is swollen and heterogeneous. **b** Sagittal scan of traumatized testis. **c** Sagittal scan of normal testis

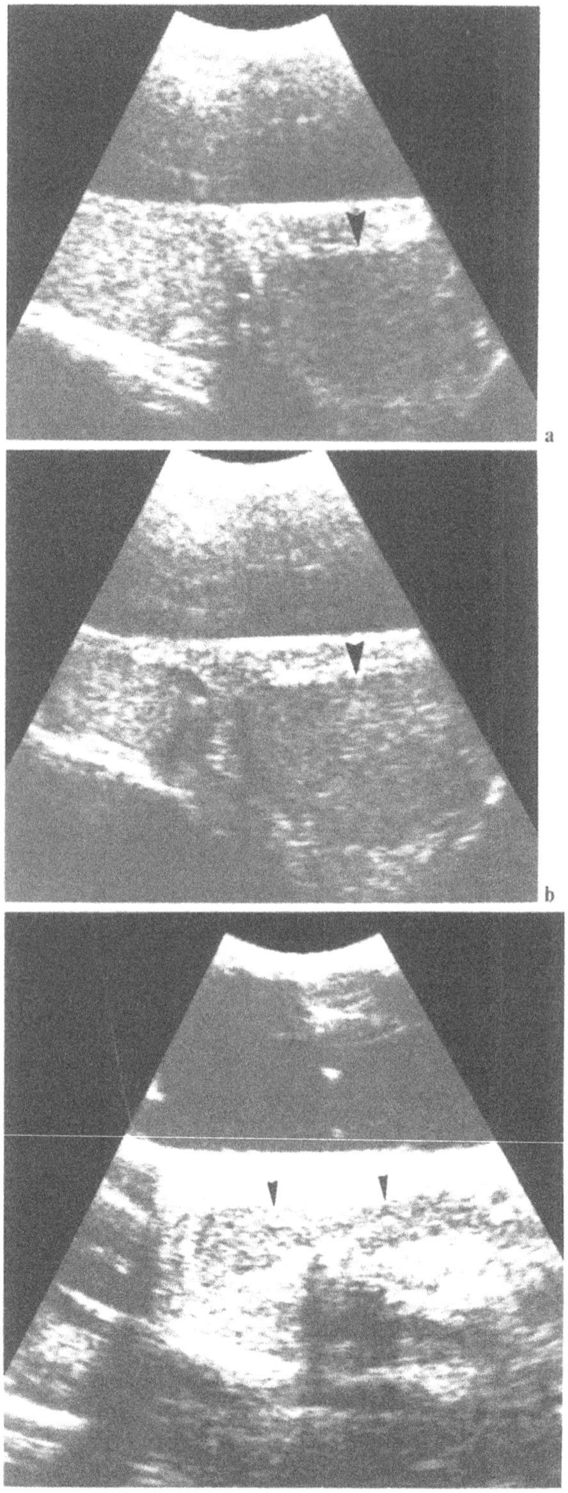

Fig. 12.49 a–c. Inflammatory processes: **a, b** Orchitis. **a** Transverse scan of both glands. Swollen left testis is sonotransparent (*arrowhead*). **b** Sagittal scan. **c** Epididymitis: *arrowheads* indicate swollen epididymis

Orchitis and Epididymitis

Orchitis gives rise to nonspecific images of sonotransparent global swelling (Fig. 12.49 a, b). Epididymitis is characterized by supratesticular swelling (Fig. 12.49 c).

Tumors

Tumors do not possess a specific pattern: any heterogeneity, any nodular pattern is consistent with a tumoral process (GLAZER 1982). Such abnormalities are encountered either in the context of the evaluation of a swollen testis (Fig. 12.50), or while assessing the testis after discovery of nonlymphomatous retroperitoneal lymph nodes in young male patients. Testicular scans can show a mere scar image. Systematic screening of the testis, is also carried out in acute lymphomas, whether Hodgkinion or not (PORTALEZ 1982; LUPETIN 1983).

Scrotal hernias should not be confused with testicular tumors (Fig. 12.51). Since we are dealing with pitfalls, please take note of Fig. 12.52.

Of the previous features, we can retain the following as indications for testicular sonography: (1) location of the undescended testis; (2) trauma; (3) morphological analysis of the swollen scrotum, in order to differentiate the pathology of the covering from epididymal or testicular swellings; and (4) systematic screening for small testicular tumors or deposits, after discovery of retroperitoneal lymph nodes, or in the presence of acute lymphoma.

The lack of specificity of testicular pathological images must, however, be emphasized: there, as elsewhere, we only see images. The definite diagnosis relies on biopsy.

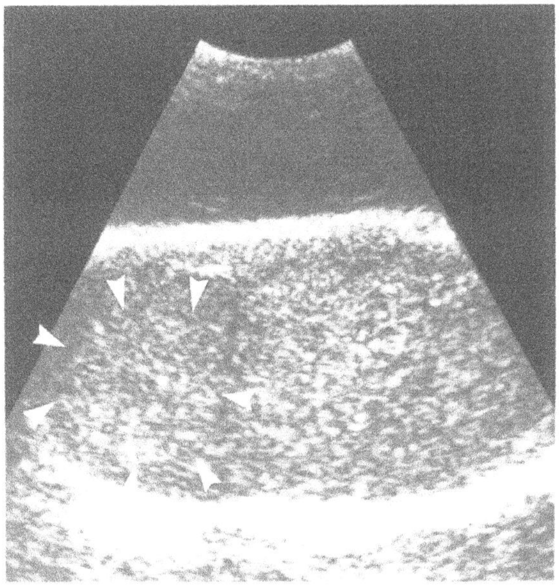

Fig. 12.50. Dysembryoma: sagittal scan shows round heterogeneous nodule (*arrowheads*)

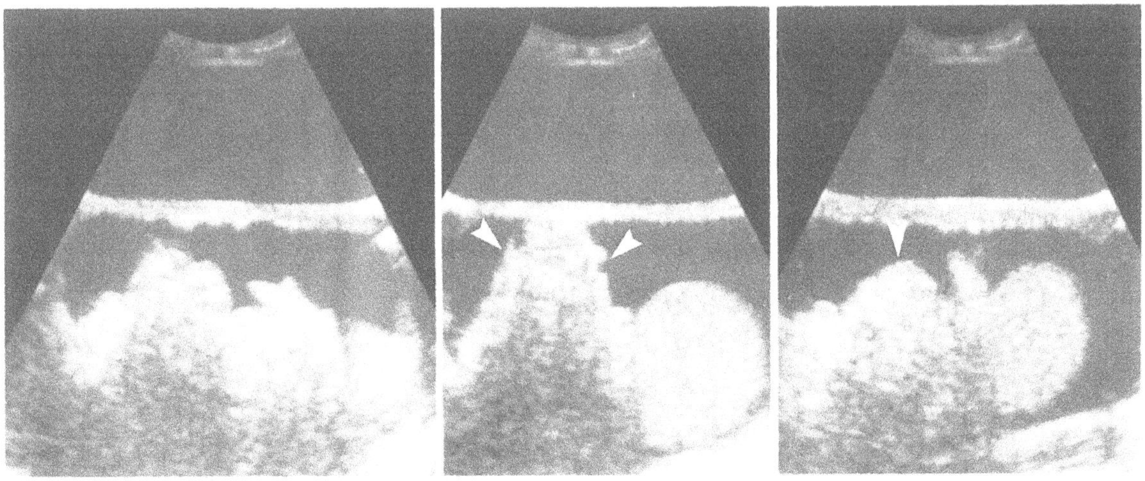

Fig. 12.51 a–c. Right scrotal hernia (*arrowhead*) and hydrocele. Two transverse scans. (Courtesy of Dr. R. Costaz, Besançon)

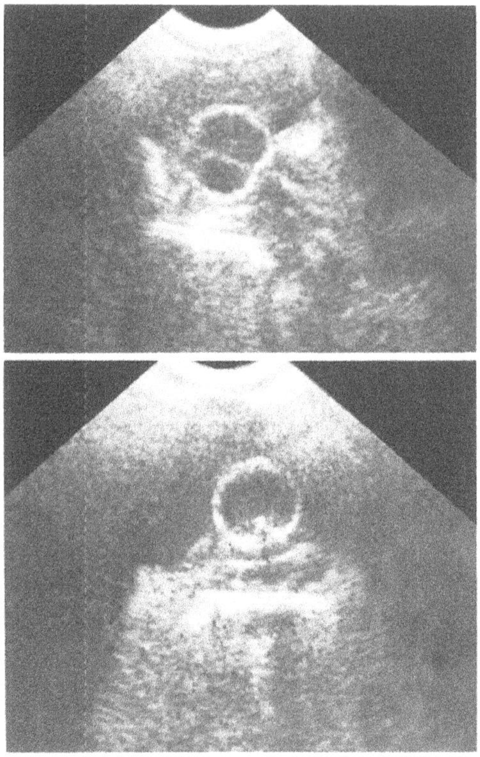

a

b

Fig. 12.52 a, b. To what lesion does this bizarre pattern correspond? Simply, of course, to Fowley's balloon in urinary bladder. **a** Sagittal scan; **b** transverse scan

References

Chapter 1

Barnett E, Morley P (1971) Ultrasound in the investigation of space occupying lesions of the urinary tract. Br J Radiol 44:733

Barnett E, Morley P (1974) Abdominal echography. Butterworth, Burrough Green

Brun PH (1979) Etude topographique (par coupes ultrasonores et dissections) des rapports de la région corporeocaudale du pancréas avec le pédicule vasculaire rénal gauche. Thèse, Université de Besançon

Callen PW, Filly RA, Sarti DA, Sample FW (1979) Ultrasonography of the diaphragmatic crura. Radiology 130:721–724

Cook JH, Rosenfield AT, Taylor KS (1977) Ultrasonic demonstration of intrarenal anatomy. AJR 129:831–835

Cronan JJ, Yoder IC, Amis ES, Pfister RC (1982) The myth of anechoic renal sinus fat. Radiology 144:149–152

Damascelli B, Lattuada A, Musumeci R, Severini A (1968) Two dimensional ultrasonic investigation of the urinary tract. Br J Radiol 41:837

Dubbins P (1986) Renal artery stenosis: duplex Doppler evaluation. Br J Radiol 59:225–230

Goldberg BB, Kotler MN, Ziskin MC, Waxham RD (1975) Diagnostic uses of ultrasound. Grune & Stratton, New York

Gray H, Goss CM (1966) Anatomy of the human body. Lea & Febiger, Philadelphia

Green WM, King DL (1976) Diagnostic ultrasound of the urinary tract. JCU 4/1:55–64

Hassani N (1976) Ultrasonography of the abdomen. Springer, Berlin Heidelberg New York

Hidalgo H, Dunnik NR, Rosenberg ER, Ram PC, Korobkin M (1982) Parapelvic cysts: appearance on CT and sonography. AJR 138:667–671

Holm HH, Kristensen JK, Rasmussen SN, Pedersen JF, Hancke S (1976) Abdominal ultrasound, Munksgaard, Copenhagen

Holmes JH (1965) Applications of ultrasound to the detection of lesions in the bladder and kidney. In: Grossmann C, Holmes H, Joyner C, Purnell E (eds) Proceedings of the first international conference on diagnostic ultrasound. University of Pittsburgh Press, New York, p 519

Holmes JH (1966) Ultrasonic studies of the bladder and kidney. In: Grossman C, Joyner C, Holmes JH, Purnell EW (eds) Diagnostic ultrasound. Plenum, New York

Leopold GR (1975) Gray scale ultrasonic angiography of the upper abdomen. Radiology 117:665–671

Kunin M (1986) Bridging septa of the perinephric space: anatomic, pathologic and diagnostic considerations. Radiology 158:361–365

Leopold GR, Asher WM (1975) Fundamentals of abdominal and pelvic ultrasonography. Saunders, Philadelphia

Meire HB (1979) Review article. Diagnostic ultrasound. Br J Radiol 52:621, 685–703

Meschan I (1966) Roentgen signs in clinical practice: Vol II, Radiology of the chest, genito-urinary system and gastrointestinal tract. Saunders, Philadelphia

Meyers MA (1976) Dynamic radiology of the abdomen. Normal and pathologic anatomy. Springer, Berlin Heidelberg New York

Morin ME, Baker DA (1979) The influence of hydration and bladder distension on the sonographic diagnosis of hydronephrosis. JCU 7/3:192–194

Moskowitz PS, Caroll BA, McCoy JM (1980) Ultrasonic renal volumetry in children. Radiology 134:61–64

Pourcelot LG (1979) Vascular imaging. 2nd Meeting of WFUMB, July 22–27, 1979, Miyazaki, Japan

Pourcelot LG, Besse D, Pejot C, Planiol Th (1979) Real time Doppler arteriography. 2nd Meeting of WFUMB, July 22–27, 1979, Miyasaki, Japan

Rastopoulos V, Kleinman PK, Marks S, Snyder M, Silverman P (1986) Renal fascial pathway posterior extension of pancreatic effusions within the anterior pararenal space. Radiology 158:367–374

Rosenfield AT (ed) (1979) Genitourinary ultrasonography. Churchill Livingstone, New York

Rosenfield AT, Taylor KJW (1978) The kidney. In: Taylor KJW (ed) Atlas of gray scale ultrasonography. Churchill Livingstone, New York

Rosenfield AT, Taylor KJW, Crade M, DeGraaf CS (1978) Anatomy and pathology of the kidney by gray scale ultrasound. Radiology 128:737–744

Rosenfield AT, Hobbins J, Taylor KJW, Cook JH III (1979) Renal ultrasound. In: Rosenfield AT, Glickman M, Hodson J (eds) Diagnostic imaging in renal disease. Appleton-Century-Crofts, New York

Rosenfield AT, Kenneth JW, Taylor PD, Jaffee CC (1980) Clinical application of ultrasound tissue characterization. Radiol Clin North Am 18:45–62

Sample WF (1977) A new technique for the evaluation of the adrenal gland with gray scale ultrasonography. Radiology 124:463–469

Sanders RC, Conrad MR (1977) The ultrasonic characteristics of the renal pelvicalyceal echo complex. JCU 5/6:372–377

Skolnick ML, Royal DR (1976) Normal upper abdominal vasculature: a study correlating contact B scanning with arteriography and gross anatomy. JCU 4/6:399

Suramo I, Päivänsalo M, Myllyla V (1983) Echo-free and relatively echo-free "renal sinus lipomatosis". Fortschr Röntgenstr 138:558–560

Taylor KJW, Carpenter BE, Hill CR, McCready VR (1976) Gray scale ultrasound imaging: the anatomy and pathology of the liver. Radiology 119:415–423

Vallance R, James W (1976) Gray scale ultrasonic imaging of the kidney. Br J Radiol 49:635–640
Von Fiegler W, Felix R (1981) Der Nierensinus im Sonogramm. Fortschr Röntgenstr 134:540–545
Von Fiegler W, Winter J (1982) Sonographische Erscheinungsformen der Fibrolipomatosis renalis. Fortschr Röntgenstr 137:656–659
Weill F (1982) Ultrasonography of digestive diseases. Mosby, St. Louis (3rd edn. 1986)
Weill F (1985) L'ultrasonographie en pathologie digestive. Vigot, Paris
Weill F, Becker JC, Kraehenbuhl JR, Heriot G, Walter JP (1973) Atlas clinique de radiographie ultrasonore. Masson, Paris
Weill F, Bihr E, Rohmer P, Eisencher A, Zeltner F (1977) Petit atlas ultrasonore des grandes branches vasculaires abdominales. Ann Radiol Paris 20/7:625–630
Weill F, Bihr E, Rohmer P, Zeltner F, Le Mouel A (1979) Une image ultrasonore piège: les pseudo-masses retro-cave d'origine rénale. Lettre, Ann Radiol (Paris) 22/7:612
Weill F, Brun Ph, Bartoli J (1980) Etude topographique des rapports vasculaires du pancréas. II: artère et veine rénale gauche. J Radiol Electrol Med Nucl 61, 2:85–87
Weill F, Le Mouel A, Bihr E, Rohmer P, Zeltner F (1980) Le signe du croissant de lune. Diagnostic ultrasonore des collections liquidiennes intra-péritonéales dans le recessus hepatorénal. J Radiol Electrol Med Nucl 61, 4:251–256
Yeh HC, Mitty HA, Wolf BS (1977) Ultrasonography of renal sinus lipomatosis. Radiology 124:799–801

Chapter 2

Albarelli JN, Lawson TL (1978) Renal ultrasonography: advantages of the decubitus position. JCU 6/2:115–116
Atkinson P, Wells PNT (1977) Pulsed Doppler ultrasound and its clinical applications. Yale J Biol Med 50:367–373
Bamber JC, Hill K (1981) Acoustic properties of normal and cancerous human liver. Ultrasound Med Biol 7:121–133, 135–144
Barnett E, Morley P (1971) Ultrasound in the investigation of space occupying lesions of the urinary tract. Br J Radiol 44:733
Barnett E, Morley P (1974) Abdominal echography. Butterworth, Burrough Green
Bartels H (1976) Indication and technic are of ultrasonically-directed kidney cyst puncture. Helv Chir Acta 43:341
Bolton WK, Tully RJ, Lewis ES, Ranniger K (1974) Localization of the kidney for percutaneous biopsy. A comparative study of methods. Ann Intern Med 81:159–164
Charbonnier A, de Boisgisson P (1979) Echographie urologique. Masson, Paris
Damascelli B, Lattuada A, Musumeci R, Severini A (1968) Two dimensional ultrasonic investigation of the urinary tract. Br J Radiol 41:837
Darby RE, Wayne RN (1974) Ultrasound diagnosis of and cyst puncture guidance for a second unilateral renal cyst. JCU 2/4:295–296
Doust BD, Maklad NF (1973) Control of renal cyst puncture by transverse ultrasonic B scanning. Radiology 109/3:679–681
Filly RA (1982) Characterization of biological fluids by ultrasound. "The leading edge in diagnostic ultrasound" Seminar. Atlantic City
Filly RA, Sommer FG, Minton AJ (1980) Characterization of biological fluids by ultrasound and computed tomography. Radiology 134:167–171
Glancy JJ, Goddard J, Pearson DE (1980) In vitro demonstration of cholesterol crystal's high echogenicity relative to protein particles. JCU 8:27–29
Goldberg BB, Pollack HM, Kellerman E (1975a) Ultrasonic localization for renal biopsy. Radiology 115:167–170
Goldberg BB, Kotler MN, Ziskin MC, Waxham RD (1975b) Diagnostic uses of ultrasound. Grune & Stratton, New York
Goldstein A, Madrazo BL (1981) Slice thickness artifacts in gray-scale ultrasound. JCU 9:365–375
Hassani N (1976) Ultrasonography of the abdomen. Springer, Berlin Heidelberg New York
Hill CR, Nicholas D, Bamber JC (1976) Practical approaches to quantitative tissue characterization. Abstract no 1120. World Federation of Ultrasound in Medicine and Biology, San Francisco
Holm HH, Pedersen JF, Kristensen S, Hancke S, Jensen F (1975) Ultrasonically guided percutaneous puncture. Radiol Clin North Am 13:493–503
Holm HH, Kristensen JK, Rasmussen SN, Pedersen JF, Hancke S (1976) Abdominal ultrasound. Munksgaard, Copenhagen
Holmes JH (1966) Ultrasonic studies of the bladder and kidney. In: Grossman C, Joyner C, Holmes JH, Purnell EW (eds) Diagnostic ultrasound. Plenum, New York
Jensen R, Kristensen JK, Holm HH (1976) Long-term results of ultrasonically guided percutaneous aspiration of renal cysts. Dan Med Bull 23/3:161
Kort A, Kronzon I (1982) Microbubble formation, in vitro and in vivo observation. JCU 10:117–120
Kossoff G (1974) Display techniques in ultrasound pulse echo investigation: a review. JCU 2:61–72
Kossoff G (1978) Principles and applications of grey scale echography. In: de Vlieger M et al. (eds) Handbook of clinical ultrasound. Wiley, New York
Kossoff G, Garret WJ (1976) Classification of soft tissues by grey scale echography. Ultrasound Med Biol 2:89–97
Kossoff G, Carpenter DA, Rodovanovich G, Robinson DE, Garett WJ (1975) Octoson: a new rapid multitransducer general purpose water-coupling echoscope. Proceedings of the 2nd European congress on ultrasonics in medicine, Munich, May 12–16
Kristensen JK, Bartels E, Jorgensen HE (1974) Percutaneous renal biopsy under the guidance of ultrasound. Scand J Urol Nephrol 8:223–226
Leopold GR, Asher WM (1975) Fundamentals of abdominal and pelvic ultrasonography. Saunders, Philadelphia
Mailloux LU, Mossey RT, McVicar MM (1978) Ultrasonic guidance for renal biopsy. Arch Intern Med 138:438
Nicholas D (1979) Ultrasonic diffraction analysis in the investigation of liver diseases. Br J Radiol 52:949–961
Nicholas D (1982) Evaluation of back scattering coefficients of excised human tissues: results, interpretation and associate measurements. Ultrasound Med Biol 8:17–28
Pedersen JF (1974) Percutaneous nephrostomy guided by ultrasound. J Urol 112:157–159
Pedersen JF, Cowan DF, Kristensen TK, Holm HH, Hancke S, Jensen F (1976) Ultrasonically-guided percutaneous nephrostomy. Radiology 119:429–431
Raskin MM, Roen SA, Serafini AN (1974) Renal cyst puncture: combined fluoroscopic and ultrasonic technique. Radiology 113/2:425–427
Rose JL, Goldberg BB (1979) Basic physics in diagnostic ultrasound. Wiley, New York

Rosenfield AT (ed) (1979) Genitourinary ultrasonography. Churchill Livingstone, New York
Rosenfield AT, Taylor KJW (1978) The kidney. In: Taylor KJW (ed) Atlas of gray scale ultrasonography. Churchill Livingstone, New York
Rosenfield AT, Hobbins J, Taylor KJW, Cook JH III (1979) Renal ultrasound. In: Rosenfield AT, Glickman M, Hodson J (eds) Diagnostic imaging in renal disease. Appleton-Century-Crofts, New York
Saitoh M, Watanabe H, Ohe H (1979a) Selective renal biopsy under ultrasonic real time guidance. 2nd Meeting of WFUMB. July 22–27, 1979, Miyasaki, Japan
Saitoh M, Watanabe H, Ohe H, Tanaka S, Itakura Y, Date S (1979b) Ultrasonic real-time guidance for percutaneous puncture. JCU 7:269–272
Sigel B (1982) Operative ultrasonography. Lea and Fibiger, Philadelphia
Sommer FG, Filly RA, Minton MJ (1979) Acoustic shadowing due to refractive and reflective effects. Am J Roentgenol 132:973–977
Tagia B, Ferrari P, Ravoni A (1977) Transparietal pyelography with ultrasonic guidance. Minerva Urol 29:29
Taylor KJW, Burns PN (1985) Duplex Doppler scanning in the pelvis and abdomen. Ultrasound Med Biol 11:643–658
Taylor KJW, Atkinson P, de Graaff CS, Dembler AG, Rosenfield AT (1978) Clinical evaluation of pulsed Doppler device linked to gray scale B scan equipment. Radiology 129:745–749
Weill F (1982) Ultrasonography of digestive diseases, 2nd edn. Mosby, St. Louis (3rd edn. 1986)
Weill F (1985) L'ultrasonographie en pathologie digestive, 3rd edn. Vigot, Paris, chaps 1, 2
Weill F, Becker JC, Kraehenbuhl JR, Heriot G, Walter JP (1973) Atlas clinique de radiographie ultrasonore. Masson, Paris
Weinstein BY, Skolnick MC (1978) Ultrasonically guided anterograde pyelography. J Urol 120:319

Chapter 3

Barnett E, Morley P (1974) Abdominal echography. Butterworth, Burrough Green
Baudain P, Marty F, Faure G, Dechelette E, Gout JP (1975) Intérêt de l'échotomographie en pathologie urogénitale chez l'enfant. Pédiatrie 30/7:745
Bryan PJ, Azimi F (1975) Ultrasound in diagnosis of congenital hydronephrosis due to obstruction of pelviureteric function. Urology 5:17–20
Cook JH III, Lytton B (1977) Intraoperative localization of renal calculi during nephrototomy by ultrasound scanning. J Urol 117:543–546
Cunningham JJ, Cunningham MA (1976) Characterization of renal stone models with gray scale echography. In vitro studies with clinical correlation. Urology 7:315
Edell SL, Zegel H (1978) Ultrasonic evaluation of renal calculi. AJR 130:261–263
Ellenbogen PH, Scheible FN, Talner LB, Leopold GR (1978) Sensivity of gray scale ultrasound in detecting urinary tract obstruction. AJR 130:731–733
Erickson LM, Nicholson SF, Lewall DB, Frischke L (1979) Ultrasound evaluation of hydronephrosis of pregnancies. JCU 7/2:128
Goldberg BB, Kotler MN, Ziskin MC, Waxham RD (1975) Diagnostic uses of ultrasound. Grune & Stratton, New York
Hasch E (1974a) Ultrasound in the investigation of disease of the kidney and urinary tract in children. Acta Paediatr Scand 63/1:42–48
Hasch E (1974b) Ultrasound in the diagnosis of hydronephrosis in infants and children. JCU 2/1:21–25
Hash E (1978) Ultrasound scanning for monitoring childhood hydronephrosis. JCU 6/3:156
Hassani N (1976) Ultrasonography of the abdomen. Springer, Berlin Heidelberg New York
Hill MC, Rich JL, Mazdial JG (1985) Finder CA Sonography VS excretory urograph in acute flank pain. AJR 144:1235–1238
Hoffman JC, Schnur MJ, Koenigsberg M (1982) Demonstration of renal papillary necrosis by sonography. Radiology 145:785–787
Holm HH, Kristensen JK, Rasmussen SN, Pedersen JF, Hancke S (1976) Abdominal ultrasound. Munksgaard, Copenhagen
Jackmann RJ, Stevens GM (1974) Benign hemorrhagic renal cyst. Radiology 110:7–13
Kane RA, Manco LG (1983) Renal arterial calcification simulating nephrolithiasis on sonography. AJR 140:101–104
Leopold GR, Asher WM (1975) Fundamentals of abdominal and pelvic ultrasonography. Saunders, Philadelphia
Mascatello VJ, Smith EH, Carrera GF, Berger M, Teele RL (1977) Ultrasonic evaluation of the obstructed duplex kidney. AJR 129:113–120
Morin ME, Baker DA (1979) The influence of hydration and bladder distension on the sonographic diagnosis of hydrophrosis. JCU 7/3:192–194
Pedersen JF, Cowan DF, Kristensen JK, Holm HH, Hancke S, Jensen F (1976) Ultrasonically-guided percutaneous nephrostomy. Report of 24 cases. Radiology 119:429–431
Pollack HM, Arger PH, Goldberg BB, Mulholland SG (1978) Ultrasonic detection of nonopaque renal calculi. Radiology 127:233–235
Rosenfield AT, Taylor KJW (1978) The kidney. In: Taylor KJW (ed) Atlas of gray scale ultrasonography. Churchill Livingstone, New York
Rosenfield AT, Taylor KJW, Crade M, De Graaf CS (1978) Anatomy and pathology of the kidney by gray scale ultrasound. Radiology 128:737–744
Rosenfield AT, Taylor KJW, Grade M (1979a) Renal ultrasound 1979: gray scale, real time, Doppler. In: Rosenfield AT (ed) Genitourinary ultrasonography. Churchill Livingstone, New York
Rosenfield AT, Hobbins J, Taylor KJW, Cook JH III (1979b) Renal ultrasound. In: Rosenfield AT, Glickman M, Hodson J (eds) Diagnostic imaging in renal disease. Appleton-Century-Crofts, New York
Sanders RC, Bearman S (1973) B scan ultrasound in the diagnosis of hydronephrosis. Radiology 108:375–382
Talner LB, Ellenbogen PH, Scheible FW, De Graaf CS (1978) Ultrasonic detection of urinary tract obstruction in renal failure. Invest Radiol 13:383
Von Christ F, Koischwitz D, Klehr HU (1982) Primäre Oxalose im Jugendalter. Fortschr Röntgenstr 136:174–177
Weill F, Becker JC, Kraehenbuhl JR, Heriot G, Walter JP (1973) Atlas clinique de radiographie ultrasonore. Masson, Paris
Winston M, Pritchard J, Paulin P (1978) Ultrasonography in the management of unexplained renal failure. JCU 6/1:23

Chapter 4

Amis ES, Cronan JJ, Yoder IC, Pfister RC, Newhouse JH (1982) Renal cysts: curios and caveats. Urol Radiol 4:199–209

Andersen BL, Curry NS, Gobien RP (1983) Sonography of evolving renal cystic: transformation associated with hemodialysis. AJR 141:1003–1004

Artaud J, Broussin B, Cadier L, Diard F (1980) Aspects echographiques des polykystoses hépatorénales récessives chez l'enfant. J Radiol 61:243–249

Barnett E, Morley P (1974) Abdominal echography. Butterworth, Borrough Green

Becker A, Schneider M (1975) Simple cyst of the kidney. Semin Roentgenol 10:103

Cho KJ, Maklad N, Curran J, Ting YM (1976) Angiographic and ultrasonic findings in infected simple cysts of the kidney. AJR 127/6:1015–1019

Fetissoff F, Boivin F, Jobard P, Allard JC (1981) Les reins polykystiques acquis de l'hémodialysé. Arch Anat Cytol Path 29:69–73

Frank B, Bolich P, Reichert J (1975) Sonographic appearance of organized blood in a cyst. Two case reports. JCU 3:233

Friday RO, Crummy AB, Malek GH (1974) Multilocular renal cyst. Angiographic, ultrasonic and cyst puncture findings. Urology 3:354–356

Goldberg BB, Kotler MN, Ziskin MC, Waxham RD (1975) Diagnostic uses of ultrasound. Grune & Stratton, New York

Green WM, Casarella WJ (1976) Differential diagnosis of echo-free renal masses. In: White D, Barnes R (eds) Ultrasound in medicine II. Plenum, New York

Grossman H, Rosenberg ER, Bowie JD, Ram P, Merten DF (1983) Sonographic diagnosis of renal cystic diseases. AJR 140:81–85

Hassani N (1976) Ultrasonography of the abdomen. Springer, Berlin Heidelberg New York

Holm HH, Kristensen JK, Rasmussen SN, Pedersen JF, Hancke S (1976) Abdominal ultrasound. Munksgaard, Copenhagen

Igawa KI, Miyagishi T (1972) The use of scintillation and ultrasonic scanning to disclose polycystic kidneys and liver. J Urol 108:685–688

Jackman RJ, Stevens GM (1974) Benign hemorrhagic renal cyst. Nephrotomography, renal arteriography and cyst puncture. Radiology 110:7–13

Kelsey JA, Bowie JD (1977) Gray-scale ultrasonography in the diagnosis of polycystic kidney disease. Radiology 122:791–795

Lawson TL, McClennan BL, Shirkhoda A (1978) Adult polycystic kidney disease: ultrasonographic and computed tomographic appearance. JCU 6:297–302

Leopold GR (1975) Gray scale ultrasonic angiography of the upper abdomen. Radiology 117:665

Leopold GR, Asher WM (1975) Fundamentals of abdominal and pelvic ultrasonography. Saunders, Philadelphia

Leopold GR, Talner LB, Asher WM, Gosink BR, Gittes RF (1973) Renal ultrasonography: an updated approach to the diagnosis of renal cyst. Radiology 109:671–678

Levine E, Grantham JJ, Slusher SL, Greathouse JL, Krohn BP (1984) CT of acquired cystic kidney disease and renal tumors in long-term dialysis patients. AJR 142:125–131

Mellins HZ (1984) Cystic dilation of the upper urinary tract: a radiologist's developmental model. Radiology 153:291–301

Monnet-Guichard M (1982) L'échotomographie dans le diagnostic et la surveillance de la maladie kystique acuise des hémodialysés chroniques. Thèse, Grenoble

Rosenfield AT, Taylor KJW (1978) The kidney. In: Taylor KJW (ed) Atlas of gray scale ultrasonography. Churchill Livingstone, New York

Rosenfield AT, Curtis AM, Putman CE et al. (1977a) Gray scale ultrasonography, computerized tomography and nephrotomography in evaluation of polycystic kidney and liver disease. Urology 9:436–438

Rosenfield AT, Siegel NS, Kappelman NB, Taylor KJW (1977b) Gray scale ultrasonography in medullary cystic disease of the kidney and congenital hepatic fibrosis with tubular ectasia. New observation. AJR 129:297–303

Rosenfield AT, Taylor KJW, Crade M, De Graaf CS (1978) Anatomy and pathology of the kidney by gray scale ultrasound. Radiology 128:734–744

Rosenfield AT, Taylor KJW, Crade M (1979a) Renal ultrasound 1979: Gray scale, real time, Doppler. In: Rosenfield AT (ed) Genitourinary ultrasonography. Churchill Livingstone, New York

Rosenfield AT, Hubbins J, Taylor KJW, Cook JH III (1979b) Renal ultrasound. In: Rosenfield AT, Glickman M, Hodson J (eds) Diagnostic imaging in renal disease. Appleton-Century-Crofts, New York

Skolnick ML, Lecky JW (1977) The ultrasonic spectrum of benign and malignant renal "cystic" masses. Differential diagnosis and diagnostic difficulties. Rev Interam Radiol 2:219

Stuck KJ, Koff SA, Silver TM (1982) Ultrasonic features of multicystic dysplastic kidney: expanded diagnostic criteria. Radiology 143:217–221

Sumner T, Friedland GW, Parker B et al. (1978) Preoperative diagnosis of unilateral multicystic kidney with hydropelvis. Urology 11:519

Taylor KJ, Kraus V (1975) Gray scale ultrasound imaging: assessment of acute hydronephrosis. Br J Urol 47:593–597

Thomas JL, Sumner TE, Crowe JE (1978) Neonatal detection and evaluation of infantile polycystic disease by gray scale echography. JCU 6:343–344

Weill F, Becker JC, Kraehenbuhl JR, Heriot G, Walter JP (1973a) Atlas clinique de radiographie ultrasonore. Masson Paris

Weill F, Gallinet D, Kraehenbuhl JR, Bittard M (1974) Fiabilité de l'exploration ultrasonore des lésions rénales. Etude statistique de 144 cas contrôlés. J Chir (Paris) 107/2:139–150

Weissberg DL, Miller RB (1983) Renal cell carcinoma and acquired cystic disease of the kidneys in a chronically dialyzed patient. J Ultrasound Med 2:191–194

Wolf B, Rosenfield AT, Taylor KJ, Rosenfield N, Gottlieb S, Hsia YE (1978) Presymptomatic diagnosis of onset of adult polycystic kidney disease by ultrasonography. Clin Genet 14:1

Yeh HC, Mitty HA, Wolf BS (1977) Ultrasonography of renal sinus lipomatosis. Radiology 124:799–801

Chapter 5

Alker DE, Barry JM, Hodges CV (1976) Angiomyolipoma: diagnosis and treatment. Urology 116:712–714

Arger PH (1976) The value of ultrasound in hypovascular hypernephromas. JCU 4/5:371

Arger PH, Mulhern CB, Pollack HM, Banner MP, Wein AJ (1979) Ultrasonic assessment of renal transitional cell carcinoma. Preliminary report. AJR 132:407–411

Astaneda-Zuniga W, Zollikofer C, Valdez-Davila O, Nath PH, Amplatz K (1979) Giant aneurysms of the renal arteries: an unusual manifestation of fibromuscular dysplasia. Radiology 133:327–330

Azimi F, Marangola JP, Kirch KH (1978) Ultrasonic diagnosis of tumor thrombosis of right renal vein. Urology 12/1:106–107

Baert AL, Wackenheim A, Jeanmart L (1980) Atlas of pathological computer tomography. Volume 2: Abdominal computer tomography. Springer, Berlin Heidelberg New York

Banner MP, Pollack HM, Chatten J, Witzleben C (1981) Multilocular renal cysts: radiologic-pathologic correlation. AJR 136:239–247

Barnett E, Morley P (1974) Abdominal echography. Butterworth, Burrough Green

Becker JA, Schneider M, Striano S, Cromb E (1974) Renal pelvic lipomatosis: a sonographic evaluation. JCU 2/4:299–301

Boisgisson Ph De, Charbonnier A, Steg A, Aboulker P (1976) L'apport de l'échotomographie dans le diagnostic des tumeurs du rein. Ann Urol 10/4:205–215

Bonavita JA, Pollack HW, Banner MP (1981) Renal onocytoma: further observations and literature review. Urol Radiol 2:229–234

Bosniak MA (1981) Angiomyolipoma (hamartoma) of the kidney: a preoperative diagnosis is possible in virtually every case. Urol Radiol 3:135–142

Boulard D (1986) Etude morphodiagnostique (échographie, scanographie, arterographie) d'une serie de 11 tumeurs bénignes du rein. Thesis, Besançon

Charboneau JW, Hattery RR, Ernst EC, James EM, Williamson B, Hartman GW (1983) Spectrum of sonographic findings in 125 renal masses other than benign simple cyst. AJR 140:87–94

Chilcote WS, Crane D (1974) Renal angiomyolipoma: ultrasound differentiation. JCU 2:226

Clayman RV, Williams RD, Fraley EF (1979) The pursuit of the renal mass. N Engl J Med 300:72

Coleman BG, Arger PH, Mulhern CB, Pollack HM, Banner MP, Arenson RL (1980) Gray-scale sonographic spectrum of hypernephromas. Radiology 137:757–765

Diamond DA, Kodroff M, Ravitz G (1977) Renal sinus angiomyolipoma. Urology 9:221–223

Duffy P, Ryan S, Aldous W (1977) Ultrasound demonstration of a 1.5 cm intrarenal angiomyolipoma. JCU 5:111–113

Felberg MAM, van Waes FGM (1982) Multilocular cystic renal cell carcinoma. AJR 138:953–955

Franken EA, Yiu-Chiu V, Smith WL, Chiu LC (1982) Nephroblastomatosis: clinicopathologic significance and imaging characteristics. AJR 138:950–952

Gates GF, Miller JH (1977) Combined radionuclide and ultrasonic assessment of upper abdominal masses in children. AJR 128:773–780

Gay BB, Dawes RK, Atkinson GO, Ball TI (1983) Wilms' tumor in horseshoe kidneys: radiologic diagnosis. Radiology 146:693–697

Goiney RC, Goldenberg L, Cooperberg PL, Charboneau JW, Rosenfield AT, Russin LD, McCarthy S, Zeman RK, Gordon PB, Rowley BA (1984) Renal oncozytoma: sonographic analysis of 14 cases. AJR 143:1001–1004

Goldberg BB, Ostrum BJ, Isard JH (1968) Nephrotomography: ultrasound differentiation of renal masses. Radiology 90/6:1113–1118

Goldberg BB, Pollack HM, Capitanio MA, Kirkpatrick JA (1975a) Ultrasonography: an aid to the diagnosis of masses in pediatric patients. Pediatrics 56:421

Goldberg BB, Kotler MN, Ziskin MC, Waxham RD (1975b) Diagnostic uses of ultrasound. Grune & Stratton, New York

Gouygen C, Mazewon E, Jardin A (1976) Bases actuelles d'approche d'une classification des tumeurs renales. Congress of the International Society of Urology. Dein, Paris 1:15–33

Green WM, Casarella WJ (1976) Differential diagnosis of echo-free renal masses. In: White D, Barnes R (eds) Ultrasound in medicine. II. Plenum, New York

Green WM, King DL, Casarella WJ (1976) A reappraisal of sonolucent renal masses. Radiology 121/1:163–171

Hansen GC, Hoffman RB, Sample WF, Becker R (1978) Computed tomography diagnosis of renal angiomyolipoma. Radiology 128:789–791

Hartman DS, Goldman SM, Friedman AC, Davis CJ, Madewell JE, Sherman JL (1981) Angiomyolipoma: ultrasonic-pathologic correlation. Radiology 139:451–458

Hartman DS, Lesar MSL, Madewell JE, Lichtenstein JE, Davis CJ (1981) Mesoblastic nephroma: radiologic-pathologic correlation of 20 cases. AJR 136:69–74

Hartman DS, Davis CH, Goldman SM, Friedman AC, Fritzsche P (1982) Renal lymphoma: radiologic-pathologic correlation of 21 cases, Radiology 144:759–766

Hassani N (1976) Ultrasonography of the abdomen. Springer, Berlin Heidelberg New York

Hill M, Sanders RC (1978) Gray scale B scan characteristics of intra-abdominal cystic masses. JCU 6/4:217

Holm HH, Kristensen JK, Rasmussen SN, Pedersen JF, Hancke S (1976) Abdominal ultrasound. Munksgaard, Copenhagen

Holmes JH (1967) Diagnosis of tumor by ultrasound. Prog Clin Cancer 1:135–150

Hunig R, Kinser J (1973) Diagnosis of Wilm's tumors by ultrasound. AJR 117/1:119–127

Kaude JV, Lacy GD (1978) Ultrasonography in renal lymphoma. JCU 6:295–382

Kristensen JK, Gammelgaard PA, Holm HH, Rasmussen SN (1972) Ultrasound in the demonstration of renal masses. Br J Urol 44:517–527

Lee TG, Henderson JC, Freeny PC, Raskin MM, Benson EP, Pearse HD (1978) Ultrasound findings of renal angiomyolipoma. JCU 6/3:150–155

Leopold GR, Asher WM (1975) Fundamentals of abdominal and pelvic ultrasonography. Saunders, Philadelphia

Levick RK (1970) La radiologie et les ultrasons dans le diagnostic de la tumeur de Wilms. Ann Radiol 13/3–4:209

Lobel B, Bellossi A, Bauchart J (1978) Cancers avasculaires du rein. Intérêt de l'échotomographie. J Urol Néphrol (Paris) 84/3:222–227

Lutz A, Lorenz D, Petzoldt R (1976) Ultrasonic diagnosis of space-occupying lesions of the kidney. Dtsch Med Wochenschr 101:1443–1448

Madewell JE, Goldman SM, Davis CJ, Hartman DS, Feigin DS, Lichenstein JE (1983) Multilocular cystic nephroma: a radiographic-pathologic correlation of 58 patients. Radiology 146:309–321

Maklad NF, Chuang VP, Doust BD, Cho KJ, Curran JE (1977) Ultrasonic characterization of solid renal lesions: echographic, angiographic and pathologic correlation. Radiology 123:733–739

Mulhern CB, Arger PH, Coleman BG, Pollack HM, Velchik M, Banner P (1982) Wilms' tumor: diagnostic therapeutic implications. Urol Radiol 4:193–198

Plainfossé MCh, Chenille E (1977) L'échographie dans l'exploration des reins muets et des masses rénales pleines. Ann Radiol (Paris) 6:563–572
Plainfossé MCh, Mercier-Pageyral B, Owczarczak W, Bacques O (1980) Echotomographie des tumeurs rénales. Valeur diagnostique. Nouv Presse Méd 9/5:295–298
Quinn MJ, Hatman DS, Firedman AC, Steinman JL, et al. (1984) Renal oncocytomas: new observations. Radiology 153:49–53
Ranniger K (1973) Ultrasonic examination of the kidney in the differential diagnosis between tumors and cysts. ROFO Suppl 35–6
Rao AKR, Kimball WR (1978) Ultrasonic appearance of an arteriovenous fistula of the kidney. JCU 6:345–346
Romeiser RS, Walls WJ, Valk WL (1974) B scan ultrasound in the evaluation of renal mass lesions. J Urol 112:8–12
Rosenfield AT (ed) (1979) Genitourinary ultrasonography. Churchill Livingstone, New York
Rosenfield AT, Taylor KJW (1977) Gray scale nephrosonography. Current status. J Urol 117/1:2–6
Rosenfield AT, Taylor KJW (1978) The kidney. In: Taylor KJW (ed) Atlas of gray scale ultrasonography. Churchill Livingstone, New York
Rosenfield AT, Hobbins J, Taylor KJW, Cook JH III (1979) Renal ultrasound. In: Rosenfield AT, Glickman M, Hodson J (eds) Diagnostic imaging in renal disease. Appleton-Century-Crofts, New York
Scheible W, Ellenbogen PH, Leopold GR, Siao NT (1978) Lipomatous tumors of the kidney and adrenal: apparent echographic specificity. Radiology 129:153–156
Shirkhoda A, Staab EV, Mittelstaedt CA (1980) Renal lymphoma imaged by ultrasound and gallium-67. Radiology 137:175–180
Silmi Moyano A, San Antonio Alvarez J, Chinchilla C (1977) The echotomographic diagnosis of renal expansive processes. J Urol Néphrol (Paris) 83:509
Smith EH, Bennett AH (1975) The usefulness of ultrasound in the evaluation of renal masses in adults. J Urol 113/4:525–529
Von Hruby W, Stellamor K, Zinner G, Marberger M (1983) Der Nierenbeckentumor im Sonogramm. RoFo 138:391–518
Von Weigert F, Ringelmann W, Voeth CH (1983) Diagnostisches Vorgehen beim solitären Angiomyolipom der Niere. RoFo 139:525–530
Weill F, Becker JC, Kraehenbuhl JR, Heriot G, Walter JP (1973) Atlas clinique de radiographie ultrasonore. Masson, Paris
Weill F, Gallinet D, Kraehenbuhl JR, Bittard M (1974) Fiabilité de l'exploration ultrasonore des lésions rénales. Etude statistique de 144 cas contrôlés. J Chir (Paris) 107/2:139–150
Weill E, Scherer K, Vogel HM (1979) Sonography, computer tomography and angiography in the diagnosis of an haemangioma of the renal pelvis. RoFo 130:5
Wills JS (1983) Cystic ademocarcinoma of the kidney mimicking multilocular renal cyst. Urol Radiol 5:51–53
Yeh HC, Mitty HA, Wolf BS (1977) Ultrasonography of renal sinus lipomatosis. Radiology 124:799–801

Chapter 6

Azimi F, Marangola JP, Kirch KH (1978) Ultrasonic diagnosis of tumor thrombosis of right renal vein. Urology 12/1:106–107
Barnett E, Morley P (1974) Abdominal echography. Butterworth, Burrough Green
Bernardino ME, Green B, Goldstein H (1975) Ultrasonography in the evaluation of post-nephrectomy renal cancer patients. Radiology 128:455–458
Bowie JD, Bernstein JR (1976) Retroperitoneal fibrosis: ultrasound findings and case report. JCU 4/6:435–437
Braschо DJ, Durant JR, Green LE (1977) The accuracy of retroperitoneal ultrasonography in Hodgkin's disease and non Hodgkin's lymphoma. Radiology 125:485–487
Bree RL, Green B (1978) The gray scale sonographic appearance of intra abdominal mesenchymal sarcoma. Radiology 128:193–197
Cadier L, Broussin B, Calabet A, Baudain P, Diard F (1982) Apport de l'échographie dans l'étude des tumeurs rétropéritonéales de l'enfant. J Radiol 63:15–23
Cooperberg PL (1977) Retroperitoneal fibrosis. A.I.U.M., Seminar of Ultrasound, Banff, Mars 1977
Cornud FR, Blandy S, Sibert A, Benacerraf R (1983) L'échographie abdominale dans le diagnostic et la surveillance des fibroses rétropéritonéales. A propos de 2 observations. J Radiol 64:111–115
Cunningham JJ (1978) Gray scale echography evaluation of hepatorenal relationship. Urology 11/6:652–656
Eisenscher A, Bartoli J (1979) Visualisation ultrasonore de la veine ovarienne gauche dilatée. Ann Radiol (Paris) 22/1:23
Fagan CJ, Larrieu AJ, Amparo E (1979) Retroperitoneal fibrosis. Ultrasound and CT features. AJR 133/2:239–243
Goldberg BB, Kotler MN, Ziskin MC, Waxham RD (1975) Diagnostic uses of ultrasound. Grune & Stratton, New York
Goldstein HM, Green B, Weaver RM (1978) Ultrasonic detection of renal tumor extension into the inferior vena cava. AJR 103/6:1083–1085
Gosink BB (1978) The inferior vena cava: mass effects. AJR 130:533–536
Greene D, Steinbach HL (1975) Ultrasonic diagnosis of hypernephroma extending into the inferior vena cava. Radiology 115/3:679–680
Hassani N (1976) Ultrasonography of the abdomen. Springer, Berlin Heidelberg New York
Holm HH, Kristensen JK, Rasmussen SN, Pedersen JF, Hancke S (1976) Abdominal ultrasound. Munksgaard, Copenhagen
Jacobson JB, Redman HC (1974) Ultrasound findings in a case of retroperitoneal fibrosis. Radiology 113/2:423–424
Kristensen JK, Gammelgaard PA, Holm HH, Rasmussen SN (1972) Ultrasound in the demonstration of renal masses. Br J Urol 44:517–527
Leopold GR, Asher WM (1975) Fundamentals of abdominal and pelvic ultrasonography. Saunders, Philadelphia
Lutz H, Lorenz D, Petzoldt R (1976) Ultrasonic diagnosis of space-occupying lesions of the kidney. Dtsch Med Wochenschr 101:1443
Madayag MA, Ambos MA, Lefleur RS, Bosniak MA (1979) Involvement of the inferior vena cava in patients with renal cell carcinoma. Radiology 133:321–326
Nes RD, Frawley J, Palmer J (1974) The use of ultrasound in the diagnosis of extension of malignant renal tumors into the inferior vena cava. J Urol 46:120–121
Ney C (1976) Thrombosis of inferior vena cava associated with malignant renal tumors. J Urol 55:583–590
Pietri H, Sahel J, La Bella A, Aimino R, Maurin P, Serafino X (1979) Ultrasonography applied to study of hepatic metastases. AJR 133:972

Rosenfield AT (ed) (1979) Genitourinary ultrasonography. Churchill Livingstone, New York Edinburgh London
Rosenfield AT, Taylor KJW (1978) The kidney. In: Taylor KJW (ed) Atlas of gray scale ultrasonography. Churchill Livingstone, New York
Rosenfield AT, Hobbins J, Taylor KJW, Cook JH III (1979) Renal ultrasound. In: Rosenfield AT, Glickman M, Hodson J (eds) Diagnostic imaging in renal disease. Appleton-Century-Crofts, New York
Sanders RC, Duffy T, McLoughlin MA, Walsh PC (1977) Sonography in the diagnosis of retroperitoneal fibrosis. J Urol 118:944–946
Slovis TL, Phillipart AL, Cushing B, Das L, Perlmutter AD, Reed JO, Wilner HI, Kroovand RL, Farooki ZQ (1981) Evaluation of the inferior vena cava by sonography and venography in children with renal and hepatic tumors. Radiology 140:767–772
Taylor KJW (1975) Ultrasonic investigation of inferior vena cava obstruction. Br J Radiol 48:1024
Taylor KJW, Viscomi GN (1979) Spectrum of ultrasonic appearances of liver metastases. Accuracy of the techniques. AJR 133:972
Von Schulze K, Thämmig R, Duvenbeck H (1982) Sonographischer Nachweis tumorbedingter Nierenvenenthrombosen. RoFo 136:117–236
Weill F (1982) Ultrasonography of digestive diseases. Mosby, St. Louis (3rd edn. 1986)
Weill F, Becker JC, Kraehenbuhl JR, Heriot G, Walter JP (1973) Atlas clinique de radiographie ultrasonore. Masson, Paris
Weill F, Rohmer P, Zeltner F, Bihr E (1978) Diagnostic ultrasonore des adénopathies lymphomateures retropéritonéales. Le signe de la veine mésentérique. Ann Radiol (Paris) 21/7:531–537

Chapter 7

Angelli G, Mossa A, Garribba P, Pagliarulo A (1983) L'échographie dans l'étude de la tuberculose rénale. J Radiol 64:99–102
Barnett E, Morley P (1974) Abdominal echography. Butterworth, Burrough Green
Cacchiarelli AA, Young N, Levine AJ (1978) Gray scale ultrasonic demonstration of nephrocalcinosis. Radiology 128:459–460
Coleman BG, Arger PH, Mulhern CB, Pollack HM, Banner MP (1981) Pyonephrosis: sonography in the diagnosis and management. AJR 137:939–943
Conrad MR, Sanders RC, Mascardo AD (1977) Perinephric abscess aspiration using ultrasound guidance. AJR 128/3:459–463
Davidson AJ (1977) Radiologic diagnosis of renal parenchymal disease. Saunders, Philadelphia, pp 162–191
Dinkel E, Orth S, Dittrich M, Schulte-Wissenmann H (1986) Renal sonography in the differentiation of upper from lower urinary tract infection. AJR 146:775–780
Edell SL, Bonavita SA (1979) The sonographic appearance of acute pyelonephritis. Radiology 132:683–685
Gelman ML, Stone LB (1976) Renal carbuncle: early diagnosis by retroperitoneal ultrasound. Urology 7:103–107
Glazer GM, Callen PW, Filly RA (1982) Medullary nephrocalcinosis: sonographic evaluation. AJR 138:55–57
Goldberg BB, Kotler MN, Ziskin MC, Waxham RD (1975) Diagnostic uses of ultrasound. Grune & Stratton, New York
Goldman SM, Minkin SD, Naravol DC, Diamond AB, Pion SJ, Meringoff BN, Sidh SM, Sanders RC, Cohen SP (1977) Renal carbuncle: The use of ultrasound in its diagnosis and treatment. J Urol 118:525–528
Hassani N (1976) Ultrasonography of the abdomen. Springer, Berlin Heidelberg New York
Hietala SO, Beachley MC, Girevenduls A, Weeler WE (1977) Combined radiographic and ultrasonographic approach in diagnosis of renal inflammatory lesions. Urology 10/5:486–495
Hoddick W, Brooke Jeffrey R, Goldberg H, Federle MP, Laing FC (1983) CT and sonography of severe renal and perirenal infections. AJR 140:517–520
Holm HH, Kristensen JK, Rasmussen SN, Pedersen JF, Hancke S (1976) Abdominal ultrasound. Munksgaard, Copenhagen
Hricak H, Cruy C, Romanski R, Uniewski MH, Levin NW, Madrazo BL, Sandler MA, Eyler WR (1982) Renal parenchymal disease: sonographic-histologic correlation. Radiology 144:141–147
Kay CJ, Rosenfield AT, Taylor KJW, Rosenberg MA (1979) Ultrasonic characteristics of chronic atrophic pyelonephritis. AJR 132:47–49
Kirk OC Van, Go RT, Wedel VJ (1980) Sonographic features of xantogranulomatous pyelonephritis. AJR 134:1035–1039
Kressel HY, Filly RA (1978) Ultrasonic appearance of gas containing abscesses in the abdomen. AJR 130:71–74
Laing FC, Salobs RP (1977) Value of ultrasonography in the detection of retroperitoneal inflammatory masses. Radiology 123:169–172
Lee KT, McClennam BL, Melson GL, Stanley BJ (1980) Acute focal bacterial nephritis. Emphasis on gray scale sonography and CT. AJR 135:87–92
Leopold GR, Asher WM (1975) Fundamentals of abdominal and pelvic ultrasonography. Saunders, Philadelphia
Pfister RC, Stanley RJ, Geisse G, Yoder FC, Newhouse JH (1977) Percutaneous aspiration of inflammatory renal masses: separation of medical from surgical disease. AJR 128:522
Plainfossé MCh, Mercier-Pageyral B, Bacques O, Vital JL (1980) Apport de l'échotomographie dans le diagnostic des abcès du rein, à propos de treize observations. Ann Radiol (Paris) 23/1:7–13
Quesne GW Le (1978) Ultrasonic detection of glomerular disease (abstr). AJR 130:96
Rochester D, Aronson AJ, Bowie JD, Kunzman A (1978) Ultrasonic appearance of acute poststreptococcal glomerulonephritis. JCU 6/1:49–50
Rosenfield AT, Taylor KJW (1978) The kidney. In: Taylor KJW (ed) Atlas of gray scale ultrasonography. Churchill Livingstone, New York
Rosenfield AT, Taylor KJW, Crade M, de Graaf CS (1978) Anatomy and pathology of the kidney by grayscale ultrasound. Radiology 128:737–744
Rosenfield AT, Taylor KJW, Crade M (1979a) Renal ultrasound 1979: gray scale, real time, Doppler. In: Rosenfield AT (ed) Genitourinary ultrasonography. Churchill Livingstone, New York
Rosenfield AT, Hobbins G, Taylor KJW, Cook JH III (1979b) Renal ultrasound. In: Rosenfield AT, Glickman M, Hodson J (eds) Diagnostic imaging in renal disease. Appleton-Century-Crofts, New York
Sagel SS, Stanley RJ, Levitt RG, Geisse G (1977) Computed tomography of the kidney. Radiology 124:359–370

Schneider M, Becker JA, Staiano S, Campos E (1976) Sonographic-radiographic correlation of renal and perirenal infections. AJR 127/6:1007–1014
Sefczek RJ, Beckman I, Lupetin AR, Dash N (1984) Sonography of acute cortical necrosis. AJR 142:553–554
Siegel MJ, Glasier CM (1981) Acute focal bacterial nephritis in children: significance of ureteral reflux. AJR 137:257–260
Weill F (1982) Ultrasonography of digestive diseases. Mosby, St. Louis (3rd edn. 1986)
Weill F, Becker JC, Kraehenbuhl JR, Heriot G, Walter JP (1973) Atlas clinique de radiographie ultrasonore. Masson, Paris

Chapter 8

Artaud J, Broussin A, Cadier LL, Diard F (1981) Aspects échographiques des polykystoses hépatorénales récessives chez l'enfant. J Radiol Electrol Med Nucl
Barnett E, Morley P (1974) Abdominal echography. Butterworth, Burrough Green
Bartrum RJ, Smith EH, d'Orsi CJ, Dantono J (1974) The ultrasonic determination of renal transplant volume. JCU 2/4:281–285
Bartrum RJ, Smith EH, d'Orsi CJ, Tilney NL, Dantono J (1976) Evaluation of renal transplants with ultrasound. Radiology 118:405–410
Berg E, Fischer R (1978) The importance of echography in the differential diagnosis of renal insufficiency. Münch Med Wochenschr 102/31:1023–1026
Boineau FG, Rothman J, Lewy JE (1975) Nephrosonography in the evaluation of renal failure and masses in infants. J Pediatr 87/2:195–201
Bullet J (1984) La surveillance échographique du rein transplanté (étude personnelle, 48 cas). Thèse, Besançon
Cahill PH, Cochran S, Sample WF (1977) Conventional radiographic and ultrasonic imaging in renal transplantation. Urology 10:33–42
Conrad MR, Dickerman R, Love IL, Curry T, Peters P, Hull A, Lerman M, Helderman H (1978) New observations in renal transplants using ultrasound. AJR 131:851–855
Coyne SS, Walsh JW, Tisnado J, Brewer WH, Sharpe AR, Armendola MA, Mendez-Picon G, Lee HM (1981) Surgically correctable renal transplant complications. An integrated clinical and radiologic approach. Radiology 138:145–151
Curran JE, Maklad NF, Baum JK (1976) Ultrasonic diagnosis of lymphocele complicating renal transplantation. Austral. Radiol 20:69
Daval JM, Fontaine P, Campion JP (1975) Echotomographic survey in human kidney transplantation. Excerpta Medica 222:7
Erwin BC, Carroll BA, Walter JF, Sommer FG (1982) Renal infarction appearing as an echogenic mass. AJR 138:759–761
Fowler JE, Paciulli J (1977) Renal vein thrombosis: diagnosis by B scan ultrasonography. Urology 118:849–850
Fried AM, Woodring JH, Lucas BA, Kryscio RJ (1983) The medullary pyramid index: an objective assessment of prominence in renal transplant rejection. Radiology 149:787–791
Glazer GM, Callen PW, Filly RA (1982) Medullary nephrocalcinosis: sonographic evaluation. AJR 138:55–57
Goldberg BB (1979) Renal sonography. Symposium on Ultrasound in Medicine. Tokio, Satellite meeting to the 2nd meeting of WFUMB, July 20, 1979
Goldberg BB, Kotler MN, Ziskin MC, Waxham RD (1975) Diagnostic uses of ultrasound. Grune & Stratton, New York
Hartman BS, Davis CJ, Lichtenstein JE, Goldman SM (1980) Renal parenchymal malacoplakia. Radiology 136:1, 33–42
Hassani N (1976) Ultrasonography of the abdomen. Springer, Berlin Heidelberg New York
Holm HH, Kristensen JK, Rasmussen SN, Pedersen JF, Hancke S (1976) Abdominal ultrasound. Munksgaard, Copenhagen
Hricak H, Cruz C, Eyler WR, Madrazo BL, Romanski R, Sandler MA (1981) Acute post-transplantation renal failure: differential diagnosis by ultrasound. Radiology 139:441–449
Hricak H, Romanski RN, Eyler WR (1982) The renal sinus during allograft rejection: sonographic and histopathologic findings. Radiology 142:693–699
Kaude JV, Lacy GD (1978) Ultrasonography in renal lymphoma. JCU 6:295–382
Koehler PR, Kanemoto HH, Maxwell JG (1976) Ultrasonic B scanning in the diagnosis of complications in renal transplant patients. Radiology 119:661–664
Lamb GH, Ayers AB (1977) Ultrasound findings in a case of renal malacoplakia. Br J Radiol 50:753
Leapman SB, Vidne BA, Butt KMH et al. (1976) Nephrolithiasis and nephrocalcinosis after renal transplantation: a case report and review of the literature. J Urol 115:129–132
Leopold GR (1970) Renal transplant size measured by reflected ultrasound. Radiology 95:687–689
Leopold GR, Asher WM (1975) Fundamentals of abdominal and pelvic ultrasonography. Saunders, Philadelphia
McDonald DG, Livertino JA (1976) Ultrasound in diagnosis and evaluation of lymphoceles after renal transplantation. Urology 7:216–218
Mindell HS, Kupic EA (1977) Horseshoe kidney: ultrasonic demonstration. AJR 129:526–527
Morley P, Barnett E, Bell PR, Briggs JK, Calman KC, Hamilton DN, Paton AM (1975) Ultrasound in the diagnosis of fluid collections following renal transplantation. Clin Radiol 26:199
Nesbit R, Blake DD, Ekstrand K, James PM Jr (1976) Lymphocele following renal transplantation: value of ultrasonography in diagnosis and follow up studies. South Med J 69:303
Ogata ES, Gooding CA, Phibbs RH (1975) Angiographic and ultrasonographic appearance of renal cortical and medullary necrosis in the newborn. Pediatr Radiol 3:226
Petrek J, Tilney NL, Smith EH, Williams JS, Vineyard GC (1977) Ultrasound in renal transplantation. Ann Burg 185:441–447
Phillips JF, Neiman HL, Brown TL (1976) Ultrasound diagnosis of post-transplant renal lymphocele. AJR 126:1194–1196
Plainfossé MC (1979) Etude dopplérographique du débit de l'artère rénale du rein greffé. Journées Frainçaises de Radiologie (groupement de radiologie ultrasonore), Paris, November 15, 1979
Rabad AM, Silmi A, Chinchilla C, Somacarrera E, Resel L, Leiva O, Antonio JJ (1975) Use of echotomography in the evolution of renal transplantations. Rev Clin Esp 137:327
Rifkin MD, Pasto ME, Goldberg B (1985) Duplex Doppler examination in renal disease: evaluation of vascular involvement. Ultrasound Med Biol 11:341–346
Rigsby CM, Taylor KI, Welting AL, Burns PN, et al. (1986) Renal allografts in acute infection: evaluation using Duplex sonography. Radiology 158:375–378

Rosenfield AT, Siegel NJ (1981) Renal parenchymal disease: histopathologic-sonographic correlation. AJR 137:793–798
Rosenfield AT, Taylor KJW (1976) Obstructive uropathy in the transplanted kidney: evaluation by grayscale sonography. J Urol 116:101–102
Rosenfield AT, Taylor KJW (1978) The kidney. In: Taylor KJW (ed) Atlas of gray scale ultrasonography. Churchill Livingstone, New York
Rosenfield AT, Siegel NJ, Kapellman NB, Taylor KJW (1977) Gray scale ultrasonography in medullary cystic disease of the kidney and congenital hepatic fibrosis with tubular ectasia: new observation. AJR 129:297–303
Rosenfield AT, Taylor KJW, Crade M, de Graaf CS (1978) Anatomy and pathology of the kidney by gray scale ultrasound. Radiology 128:737–744
Rosenfield AT, Taylor KJW, Crade M (1979a) Renal ultrasound 1979: gray scale, real time, Doppler. In: Rosenfield AT (ed) Genitourinary ultrasonography. Churchill Livingstone, New York
Rosenfield AT, Hobbins J, Taylor KJW, Cook JH III (1979b) Renal ultrasound. In: Rosenfield AT, Glickman M, Hodson J (eds) Diagnostic imaging in renal disease. Appleton-Century-Crofts, New York
Rosenfield AT, Zeman RK, Cronan JJ, Taylor KJW (1980) Ultrasound in experimental and clinical renal vein thrombosis. Radiology 137:735–741
Sanders RC, Jeck DL (1976) B scan ultrasound in the evaluation of renal failure. Radiology 119:199–202
Sefczek RJ, Beckman I, Lupetin AR, Dash N (1984) Sonography of acute cortical necrosis. AJR 142:553–554
Spies JB, Hricak H, Stemmer TM, Zeineh S, Alpers CH, Zayat P, Lue TF, Kerlan RK, Madrazo BL, Sandler MA (1984) Sonographic evaluation of experimental acute renal arterial occlusion in dogs. AJR 142:341–346
Spigos DC, Tan W, Pavel DG, Mozes M, Jonasson O, Capek V (1977) Diagnosis of urine extravasation after renal transplantation. AJR 129:409–413
Subramanyam BR (1981) Renal amyloidosis in juvenile rheumatoid arthritis: sonographic features. AJR 136:411–412
Toomey FB, Fritzsche P, Carlsen E, Caggiano H, Vyhmeister N, Kullman V (1977) Application of aortography and ultrasound in evaluation of renal agenesis. Pediatr Radiol 6:168
Trackler RT, Resnick ML, Leopold GR (1978) Pelvic horseshoe kidney: ultrasound findings and case report. JCU 6/1:51–52
Von Wernecke K, Heckemann R, Jakubowski HD (1982) Perirenale Raumforderungen nach Nierentransplantation. RoFo 137:403–409
Weill F, Becker JC, Kraehenbuhl JR, Heriot G, Walter JP (1973) Atlas clinique de radiographie ultrasonore. Masson, Paris
Winston M, Pritchard J, Paulin P (1978) Ultrasonography in the management of unexplained renal failure. JCU 6/1:23

Chapter 10

Barnett E, Morley P (1974) Abdominal echography. Butterworth, Borrough Green England
Belloir A, Didier D, Weill FS (1983) Etude ultrasonographique des hématomes rétropéritonéaux et abdomino-pelviens. J Radiol 64:621–625
Elbadani A, Linke CA, Carstensen EL et al. (1976) Histomorphologic features of ultrasonic renal injury. Arch Pathol Lab Med 100:199
Goldberg BB, Kotler MN, Ziskin MC, Waxham RD (1975) Diagnostic uses of ultrasound. Grune & Stratton, New York
Hassani N (1976) Ultrasonography of the abdomen. Springer, Berlin Heidelberg New York
Healy ME, Stephen ST, Moss AA (1984) Uriniferous pseudocysts: CT findings. Radiology 153:757–762
Holm HH, Kristensen JK, Rasmussen SN, Pedersen JF, Hancke S (1976) Abdominal ultrasound. Munksgaard, Copenhagen
McCullough DL, Leopold GR (1976) Diagnosis of retroperitoneal fluid collections by ultrasonography: signs of surgically proved cases. J Urol 115/6:656–659
Rosenfield AT (ed) (1979) Genitourinary ultrasonography. Churchill Livingstone, New York
Rosenfield AT, Taylor KJW (1978) The kidney. In: Taylor KJW (ed) Atlas of gray scale ultrasonography. Churchill Livingstone, New York
Rosenfield AT, Taylor KJW, Crade M, De Graaf CS (1978) Anatomy and pathology of the kidney by gray scale ultrasound. Radiology 128:737–744
Rosenfield AT, Hobbins J, Taylor KJW, Cook JH III (1979) Renal ultrasound. In: Rosenfield AT, Glickman M, Hodson J (eds) Diagnostic imaging in renal disease. Appleton-Century-Crofts, New York
Schaner EG, Ballow JE, Doppman JL (1977) Computed tomography in the diagnosis of subcapsular and perirenal hematomas. AJR 129:83–88
Vickery FR, Shirley IM, Cusick G (1977) Ultrasound and renal hematoma. J Belge Radiol 60:271
Von Nebel G, Lingg G, Berg E, Fischer R (1982) Zum computertomographischen und sonographischen Nachweis von renalen Hämatomen nach perkutaner Nierenbiopsie. Fortschr Roentgenstr 136:413–416
Weill FS (1982 Ultrasonography in digestive disease, 2nd edn. Mosby, St. Louis (3rd edn. 1986)
Weill FS (1985) L'ultrasonographie la pathologe digestive. Vigot, Paris, chaps 14, 29
Weill F, Becker JC, Kraehenbuhl JR, Heriot G, Walter JP (1973a) Atlas clinique de radiographie ultrasonore. Masson, Paris
Weill F, Kraehenbuhl JR, Bittard M, Vichard P (1973b) Les épanchements liquidiens pleuraux. J Chir (Paris) 105:469–474
Weill F, Gallinet D, Aucant D, Kraehenbuhl JR, Vichard P (1974) Le diagnostic tomoéchographique des hématomes périrénaux. Concours Médical 96:6835–6845
Weill F, Le Mouel A, Bihr E, Rohmer P, Zeltner F (1980) Ultrasonographie des petites collections péritonéales dans le recessus hépatorénal (le signe du croissant de lune). J Radiol Electrol Med Nucl 61,4:251–256
Weill F, Rohmer P, Belloir A, Bagni P (1983) The butterfly sign; an indicator of fluid within both the greater peritoneal cavity and the lesser omental bursa. J Ultrasound Med 2:161–164

Chapter 11

Ambos MA, Bosniak MA, Lefleur RS, Mitly HA (1981) Adrenal adenoma associated with renal cell carcinoma. AJR 136:81–84

Baert AL, Wackenheim A, Jeanmart L (1980) Atlas of pathological computer tomography. Volume 2: Abdominal computer tomography. Springer, Berlin Heidelberg New York
Barnett E, Morley P (1974) Abdominal echography. Butterworth, Burrough Green
Behan M, Martin EC, Muecke C, Kazam E (1977) Myelolipoma of the adrenal: two cases with ultrasound and CT findings. AJR 129:993–996
Bell RL (1977) Ultrasound of a pheochromocytoma. J Tenn Med Assoc 70:111
Bernardino ME, Goldstein HM, Green B (1978) Gray scale ultrasonography of adrenal neoplasms. AJR 130:741–744
Bernardino ME, Libshitz HI, Green N, Goldstein HM (1978) Ultrasonic demonstration of inferior vena cava involvement with right adrenal gland masses. JCU 6/3:167
Birnholz JC (1973) Ultrasound imaging of adrenal mass lesions. Radiology 109:163–166
Bowerman RA, Silver TM, Jaffe MH, Stuck KJ, Ninerman DL (1981) Sonography of adrenal pheochromocytomas. AJR 137:1227–1231
Crade M, Taylor KJW, Rosenfield AT (1978) Discovery of an adrenal tumor by ultrasound: case report. JCU 6/3:191–192
Davidson JK, Morley P, Hurley GD, Holford NGH (1975) Adrenal venography and ultrasound in the investigation of the adrenal gland: an analysis of 58 cases. Br J Radiol 48:435–450
Forsythe JR, Gosink BB, Leopold GR (1977) Ultrasound in the evaluation of adrenal metastases. JCU 5/4:31–34
Gee WF, Chikos PM, Greaves JP et al. (1975) Adrenal myolipoma. Urology 5:562–566
Ghorashi B, Holmes JH (1976) Gray scale sonographic appearance of an adrenal mass: a case report. JCU 4:121–123
Goldberg BB, Pollack HM, Capitanio MA, Kirkpatrick JA (1975 a) Ultrasonography: an aid in the diagnosis of masses in pediatric patients. Pediatrics 56:421–428
Goldberg BB, Kotler MN, Ziskin MC, Waxham RD (1975 b) Diagnostic uses of ultrasound. Grune & Stratton, New York
Hassani N (1976) Ultrasonography of the abdomen. Springer, Berlin Heidelberg New York
Holm HH, Kristensen JK, Rasmussen SN, Pedersen JF (1972) Ultrasonic diagnosis of juxtarenal masses. Scand J Urol Nephrol 15:83–88
Holm HH, Kristensen JK, Rasmussen SN, Pedersen JF, Hancke S (1976) Abdominal ultrasound. Munksgaard, Copenhagen
Lawson EE, Teele RL (1978) Diagnosis of adrenal hemorrhage by ultrasound. J Pediatr 92:423–426
Leopold GR, Asher WM (1975) Fundamentals of abdominal and pelvic ultrasonography. Saunders, Philadelphia
Marchal G, Baert AL (1976) Echography of suprarenal masses. Radiology 6:337
Mitty HA, Yeh HC, Rose J, Wolf BS (1977) Adrenal imaging: correlation of ultrasonography with urography, angiography, and body scanning. AJR 128/3:523
Morley P (1976) Ultrasound in the investigation of the adrenal glands and the kidneys. Neth J Med 19:74
Oppenheimer DA, Carroll BA, Yousem S (1983) Sonography of the normal neonatal adrenal gland. Radiology 146:157–160
Pery M, Kaftori JK, Bar-Maor JA (1981) Sonography for the diagnosis and follow-up of neonatal adrenal hemorrhage. JCU 9:397–401
Pond GD, Haber K (1976) Echography: a new approach to the diagnosis of adrenal hemorrhage of the newborn. J Can Assoc Radiol 27:40–44
Rao AKR, Silver TM (1976) Normal pancreas and splenic variants simulating suprarenal and renal tumors. AJR 126:530–537
Rosenfield AT (ed) (1979) Genitourinary ultrasonography. Churchill Livingstone, New York
Rosenfield AT, Taylor KJW (1978) The kidney. In: Taylor KJW (ed) Atlas of gray scale ultrasonography. Churchill Livingstone, New York
Rosenfield AT, Hobbins J, Taylor KJW, Cook JH III (1970) Renal ultrasound. In: Rosenfield AT, Glickman M, Hodson J (eds) Diagnostic imaging in renal disease. Appleton-Century-Crofts, New York
Rubin HB, Hirose F, Benfield JR (1975) Myelolipoma of the adrenal gland. Am J Surg 130:354–358
Sabatier JC, Metton G, Portalez D, Marty MJ, Joffre F (1980) Apport de l'échographie dans le diagnostic des tumeurs surrénaliennes. J Radiol 61/1:769–771
Sample WF (1977) A new technique of the evaluation of the adrenal gland with gray scale ultrasonography. Radiology 124:463–469
Sample WF (1978) Adrenal ultrasonography. Radiology 127:461–466
Sample WF, Sarti DA (1978) Computed tomography and gray scale ultrasonography of the adrenal gland: a comparative study. Radiology 128:377–383
Scheible W, Ellenbogen PH, Leobold GR, Siao NT (1978) Lipomatous tumors of the kidney and adrenal: apparent echographic specificity. Radiology 129:153–156
Von Georgi M, Weiss H, Trede M, Saeger HD, Bleyl U, Mittelstaedt GV (1982) Radiologische Differentialdiagnostik zystischer Nebennierenprozesse. Röntgenstr 137:637–646
Weill F, Becker JC, Kraehenbuhl JR, Heriot G, Walter JP (1973) atlas clinique de radiographie ultrasonore. Masson, Paris
Yeh HC (1980) Sonography of the adrenal glands – normal glands and small masses. AJR 135:1167–1177
Yeh HC, Mitty HA, Rose J, Wolf BS, Gabrilove JL (1978 a) Ultrasonography of adrenal masses: usual features. Radiology 127:467–474
Yeh HC, Mitty HA, Rose J, Wolf BS, Gabrilove JL (1978 b) Ultrasonography of adrenal masses: unusual manifestations. Radiology 127:475–483
Zappasodi F, Derchi LE, Rizzato G (1986) Ultrasonography of the normal adrenal glands. Br J Radiol 59:759–764

Chapter 12

Banner M (1981) Prospective analysis of the value of scrotal ultrasound. Radiology 141:763–766
Barnett E, Morley P (1974) Abdominal echography. Butterworth, Burrough Green
Berger RB, Taylor KJW, Rosenfield AT (1982) Pelvic varices stimulating cystic ovaries: differentiation by pulse doppler. JCU 10:186–189
Blei L, Sihelnik S, Bloom D, Stutzman R, Chiadis J (1983) Ultrasonographic analysis of chronic intratesticular pathology. J Ultrasound Med 2:17–23
Bouvier JF, Pascand E, Marlhes F, Pascand JL, Hummel P, Rousseau J (1984) Urachal cyst in the adult. Ultrasound diagnosis. JCU 12:48–50

Brandt TD, Neiman HL, Calenoff L, Greenberg M, Kaplan PE, Nanninga JB (1981) Ultrasound evaluation of the urinary system in spinal-cord-injury patients. Radiology 141:473–477
Bree RL, Silver TM (1981) Sonography of bladder and perivesical abnormalities. AJR 137:1101
Bree RL, Silver TM (1982) Nongynecologic bladder and perivesical ultrasound. Urol Radiol 4:135–145
Brooke Jeffrey R, Laing FC, Hricak H, McAninch JW (1983) Sonography of testicular trauma. AJR 141:993–995
Carroll BA, Gross DM (1983) High frequency scrotal sonography. AJR 140:511–515
Cunningham JJ (1983) Sonographic findings in clinically unsuspected acute and chronic scrotal hematoceles. AJR 140:749–752
Dahnert WF, Hamper UM, Enggleston PW, Sanders RC (1986) Evaluation of prostate by transrectal sonography with histopathologic correlations: The echogenic appearance of early carcinoma. Radiology 158:97–102
Declercq G, Denis L (1978) Ultrasonic assessment of prostatic masses. Acta Urol Belg 46:74–79
Fornage B (1979) L'ultrasonographie de la protaste. Mémoire pour l'obtention du C.E.S. de Radiologie option diagnostic. Université de Paris V, René Descartes. U.E.R. Cochin
Fornage B (1985) L'échographie de la prostate, 1st edn. Vigot, Paris
Frentzel-Beyme B (1985) Die transrektale Prostatsonographie. Auswertung einer Pilotstudie. RoFo 142:296–298
Fulmer LR, Fye C (1982) Elephantiasis of the scrotum. JCU 10:143–144
Gilsanz V, Miller JH, Reid BS (1982) Ultrasonic characteristics of posterior urethral valves. Radiology 145:143–145
Glazer HS, Lee JKT, Leland Melson G, McClennan BL (1982) Sonographic detection of occult testicular neoplasms. AJR 138:673–675
Goldberg BB, Kotler MN, Ziskin MC, Waxham RD (1975) Diagnostic uses of ultrasound. Grune & Stratton, New York
Gotoh K, Nishi M (1975) Ultrasonic diagnosis of prostatic cancer. Acta Urol Jap 11:87
Greenberg M, Neiman HL, Brandt TD, Falkowski W, Carter M (1981) Ultrasound of the prostate. Radiology 141:757–762
Greiner von KG, Jacob B, Slosek D, Schwartz R (1983) Sicherung der T-Klassifikation von Harnblasentumoren durch transkutane Sonographie intravesikale Sonographie und CT. RoFo 139:510–515
Harada K, Igari D, Tanahashi Y (1976) Transrectal ultrasonography and pathological staging of bladder tumors. Abstracts World Federation of Ultrasound in Medicine and Biology. 2nd congress, San Francisco USA
Harada K, Igari D, Tanahashi Y, Watanabe H, Saitoh M, Mishina T (1977) Staging of bladder tumors by means of transrectal ultrasonography. JCU 5:388–392
Harada K, Igari D, Tanahashi Y (1979) Gray scale transrectal ultrasonography of the prostate. JCU 7/1:45–49
Hassani N (1976) Ultrasonography of the abdomen. Springer, Berlin Heidelberg New York
Holm HH, Northeved A (1974) A transurethral ultrasonic scanner. J Urol 3:238
Holm HH, Kristensen JK, Rasmussen SN, Pedersen JF, Hancke S (1976) Abdominal ultrasound. Munksgaard, Copenhagen
Kremer H, Dobrinski W, Mikyska M, Baumgartner M, Zollner N (1982) Ultrasonic in vivo and in vitro studies on the nature of the ureteral jet phenomenon. Radiology 142:175–177
Lee F, Gray IM, McLeary RD, Lee F, jr, et al. (1986) Prostatic evaluation by transrectal sonography: criteria for diagnosis of early carcinoma. Radiology 158:91–95
Leopold GR, Asher WM (1975) Fundamentals of abdominal and pelvic ultrasonography. Saunders, Philadelphia
Lupetin AR, King W, Rich P, Lederman RB (1983) Ultrasound diagnosis of testicular leukemia. Radiology 146:171–172
Marchal GJ, Van Dijck XM, Kint EJ, Peeters SR, Baert AL, Goddeeris P (1982) The sonographic visualization of the vesico-ureteral junction. CT-Sonographie 2:62–67
Miller S, Garvie W, Christie A (1973) The evaluation of prostate size by ultrasonic scanning: a preliminary report. Br J Urol 48:187
Mittelstaedt CA, Gosink BB, Leopold GR (1977) Gray scale patterns of pelvic disease in the male. Radiology 123/3:727–732
Miyazaki Y, Yamaguchi A, Hara S (1979) Ultrasonographic pathomorphology of the prostate. 2nd Meeting of WFUMB, July 22–27, Miyazaki, Japan
Morley P (1978) Clinical staging of epithelial bladder tumors by echotomography. In: Hill CR, McReady VR, Cosgrove D (ed) Ultrasound in tumour diagnosis. Pitmans, London
Morley P (1979) The Bladder. In: Rosenfield AT (ed) Genitourinary ultrasonography. Churchill Livingstone, New York
Portalez D, Song MY, Marty MH, Joffre F (1982) Ultrasonography patterns of testicular non-Hodgkin's lymphoma. Eur J Radiol 2:222–225
Resnick MI, Willard JW, Boyce WH (1977) Recent progress in ultrasonography of the bladder and prostate. J Urol 117:444–446
Resnick MI, Willard JW, Boyce WH (1978) Ultrasonic evaluation of the prostatic nodule. J Urol 120:86
Rifkin MD, Kurtz AB, Pasto ME, Goldberg BB (1983) Unusual presentation of cystitis. J Ultrasound Med 2:25–28
Rifkin MD, Firedland GW, Shorthill L (1986) Prostatic evaluation by transrectal endosonography: detection of carcinoma. Radiology 158:85–90
Rizzato G, Basadonna P, Del Zotto A, Lombardo VL, Petz G (1982) Pelvic lipomatosis. Diagnostic role of ultrasonography and case report. Eur J Radiol 2:313–316
Rosenfield AT, Taylor KJW (1978) The kidney. In: Taylor KJW (ed) Atlas of gray scale ultrasonography. Churchill Livingstone, New York
Rosenfield AT, Hobbins J, Taylor KJW, Cook JH III (1979a) Renal ultrasound. In: Rosenfield AT, Glickman M, Hodson J (eds) Diagnostic imaging in renal disease. Appleton-Century-Crofts, New York
Rosenfield AT, Taylor KJW, Weiss RM (1979b) Ultrasonic evaluation of bladder. J Urol 121:119–120
Saitoh H, Watanabe H, Igari D, Tanahashi Y, Harada K (1974) Ultrasonography of the prostate. Detection of prostatic calculi associated with benign prostatic hypertrophy and prostatic cancer. Arch Jpn Soc Ultrasonics Med 25:43
Saito T, Iwata Y, Yoshiba H, Imamura K (1979) Morphological changes of the prostate observed with ultrasonotomography in anti-androgenic therapy of the prostatic hypertrophy. 2nd Meeting of WFUMB, (4th World Congress on Ultrasonics in Medicine-Abstract. Free Communication 179 p 326) July 22–27, 1979, Miyazaki, Japan
Shapeero LG, Friedland GW, Perkash I (1983) Transrectal sonographic voiding cystourethrography: studies in neuromuscular bladder dysfunction. AJR 141:83–90

Spataro RF, Davis RS, McLachlan MSF, Linke CA, Barbaric ZL (1983) Urachal abnormalities in the adult. Radiology 149:659–663

Takahashi H, Ouchi T (1964) The ultrasonic diagnosis in the field of urology on the diagnosis of prostate disease. In: Proceedings of the 4th Meeting of the Japanese Society of Ultrasonics in Medicine, Osaka 2:35

Taylor KJW (ed) (1978) Atlas of gray scale ultrasonography. Churchill Livingstone, New York

Von Egender G, Goidinger K, Jakse G (1982) Klassifikation der Harnblasentumoren durch die Sonographie. Fortsch Röntgenstr 136:416–420

Von Greiner KG, Jacob F, Klose KC, Schwartz R (1983) Sicherung der T-Klassifikation von Harnblasentumoren durch transkutane Sonographie, intravesikale Sonographie und Computertomographie. Fortsch Röntgenstr 139:510–515

Watanabe H (1979) Prostatic ultrasound. In: Rosenfield AT (ed) Genitourinary ultrasonography. Churchill Livingstone, New York

Watanabe H, Katoh H, Katoh T et al. (1968) Diagnostic application of the ultrasonography for the prostate. Jpn J Urol 59:273

Watanabe H, Kaiho H, Tanaka M, Terasawa Y (1971) Diagnostic application of ultrasonography to the prostate. Invest Urol 8:548–559

Watanabe H, Igari D, Tanahashi Y, Harada K, Saitoh M (1974) Development and application of new equipment for transrectal ultrasonography. JCU 2:91–98

Watanabe H, Igari D, Tanahashi Y, Harada K, Saitoh M (1975) Transrectal ultrasonography of the prostate. J Urol 114:734–739

Watanabe H, Saitoh M, Igari D, Tanahashi Y, Harada K, Hisamichi S (1977) Mass screening program for prostatic diseases with transrectal ultrasonography. J Urol 117:746–748

Weill F, Becker JC, Kraehenbuhl JR, Heriot G, Walter JP (1973) Atlas clinique de radiographie ultrasonore. Masson, Paris

Whitley Vick C, Bird KI, Rosenfield AT, Richter J, Taylor KJW (1982) Ultrasound of the scrotal contents. Urol Radiol 4:147–153

Williams DBD, Fisk JD (1981) Sonographic diagnosis of giant urachal cyst in the adult. DAJR 136:417–418

Wolverson MK, Houttuin E, Heiberg E, Sundaram M, Gregory J (1983) High-resolution real time sonography of scrotal varicocele. AJR 141:775–779

Wolverson MK, Houttuin E, Heiberg E, Sundaram M, Shields JB (1983) Comparison of computed tomography with high-resolution real-time ultrasound in the localization of the impalpable undescended testis. Radiology 146:133–136

Subject Index

www.ingramcontent.com/pod-product-compliance
Ingram Content Group UK Ltd.
Pitfield, Milton Keynes, MK11 3LW, UK
UKHW051509290926
15471UKWH00008B/1509
* 9 7 8 3 6 4 2 7 0 4 1 9 2 *